# Minimally Invasive Percutaneous Nephrolithotomy

Madhu S. Agrawal • Dilip K. Mishra
Bhaskar Somani
Editors

# Minimally Invasive Percutaneous Nephrolithotomy

Springer

*Editors*
Madhu S. Agrawal
Professor and Head, Department of Urology
Global Rainbow Healthcare
Agra, Uttar Pradesh, India

Dilip K. Mishra
Head, Department of Urology
Pushpanjali Hospital and Research Center
Agra, Uttar Pradesh, India

Bhaskar Somani
Professor and Consultant Urological Surgeon
University Hospital Southampton
Hampshire, UK

ISBN 978-981-16-6000-9 ISBN 978-981-16-6001-6 (eBook)
https://doi.org/10.1007/978-981-16-6001-6



This Springer imprint is published by the registered company Springer Nature Singapore Pte Ltd.
The registered company address is: 152 Beach Road, #21-01/04 Gateway East, Singapore 189721, Singapore

# Foreword

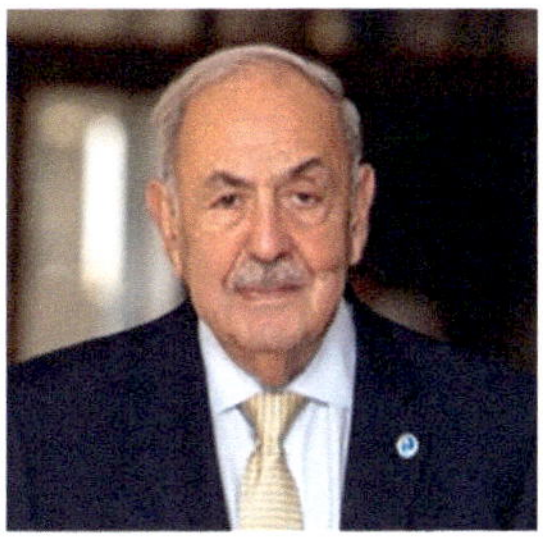

With the advent of percutaneous access to the kidney in the 1980s, Kurt Amplatz developed a dilating system. I believed, at that time, that the tract size should allow the percutaneous removal of a 10 mm stone, which would allow us to use strong forceps through the scope to effectively grasp the stone. Empirically, it was decided that the largest Amplatz sheath would have an inner circumference of 30 mm.

Industry has now developed effective lithotripters and most fragments can be easily irrigated following fragmentation and larger fragments can be grasped with more delicate instruments. This allows sheaths with a smaller inner circumference to be used effectively.

Any changes in instrumentation and techniques that diminish morbidity in percutaneous renal surgery are welcome. Some studies have shown decreased blood loss with smaller tracts while others have shown no difference in the incidence of blood transfusion. Smaller scopes have a smaller field of vision and usually the procedures take longer. However, if the morbidity is less, it is time well spent.

Dr Agrawal and his co-editors are very experienced endourologists and they have compiled an excellent book covering all aspects of "Mini-PCNL". They have selected authorities in the field to write the various chapters and I highly recommend this book to all endourologists. It not only covers all the basic techniques, but in addition it elucidates the latest technology. It is so thorough that it will be a text that you will use repeatedly in your career as you encounter the various problems that we all experience in the treatment of difficult stones.

Arthur D. Smith, MD
Long Island Jewish Medical Center
New York, USA

Donald and Barbara Zucker School
of Medicine at Hofstra/Northwell
New York, USA

Northwell Health Urology at the Center for Advanced Medicine
New Hyde Park, NY, USA
ASmith1@northwell.edu

# Foreword

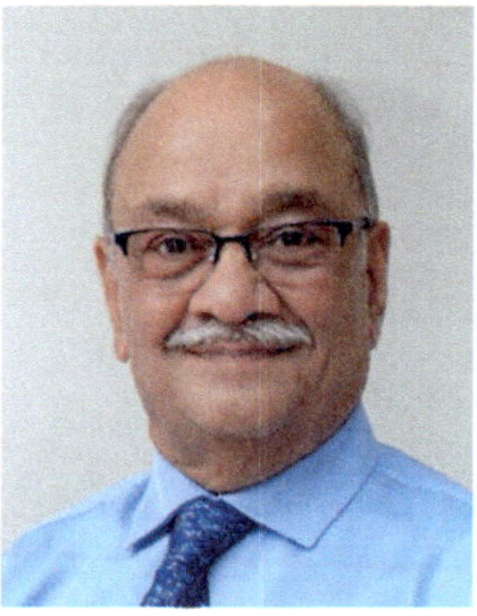

Stone disease is a global disease affecting all people of all ethnicity and gender. There are around 50% chance of recurrent stone formation in a patient with stone disease. The stone disease may hamper kidney health and may even lead to renal failure.

Over decades, there has been a paradigm shift from high stone bulk like staghorn stones to lower stone bulk. There is early detection of smaller stones due to current imaging modalities. There have been technical advancements in stone management from open approach to minimally invasive endourological approach. The endourological management of kidney stone disease has undergone significant improvements from a large bore approach like standard PCNL to a very small-bore approach like Microperc. There have been improvements in the energy source technology as well. There has been shift in intra-corporeal lithotripsy from low-power laser to high-power laser and shift from traditional pneumatic to combined ultrasonic and pneumatic lithotripsy along with integrated suction. Newer ideas are being explored in stone management like addition of suction to the PCNL sheath. These advancements have led to miniaturisation of PCNL tract leading to increased implications of mini-PCNL in all stone scenarios.

This book focussing on mini-PCNL has thrown light on all aspects right from surgical anatomy of kidney, various patient positions, anaesthesia challenges, renal imaging and access, lithotripsy modalities, newer advances in the energy sources, and challenging situations in Mini-PCNL. I would take this opportunity to congratulate Dr Madhu S. Agrawal and his team for addressing each aspect of mini-PCNL and inviting expert global faculties for their contributions. It would be an excellent piece of work for residents and endourologists.

Mahesh Desai, MS, FRCS, FRCS, FACS
Muljibhai Patel Urological Hospital
Nadiad, Gujarat, India

# Preface

The treatment of stone disease has undergone dramatic changes with the introduction of minimally invasive technology. Percutaneous Nephrolithotomy (PCNL) has become the mainstay of surgical treatment for large volume nephrolithiasis in the present time. Percutaneous stone surgery has also evolved from large tracts to smaller tracts over a period of time. This monograph on Mini-PCNL has been prepared to cover all aspects and latest advances in this exciting field of minimally invasive percutaneous surgery with an honest overview from the leading world experts.

The book is composed of 30 chapters divided into 8 sections, which help maintain the flow. Section 1 deals with the history and anatomical principles of m-PCNL including the ALARA principle of reducing radiation. Section 2 covers the armamentarium for m-PCNL including the fragmentation devices used with it. Section 3 looks into the anaesthetic considerations and the positioning of the patient for this procedure. Section 4 covers all aspects of renal access for the m-PCNL. Section 5 covers the nuances of the procedure including tract dilatation, intrarenal pressure, fluid management, and exit strategy. Section 6 investigates the modern aspects of m-PCNL including the variations of m-PCNL including the micro, ultra-mini, super-mini, and ECIRS techniques. Section 7 covers special situations of doing m-PCNL including bilateral procedures, renal anomalies, renal transplant, obese and paediatric patients. Section 8, which is the last section, looks into the complications and outcomes of m-PCNL.

The book covers all aspects of m-PCNL and will be a good guide to new endourology trainees as well as a refresher and update for experienced endourologists. The use of figures and tables allows the reader to understand and comprehend the message well. This summarises all aspects of m-PCNL including the future aspects of technological advances. We hope all urologists will enjoy reading this, also that this monograph will encourage safe and standardised uptake of m-PCNL.

We are grateful to all authors for their contribution and support in this endeavour. We would also like to take this opportunity to thank our families for their support, our office staff for their help in preparation of the manuscript, and the publishers Springer Nature and their team for their help and cooperation in making this project successful.

## Editors

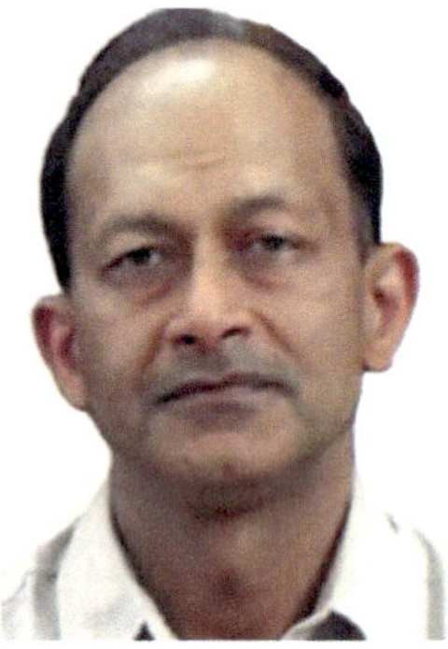 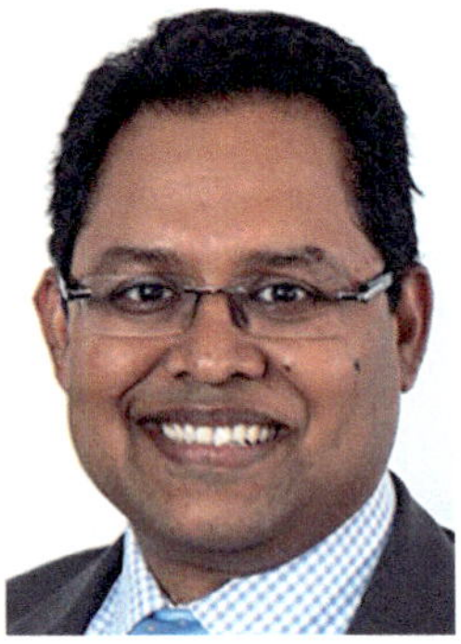 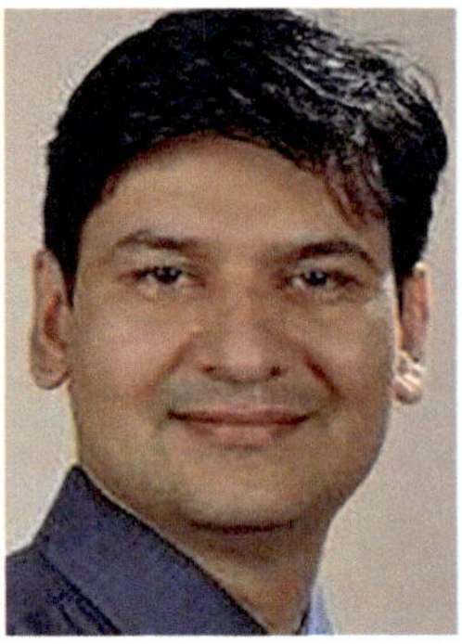

Agra, India — Madhu S. Agrawal
Hampshire, UK — Bhaskar Somani
Agra, India — Dilip K. Mishra

# Contents

# Contributors

**Mayank Agrawal, MBBS, MS, DNB (General Surgery)** Department of Urology, Grant Government Medical College and Sir JJ Group of Hospitals, Mumbai, Maharashtra, India

**Madhu S. Agrawal, MS, MCh (Urol), FRCS** Professor and Head, Department of Urology, Global Rainbow Healthcare, Agra, Uttar Pradesh, India

SN Medical College, Agra, Uttar Pradesh, India

**Amandeep M. Arora, MS, MCh (Urol), DNB** Tata Memorial Hospital, Mumbai, Maharashtra, India

**Nabil Atassi, MD** Department of Urology, Klinikum Sindelfingen, Böblingen, Germany

**Mario Basulto-Martínez, MD** European Training Center in Endourology, Department of Urology, IRCCS Ospedale San Raffaele, Milan, Italy

**Taif Bendigeri, MS, M.Ch (Urology)** Asian Institute of Nephro-Urology (AINU), Hyderabad, India

**Ajay Bhandarkar, MCh, DNB (Urology)** Sujay Urological Hospital, Vadodara, Gujarat, India

**Anna Brewin, MRCS** University Hospital Southampton NHS Trust, Southampton, UK

**Ramandeep S. Chalokia, MRCS** Warrington and Halton Teaching Hospitals, NHS Foundation Trust, Warrington, UK

**Cecilia Maria Cracco, MD, PhD** Department of Urology, Cottolengo Hospital, Torino, Italy

**Janak Desai, MS, M.Ch (Urology)** Samved Hospital, Ahmedabad, Gujarat, India

**Sudheer Kumar Devana, MS, MCh (Urology)** Department of Urology, Post Graduate Institute of Medical Education and Research, Chandigarh, India

**Saman Farshid, MD** Clinical Research Development Unit, Imam Khomeini Hospital, Urumieh University of Medical Sciences, Urumieh, Iran

**Mehmet Ferhat, MD** Department of Urology, Bahcelievler Medicana Hospital, Istanbul, Turkey

**Venkat Arjunrao Gite, MS, DNB (Urology), MNAMS** Department of Urology, Grant Government Medical College and Sir JJ Group of Hospitals, Mumbai, Maharashtra, India

**Guido Giusti, MD, PhD** European Training Center in Endourology, Department of Urology, IRCCS Ospedale San Raffaele, Milan, Italy

**Rahul Jena, MS, MCh (Urol)** Department of Urology and Renal Transplant, Sanjay Gandhi Postgraduate Institute of Medical Sciences, Lucknow, Uttar Pradesh, India

**Alok Kumar Jha, MS, DNB (Urology), MNAMS** SSB Heart and Multispeciality Hospital, Faridabad, Haryana, India

**Patrick Juliebø-Jones, MRCS** Department of Urology, Haukeland University Hospital, Bergen, Norway

**Panagiotis Kallidonis, MD, PhD, FEBU** Department of Urology, University of Patras, Patras, Greece

**Amir H. Kashi, MD** Urology and Nephrology Research Center (UNRC), Shahid Labbafinejad Hospital, Shahid Beheshti University of Medical Sciences (SBMU), Tehran, Iran

**Thomas Knoll, MD, PhD, MSc** Department of Urology, Klinikum Sindelfingen, Böblingen, Germany

**Handattu M. Krishna, MD** Department of Anesthesiology, Kasturba Medical College, Manipal, Manipal Academy of Higher Education, Manipal, Karnataka, India

**Rajesh A Kukreja, DNB (Urology), Fellow World Endourology Society** Urocare Hospital, Indore, India

**Evangelos Liatsikos, MD, PhD** Department of Urology, University of Patras, Patras, Greece

**Despoina Liourdi, MD** Department of Internal Medicine, General Hospital of Patras "Ag. Andreas", Patras, Greece

**Pankaj N. Maheshwari, MS, DNB, MCh (Urology)** Fortis Hospital Mulund, Mumbai, Maharashtra, India

Department of Urology, Grant Government Medical College and Sir JJ Group of Hospitals, Mumbai, Maharashtra, India

**C. Mallikarjuna, MS, MCh (Urology)** Asian Institute of Nephro-Urology (AINU), Hyderabad, India

**Dilip K. Mishra, MS, MRCS, FICS, MCh (Urology)** Kasturba Medical College, Manipal, Karnataka, India

Head, Department of Urology, Pushpanjali Hospital and Research Center, Agra, Uttar Pradesh, India

Department of Urology, Center for Minimally-Invasive Endourology, Global Rainbow Healthcare, Agra, Uttar Pradesh, India

**R. Mukhilesh, MS, MCh (Urol)** Department of Urology, KKS Hospital and Kidney Care Center, Gobichettipalayam, Erode, India

**Karthickeyan Naganathan, MS, MRCS, DNB, MCh (Urol)** Frontline Hospital, Trichy, Tamil Nadu, India

**Udo Nagele, MD** Department of Urology and Andrology, General Hospital Hall in Tirol, Hall in Tirol, Austria

Training and Research in Urological Surgery and Technology (T.R.U.S.T.)-Group, Hall in Tirol, Austria

**Savan Kumar Nagesh, MD** Department of Anesthesiology, Kasturba Medical College, Manipal, Manipal Academy of Higher Education, Manipal, Karnataka, India

**Palle Jörn Sloth Osther, M.D., Ph.D.** Department of Urology, Urological Research Center, Vejle Hospital—A Part of Hospital Littlebelt, University Hospital of Southern Denmark, Vejle, Denmark

**Susanne Sloth Osther, MD** Department of Urology, Urological Research Center, Vejle Hospital—A Part of Hospital Littlebelt, University Hospital of Southern Denmark, Vejle, Denmark

**Shashi Kiran Pal, MS, MCh (Urology)** Indraprastha Apollo Hospital, New Delhi, India

**Arabind Panda, MS, MCh (Urology)** Department of Urology, Krishna Institute of Medical Sciences (KIMS) Hospital, Secunderabad, India

**Praveen Kumar Pandey, MS, MCh, DNB (Urology)** Sahara Super-speciality Hospital, Lucknow, Uttar Pradesh, India

**Manasi Parikh, MD, MSCR** Boston University, Boston, MA, USA

**Dipen Patel, MS, DNB (Urology)** Sujay Urological Hospital, Vadodara, Gujarat, India

**Abhijit P. Patil, MS, MCh, DNB (Urology)** Department of Urology, Muljibhai Patel Urological Hospital (MPUH), Nadiad, Gujarat, India

**Ashish V. Rawandale-Patil, MS, MCh (Urol)** Institute of Urology, Dhule, Maharashtra, India

**Lokesh G. Patni, MS, M.Ch (Urology)** Institute of Urology, Dhule, Maharashtra, India

**Silvia Proietti, MD** European Training Center in Endourology, Department of Urology, IRCCS Ospedale San Raffaele, Milan, Italy

**Rajeev TP, MS, MCh (Urology)** Department of Urology, Gauhati Medical College Hospital, Guwahati, India

**Jean de la Rosette, MD PhD** Department of Urology, Medipol Mega University Hospital, Istanbul Medipol University, Istanbul, Turkey

**Ravindra B. Sabnis, MS, MCh (Urology)** Department of Urology, Muljibhai Patel Urological Hospital (MPUH), Nadiad, Gujarat, India

**Giuseppe Saitta, MD** European Training Center in Endourology, Department of Urology, IRCCS Ospedale San Raffaele, Milan, Italy

**Kemal Sarıca, MD** Department of Urology, Medical School, Biruni University, Istanbul, Turkey

**Ulhas Sathaye, MS, MCh (Urology)** Sahayog Speciality Hospital, Jamnagar, Gujarat, India

**Cesare Marco Scoffone, MD** Department of Urology, Cottolengo Hospital, Torino, Italy

**Kaushikkumar V. Shah, MS, M.Ch (Urology)** Varun Hospital, Surat, Gujarat, India

**Milap Shah, MS, MCh (Urology)** Department of Urology, Kasturba Medical College, Manipal, Karnataka, India

**Aditya P. Sharma, MS, MCh (Urology)** Department of Urology, Post Graduate Institute of Medical Education and Research, Chandigarh, India

**Abhishek Singh, MS, MCh, DNB (Urology)** Department of Urology, Muljibhai Patel Urological Hospital (MPUH), Nadiad, Gujarat, India

**Harprit Singh, MS, DNB (Urology)** Department of Urology, Mercy Hospital, Jamshedpur, Jharkhand, India

**Bhaskar Somani, FEBU, DM, FFST, FRCS (Urol)** Professor and Consultant Urological Surgeon, University Hospital Southampton, Hampshire, UK

**Aneesh Srivastava, MS, MCh (Urology)** Department of Urology and Renal Transplant, Sanjay Gandhi Postgraduate Institute of Medical Sciences, Lucknow, Uttar Pradesh, India

**Palaniappan Sundaram, MBBS, FAMS, FRCS (Urology)** Department of Urology, Sengkang General Hospital, Singapore, Singapore

**Haresh G. Thummar, MS, DNB (Urology)** Department of Urology, Vedanta Kidney Care, Bhailal Amin General Hospital, Vadodara, Gujarat, India

**Theodoros Tokas, PhD, FEBU** Department of Urology and Andrology, General Hospital Hall in Tirol, Hall in Tirol, Austria

Training and Research in Urological Surgery and Technology (T.R.U.S.T.)-Group, Hall in Tirol, Austria

**Arman Tsaturyan, MD, MPH, PhD** Department of Urology, University of Patras, Patras, Greece

**Yuyi Yeow, MBBS, MRCS Ed, FRCS (Urol), FAMS** Department of Urology, Tan Tock Seng Hospital, Singapore, Singapore

**B. M. Zeeshan Hameed, MS, MCh (Urology)** Department of Urology, Kasturba Medical College, Manipal, Karnataka, India

**Guohua Zeng, MD** Department of Urology and Guangdong Key Laboratory of Urology, The First Affiliated Hospital of Guangzhou Medical University, Guangzhou, China

**Wei Zhu, PhD & MD** Department of Urology and Guangdong Key Laboratory of Urology, The First Affiliated Hospital of Guangzhou Medical University, Guangzhou, China

# Part I

# History, Anatomical Principles, and Imaging

# 1 Anatomy of the Kidney with Respect to Percutaneous Nephrolithotomy

Cesare Marco Scoffone and Cecilia Maria Cracco

## 1.1 Introduction

Anatomy provides the roadmap for percutaneous nephrolithotomy (PCNL).

Familiarity with gross, surgical, and radiologic anatomy of the kidney is essential in order to plan and then perform a successful percutaneous renal access, foresee possible intraoperative technical difficulties, prepare a proper and complete armamentarium of endoscopes, devices, and accessories, inform the patient about the expected success rate of the procedure, minimize the shared risk of complications and, in case of complications occur, recognize them timely and manage them efficiently [1].

In the past, the knowledge of renal anatomy for PCNL could count on books and atlases, the study of formalin-fixed human cadavers, the observation of open surgeries, imaging from intravenous urography and retrograde pyelography, resin casts of the renal collecting system [2].

Nowadays, we can count on additional tools like freshly frozen [3] or embalmed [4] human cadavers for surgical training, the Anatomage virtual dissection table [5] (Fig. 1.1), ultrathin Computerized Tomography (CT) with urography/pyelography, three-dimensional (3D) reconstructions, low-dose/ultra-low-dose protocols and the dual-energy technology [6, 7], 3D printing of the vascularization and collecting system of the kidneys [8, 9] (Fig. 1.2), intraoperative real-time endoscopic vision in high definition (HD) [10], informing us about the real-time dynamic anatomy of the collecting system [11, 12].

Thanks to all these technological advancements urologists in these days have the unique opportunity to obtain a detailed and personalized picture of the anatomy of the patient before PCNL, with particular reference to the collecting system containing the urolithiasis, the surrounding organs and the renal vascularization.

## 1.2 Renal Number

The kidneys are paired organs. A solitary kidney (1/1000 people) [13] might be congenital (unilateral aplasia/agenesis) or acquired (secondary to nephrectomy performed because of structural abnormalities, renal/pararenal tumors, outcomes of severe parenchymal infection or ureteral obstruction, renal trauma). Supernumerary kidneys are extremely rare, in fact not more than 100 cases have been reported [14].

C. M. Scoffone (✉) · C. M. Cracco
Department of Urology, Cottolengo Hospital, Torino, Italy


M. S. Agrawal et al. (eds.), *Minimally Invasive Percutaneous Nephrolithotomy*, https://doi.org/10.1007/978-981-16-6001-6_1

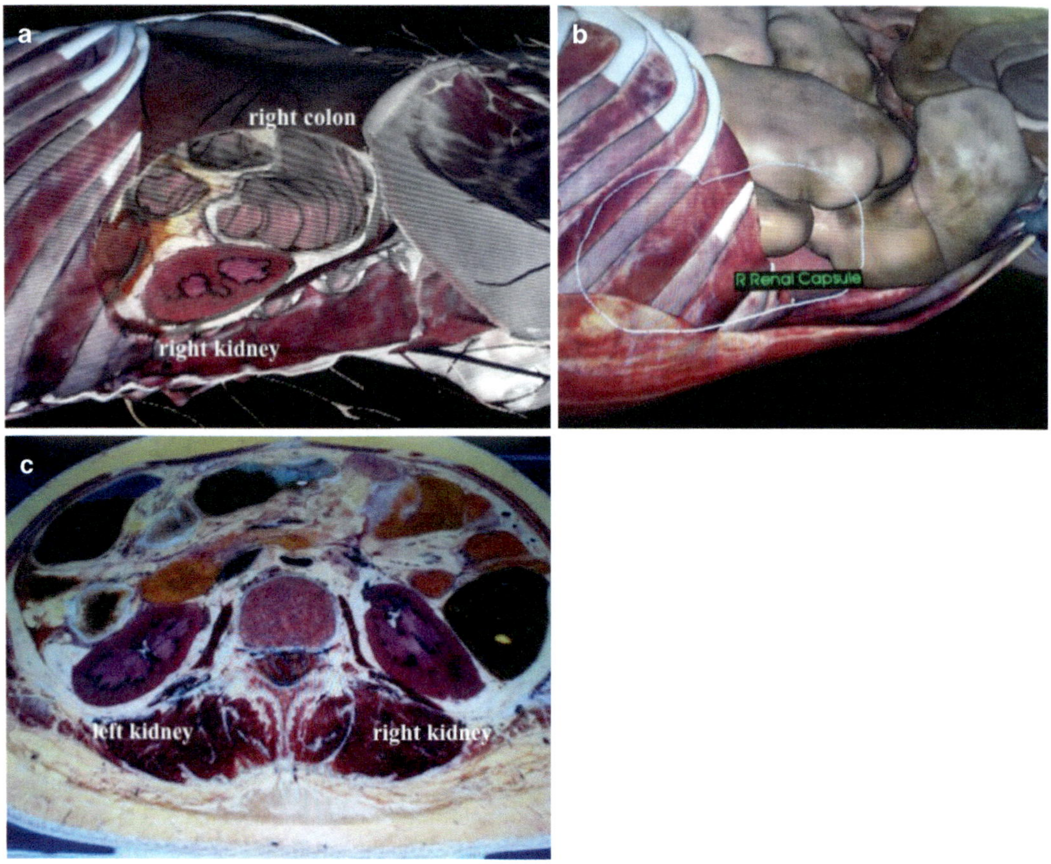


**Fig. 1.1** Anatomic details of the kidneys obtained from the Anatomage Table EDU (Anatomage Inc.), located in the Department of Neuroscience, Torino, Italy (courtesy of prof. A. Vercelli). The 3D rendering of the cadaver is from Anatomage Table. The Image sets were provided by Dr. JinSeo Park, Department of Anatomy, Dongguk University College of Medicine, and Dr. Min Suk Chung, Department of Anatomy, Ajou University School of Medicine. (**a**) Relationship between right kidney and right colon in the supine position; (**b**) Superficial projection of the right kidney covered by the renal capsule in the supine position; (**c**) Transversal section of the kidneys in supine position, similar to CT scan axial images

### 1.2.1 Clinical Implications for PCNL

A solitary kidney should be identified and adequately studied before PCNL from the anatomical and functional point of view. In fact, the choice of the percutaneous approach for the treatment of large and/or complex urolithiasis in a solitary kidney should be balanced, taking into account not only the well-known efficacy of the procedure (stone-free rates range from 67% to 97.7% with the lowest retreatment rate), but also its safety (complication rates are about 26.4%, especially bleeding in anticoagulated patients, with potential postoperative acute kidney failure) [15–17].

The extremely rare supernumerary kidneys (sometimes with abnormal size, position, and morphology) should also be recognized, defining the entity of their functional contribution as well as their exact position, in order to avoid their inadvertent lesion during the percutaneous renal puncture of the native kidney.

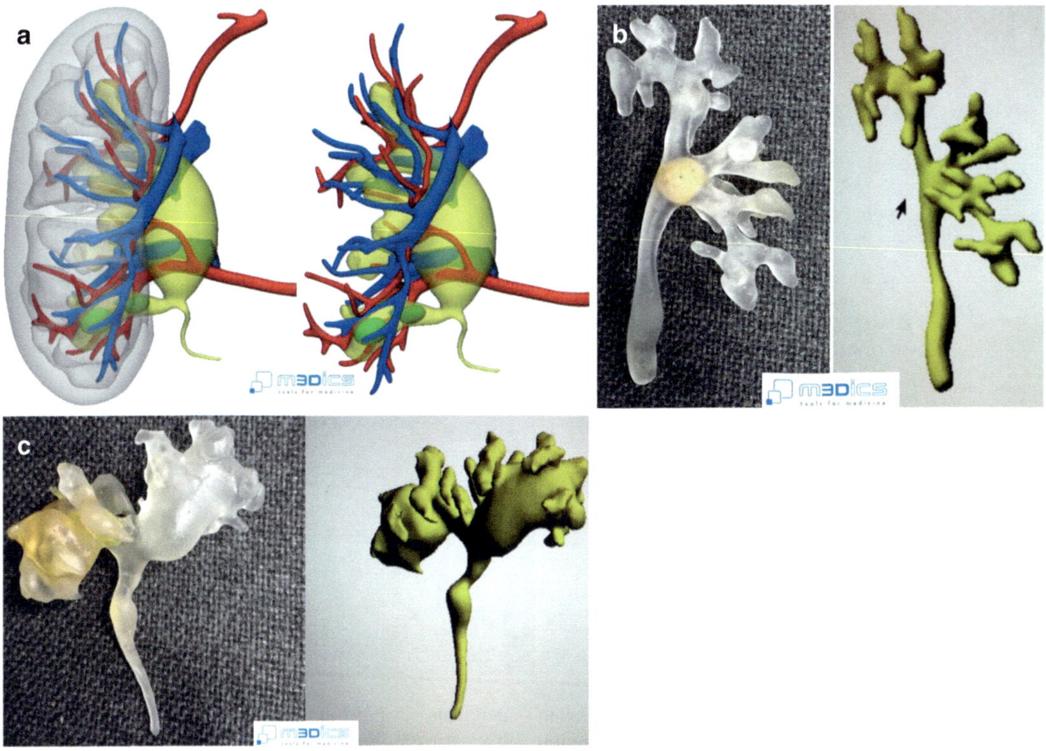


**Fig. 1.2** (**a**) 3D reconstructions of vascularization and collecting system of the kidney (Medics©, Moncalieri (Torino); Italy, permission granted); (**b**) 3D model of the collecting system from a stone patient, obtained from 3D reconstructions prepared from CT scans; (**c**) another 3D model of the collecting system of another patient, demonstrating the high anatomic variability of the upper tract

## 1.3 Renal Position

Orthotopic kidneys are normally situated in the posterior part of the abdomen in the retroperitoneum, on each side of the vertebral column. The right kidney is 1–2 centimeters lower than the left one because of the compression of the liver (extending from the top of the 1st to the bottom of the 3rd lumbar vertebra on the right, from the 12th thoracic vertebra to the 3rd lumbar vertebra on the left) [1] (Fig. 1.3).

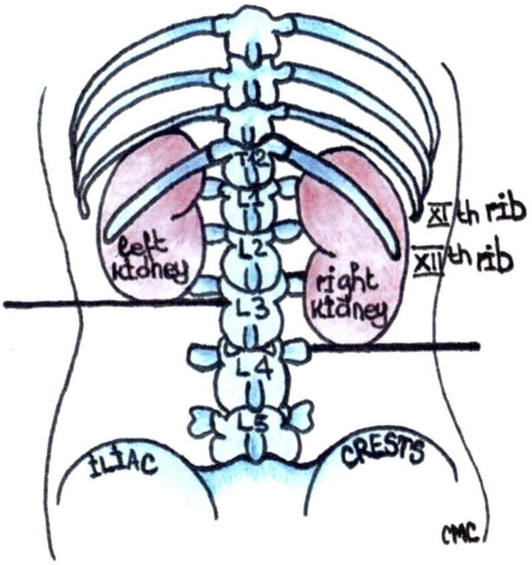


**Fig. 1.3** Drawing showing the lower position of the right kidney in comparison with the left kidney in normal conditions

### 1.3.1 Clinical Implications for PCNL

Changes in body position (supine/erect and prone/supine), physiologic respiratory movements as well as forced inspiration and expiration during general anesthesia, nephroptosis,

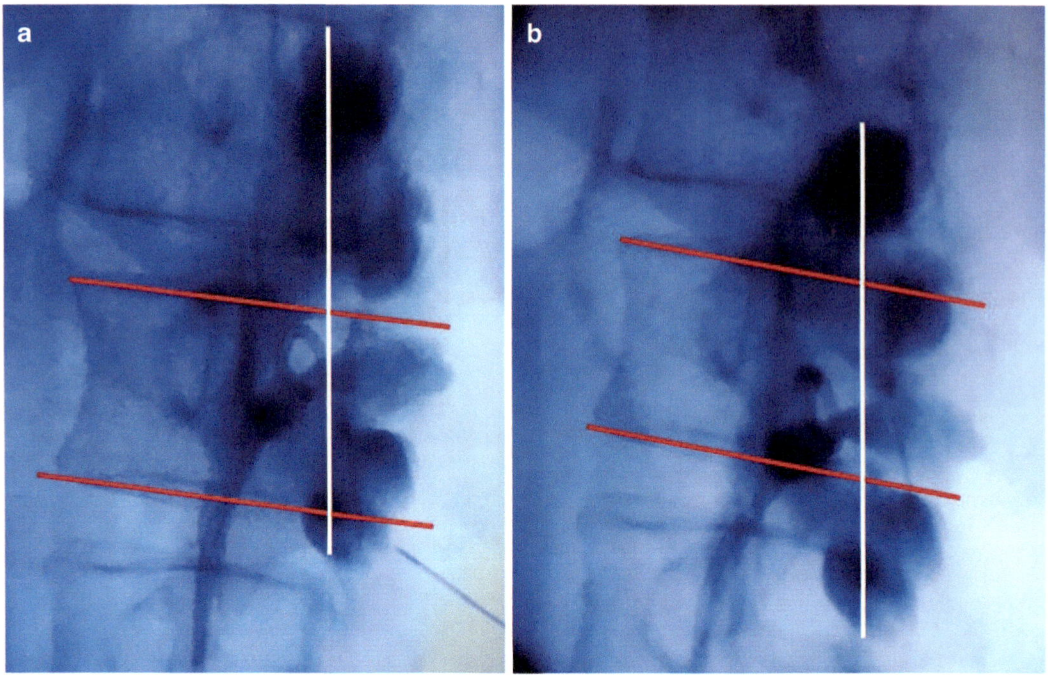


**Fig. 1.4** Retrograde pyelography (**a**) demonstrating in (**b**) the lower position of the kidney in forced inspiration during general anesthesia, which can be used for a better percutaneous puncture (*red* lines marking the same lumbar vertebra used as reference anatomic structure, *white* lines showing the level of the collecting system)

hydronephrosis with thin renal parenchyma may modify the normal position of the kidneys because of different extents of renal mobility in the various planes [18–22].

For instance, during inspiration kidneys may be displaced caudally, ventrally, and outward in a triaxial movement up to 25 mm [21] (Fig. 1.4), possibly interfering also with the complete efficacy of fusion imaging for the renal percutaneous puncture.

In prone position the nephrostomy tract length is shorter, which is considered an advantage: the nearer the fulcrum to the skin the more maneuverable the distal end of the lever will be within the collecting system. This happens because of the different compliance of posterior and anterior body walls: when the more pliable anterior body wall as opposed to the surgical bed more backpressure is placed on the kidneys, which pushes them posteriorly reducing the tract length [18]. On the other hand, in supine position the kidneys situated deeper in the abdomen have a wider access angle [19].

Ectopic kidneys (congenital, with or without fusion abnormalities, or iatrogenic like in case of renal transplant) should be ruled out by preoperative imaging, representing a therapeutic challenge [23–25].

## 1.4 Renal Morphology and Spatial Orientation

The kidneys are bean shaped, with an anterior and a posterior aspect, a lateral convex and medial/hilar concave margin, an upper and a lower pole. The right kidney is slightly shorter and wider than the left one.

Upper poles are more medial and posterior than the inferior ones, which are more lateral and anterior. The main axis is therefore directed downward, laterally and anteriorly, parallel to the oblique course of the psoas major muscles. Additionally, the medial margins are 30° anteriorly rotated if compared to the lateral margins [1] (Fig. 1.5).

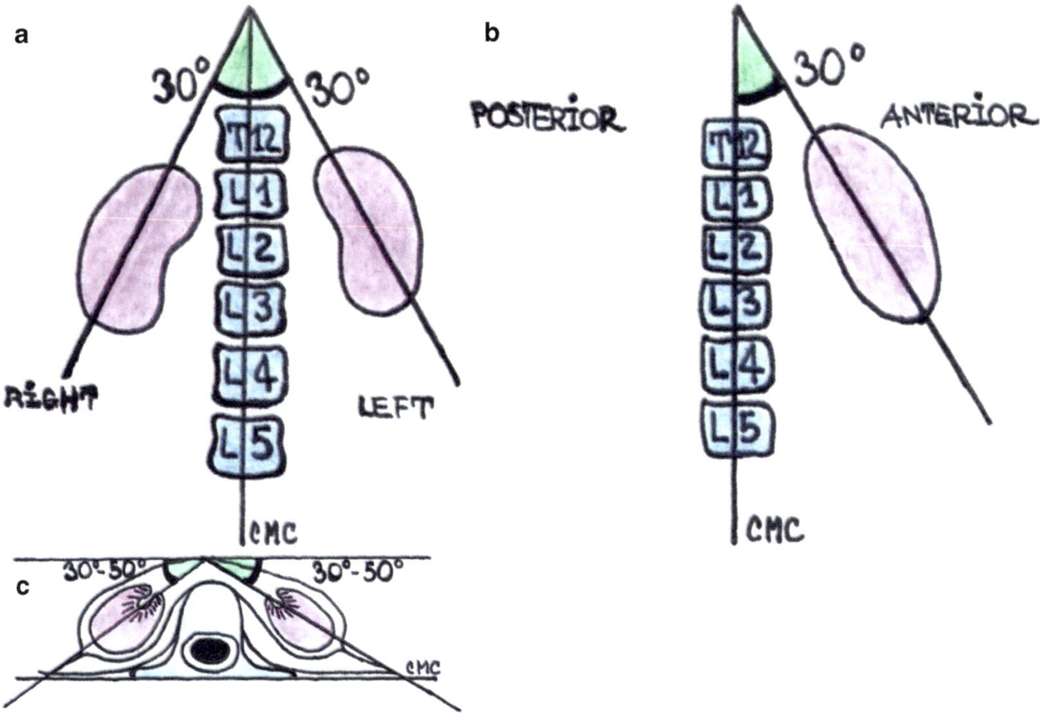


**Fig. 1.5** Drawing demonstrating the orientation of the kidneys: (**a**) in the coronal plane, (**b**) in the sagittal plane, and (**c**) in the axial plane

Congenital malrotation of the kidneys may occur, alone or conjugated with other renal anomalies like horseshoe kidneys [26, 27].

### 1.4.1 Clinical Implications for PCNL

When performing a percutaneous renal puncture it is useful to know the spatial orientation of the kidney in the three planes, but it is especially important to know which factors may possibly modify it, like the intraoperative position of the patient chosen for PCNL [18–20], the patient's body mass index (BMI) (with variable consistencies of the perirenal fat in obese patients, or an increased mobility in very slim patients where the perirenal fat is scarce, especially in the supine position and in females) [11, 12, 28–30], the respiratory movements (displacing the kidneys up to 3 cm, a distance equivalent to one vertebral body) [31] (Fig. 1.4).

Renal cysts of various sizes, renal masses of any kind, pyelonephritic scars, outcomes of previous open or endoscopic surgeries for renal stones, other anatomic anomalies like calyceal diverticula may well modify the renal morphology. A preoperative CT urography is essential in order to characterize any renal mass and define its priority relative to stone treatment; the presence of a simple renal cyst on the way of the renal puncture should be ruled out in order to manage it correctly; renal and perirenal scarring as outcomes of previous renal surgeries might also interfere with the three-dimensional renal displacement of the kidney during the access process, especially during tract dilation [28].

## 1.5 Renal Size

In the adult, each kidney measures 10–12 centimeters in length, 5–7.5 centimeters in width, 2.5–3 centimeters in thickness [1]. They are about 125–170 grams in weight, being 10–15 grams smaller in women and even smaller in children, according to age and BMI [32].

### 1.5.1 Clinical Implications for PCNL

One or both kidneys can be congenitally smaller (hypoplasia) or become smaller (hypotrophy) as a consequence of clinical conditions such as chronic obstruction, acute pyelonephritis, or vesicoureteral reflux. When facing urolithiasis in a small kidney the entity of its functional contribution should always be determined in advance, in order to decide whether it is worthwhile to treat the renal stones, or if it's better to perform a simple nephrectomy of a nonfunctioning kidney.

When dealing with a pediatric kidney, the urologist should adapt instruments and accessories to the patient and not vice versa [11, 12].

## 1.6 Relationships of the Kidney with Neighboring Organs [1]

### 1.6.1 Posterior Relationships

- Superiorly = inferior edge of the diaphragm and underlying costo-diaphragmatic sinuses, ribs (on the right the 12th rib, on the left the 11th–12th rib).
- Medially = psoas major muscle and its fascia.
- Laterally = quadratus lumborum muscle and aponeurosis of the transversus abdominis muscles.
- Obliquely across the posterior surfaces of the kidneys = subcostal nerves and vessels, iliohypogastric, and ilioinguinal nerves.

### 1.6.2 Clinical Implications for PCNL

There is the risk of pneumothorax/hemothorax/hydrothorax when puncturing above the 11th rib in the 10th intercostal space, where underlying there are the pleural cavities containing the lungs [33].

There is also the risk of injury of the posterior intercostal artery, potentially causing hemothorax, when staying attached with the needle to the inferior margin of the rib, therefore it is better to stay in the middle of the intercostal space or immediately above the upper border of the lower rib [34, 35].

### 1.6.3 Anterior Relationships (Fig. 1.6)

- Right side = liver superiorly (intraperitoneal and retroperitoneal bare area), adrenal gland superomedially, small intestine and hepatic flexure of the colon inferiorly, second portion of the duodenum and head of the pancreas medially.
- Left side = spleen and stomach superiorly, adrenal gland superomedially, pancreatic tail, jejunum and splenic vessels medially, jejunum and splenic flexure of the colon inferiorly.

### 1.6.4 Clinical Implications for PCNL

There is the theoretical risk of puncturing all these organs, especially in case of hepatomegaly/splenomegaly, or if the renal puncture is performed anteriorly to the posterior axillary line in supine (Fig. 1.7) and posteriorly in prone, and/or too deep over passing the kidney [36, 37].

Excessive traction and torquing during the procedure might damage the right hepatorenal ligament (joining upper pole of the right kidney and liver), on the left the splenorenal ligament (joining the upper pole of the left kidney and spleen), with the risk of capsular tear and consequent bleeding.

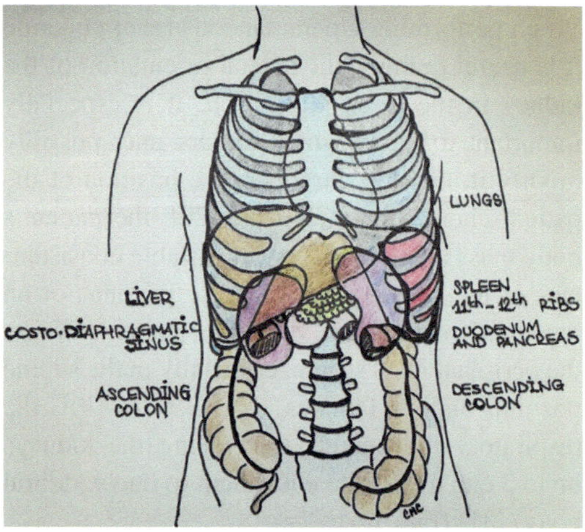


**Fig. 1.6** Drawing of the main anterior relationships of the kidneys

Retrorenal colon should be preoperatively identified by CT scan: its frequency of occurrence in supine position is 1.9%, but up to 10.0% in prone position because in this case the colon is displaced posteriorly [18, 38]. Another work demonstrated that the colon was located along the expected path of a lower pole access tract in 15% of prone CT scans and only in 6% of supine ones [39] (Fig. 1.8).

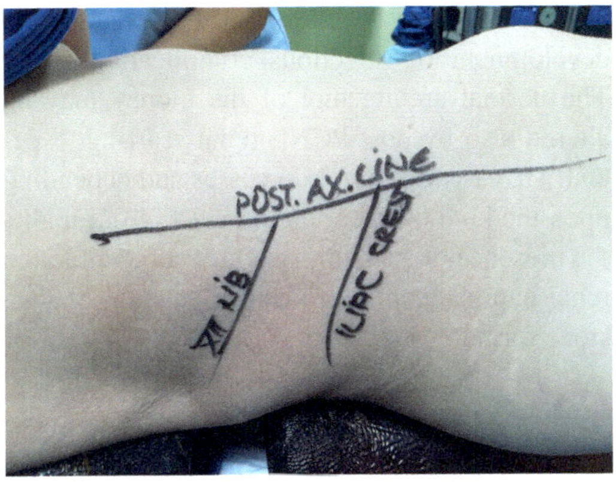


**Fig. 1.7** Reference lines for a safe percutaneous renal puncture in the Galdakao-modified supine Valdivia position: posterior axillary line, 12th rib, and iliac crest

## 1.7 Gross and Microscopic Anatomy of the Kidney

The kidneys are surrounded by a smooth, tough fibrous capsule, provided with an afferent innervation sustaining nociception in case of distension [40, 41].

Between the capsula fibrosa and the renal fascia of Gerota there is the perinephric fat, while outside the renal fascia of Gerota there is the paranephric fat. The renal fascia of Gerota constitutes an anatomic barrier, being closed superiorly (fused above the adrenal glands with the infradiaphragmatic fascia) and laterally (fused behind the ascending and descending colon), fused with the contralateral one medially, while it is open inferiorly. Anteriorly the prerenal fascia and posteriorly the retrorenal fascia fade caudally in the retroperitoneum, medially the posterior sheaths fade in the prevertebral fascia, giving rise to the Zuckerkandl's fascia, and the anterior ones join each other ventrally to the blood vessels forming the Toldt's fascia immediately below the parietal peritoneum [1] (Fig. 1.9).

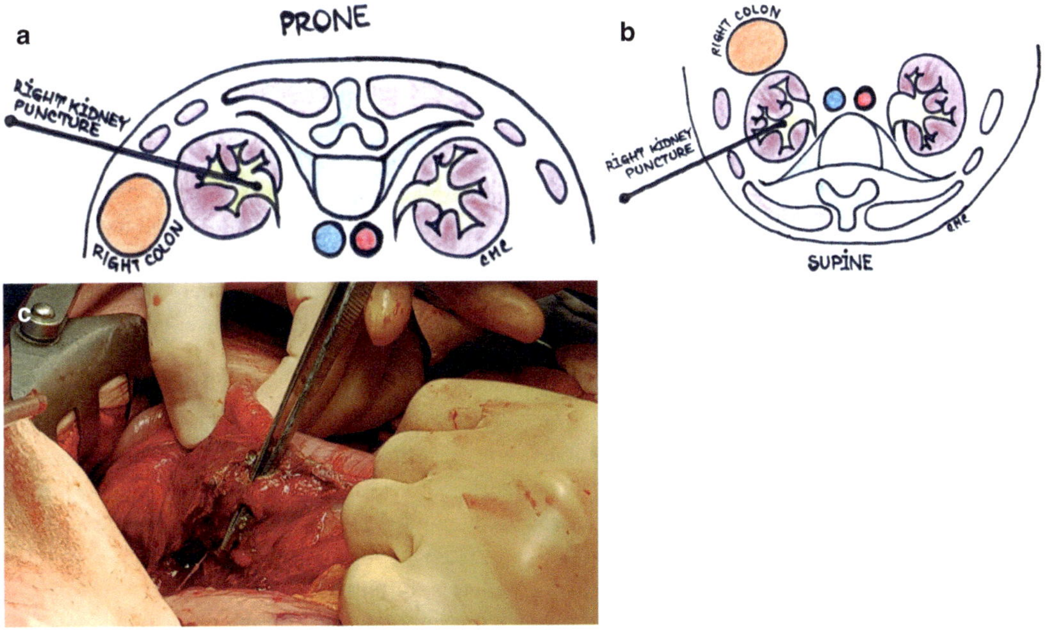


**Fig. 1.8** Drawing of the relationships of the colon with the percutaneous tract to the right kidney in prone (**a**) and supine (**b**) position; (**c**) open surgery for the repair of a left colon injury

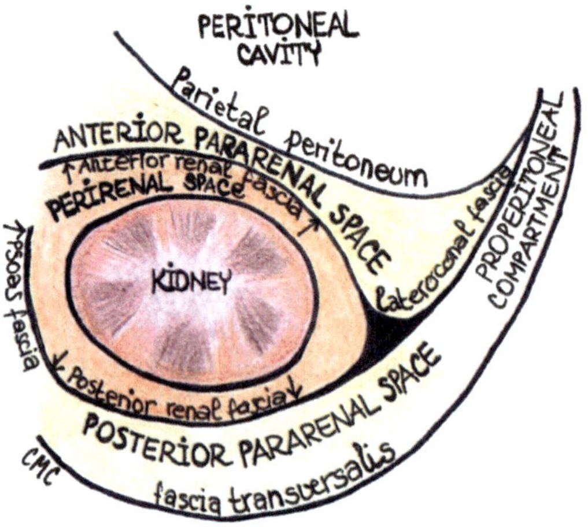


**Fig. 1.9** Drawing of the perirenal and pararenal spaces with the delimiting fascias

Two distinct regions can be identified on the cut surface of a bisected kidney: the cortex and the medulla. The renal cortex corresponds to the columns of Bertin containing glomeruli with proximal and distal convoluted tubules, the renal medulla corresponds to the 14–20 pyramids containing straight tubules, loops of Henle, and collecting ducts, joining to form about 20 papillary ducts opening at the area cribrosa papillae renalis [1].

### 1.7.1 Clinical Implications for PCNL

The renal capsule is nonelastic and provided with an afferent innervation sustaining nociception in case of acute distension of the collecting system like during a renal colic [40, 41], while a sudden increase in intrarenal pressure can break it allowing the formation of a urinoma.

The perirenal space is open inferiorly, allowing bleeding and hematomas (including those post-PCNL) to flow down along the psoas.

The perinephric fat volume of calcium oxalate kidneys seems to be significantly greater than non-stone bearing kidneys [29]. An increased para/perinephric fat could influence renal function through local mechanisms secreting paracrine substances with functional or metabolic renal action, or exerting a direct mechanical compression of the kidney causing its damage through increased interstitial hydrostatic pressure and reduced renal blood flow. It could be secondary to reduced kidney size, filling the free space left by kidneys, being an epiphenomenon of impaired renal function [30]. A certain amount of para/perinephric fat can also increase the skin-to-stone distance, which together with obesity may create the need for an extralong equipment.

High intrarenal pressures may cause pyelo-venous, pyelo-lymphatic, and pyelo-interstitial reflux of bacteria and toxins, supporting the development of infectious complications [42]. The normal architecture of the kidney may be altered also by post-PCNL renal scarring, especially in case of multiple accesses and depending upon the kind of tract dilation used [43]. Finally, the presence of Randall's plaques adherent to the renal papillae can help identify calcium oxalate stone formers [44].

## 1.8 Renal Arteries

The renal arteries arise from the aorta, being the right one longer and passing dorsally to the inferior vena cava. Renal arteries are located between the renal vein anteriorly and the renal pelvis posteriorly. There should be a single renal artery, but supernumerary renal arteries are very common (25–40% of kidneys) [1].

The renal artery gives off the inferior suprarenal artery, and then branches in an anterior and a posterior branch, the first for the anterior two-thirds of the renal parenchyma and the latter for the posterior one-third.

The anterior branch further gives rise to an apical, upper, middle, and lower branch, so in the end the segmental branches are five, also according to the classic Graves' classification. Although, the arterial segmental vasculature is often different from this description [45], with overlapping terminal vessels between the different segments reducing the potential ischemic damage.

Each segmental artery branches into lobar arteries, further subdividing into interlobar arteries progressing peripherally through the renal columns of Bertin between the pyramids. Close to the base of the pyramids they give off the arcuate arteries, from their convex side originate the interlobular arteries, which in turn originate the afferent arterioles of the glomeruli. The arterioles rectaespuriae originate from the efferent arterioles of the glomeruli; the rectaeverae originate from the concavity of the arcuate arteries [46].

### 1.8.1 Clinical Implications for PCNL

The line of Brödel (a German medical illustrator of the beginning of the twentieth century) or avascular plane is longitudinal and located between the anterior and posterior segmental arteries, just posterior to the lateral aspect of the kidney. It is always consistent at the level of the middle segment of the kidney, while it is variable at the apical, superior, and inferior segments, being 1.8–2.4 centimeters from the lateral margin of the kidney. It is absent in 20% of cases, and 4th/5th order vessels cross this line in 100% of cases at the level of the middle calyx, in 27% of cases at the level of the superior calyx and in 33% of cases at the level of the inferior calyx. For all these reasons the best calyx for the puncture seems to be the lowermost posterior calyx [47].

The architecture of the arterial vascularization of the kidney supports the rationale of the so-called "papillary puncture," reaching the tip of the renal papilla along the axis of the calyceal infundibulum where major arterial branches should be absent most of the time [48] (Fig. 1.10). In spite of this, the no-papillary puncture has also been performed safely and effectively, at least in expert hands [49]. The use of vessel-sparing technique with the aid of color Doppler ultrasound in real time may also be effective in identifying major arterial vessels within the renal parenchyma [50].

If the posterior segmental branch passes anterior to the ureter ureteropelvic junction obstruction (UPJO) may occur. It is important to remember that not all renal calcifications are stones… a thorough preoperative imaging might save the situation, for instance avoiding to perform a dangerous PCNL for a calcified pseudoaneurysm [51]. Finally, in case angioembolization for a post-PCNL arteriovenous fistula or pseudoaneurysm, have in mind the arterial architecture,

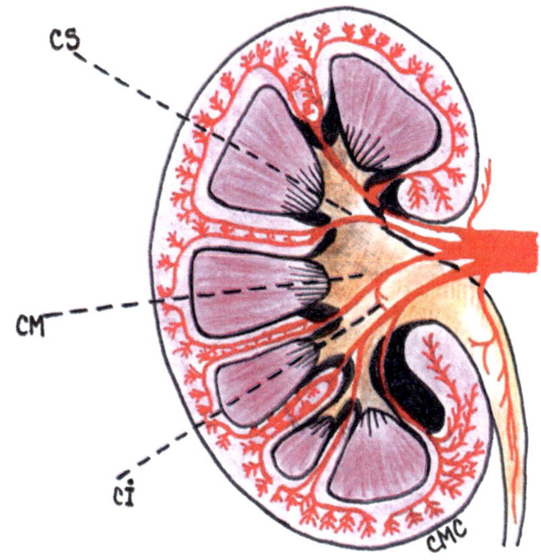


**Fig. 1.10** Drawing of the "avascular tract" followed by the so-called papillary renal puncture

in order to minimize the ischemia of the renal parenchyma [52].

## 1.9 Renal Veins

The venous drainage does not follow the segmental scheme, being diffusely anastomosed and not terminal. The cortex is drained by the stellate veins, mainly draining into the arches of the interlobular veins.

There are three systems of longitudinal free anastomotic arcades, of first, second, and third order from the periphery to the center, with anastomoses between the stellate veins (peripherally in the cortex), the arcuate veins (at the base of the pyramids), and the interlobar veins (close to the renal sinus). There are also transverse anastomoses linking ventral and dorsal veins at various levels. Around the minor calyces, there are large anastomoses forming a sort of venous collar.

The interlobar veins become lobar veins, producing two (29%) or three (54%) large venous segmental trunks, draining into the renal veins (which should be two), then into the inferior vena cava, being the left one longer and receiving the left suprarenal, gonadal, and lumbar veins [1].

Anomalies of the venous drainage are less common than those of the renal arteries.

### 1.9.1 Clinical Implications for PCNL

Injuries to the main renal vessels are uncommon, accounting for less than 0.5%. Tearing and torquing the kidney may cause lesions of the major renal veins and thus relevant bleeding. Direct injury and penetration into the vascular system with the puncturing needle, the dilators or the Amplatz sheath may cause massive hemorrhage. In any case, venous injuries during PCNL are probably underdiagnosed most of the time in absence of injection of contrast material through the nephroscope [53].

## 1.10 Renal Lymphatic Drainage

There is a superficial subcapsular plexus draining the tissue beneath the capsule, a deep hilar plexus draining interstitial fluids into 4 or 5 large trunks, and a plexus communicating with the subcapsular one but draining independently to the lateral aortic nodes. They empty into the lymph nodes associated with the renal vein. Left drainage mainly goes to the left para-aortic lymph nodes, right drainage primarily into the right interaortocaval and right paracaval lymph nodes [54].

### 1.10.1 Clinical Implications for PCNL

This compartment is not relevantly involved in PCNL. A rare case of chyluria has been reported in the literature, due to mechanical injury of one of the trunks near the renal hilus [54].

## 1.11 Renal Innervation

Innervation of the kidney includes both afferent and efferent fibers of the renal plexus. This plexus is a combination of fibers originating from the celiac plexus, intermesenteric plexus, and lumbar splanchnic nerves.

The afferent innervation is essential for nociception recognition and projects to brain regions like subfornical organs, hypothalamus, and brainstem.

The efferent innervation mainly regulates cardiovascular function and arterial pressure; it is primarily sympathetic and receives input from each contributing plexus, while little evidence exists for parasympathetic innervation of the kidney [39, 40].

### 1.11.1 Clinical Implications for PCNL

Kidneys can function well without neurologic control, as evidentiated by the successful function of transplanted kidneys.

The afferent innervation is essential for nociception recognition, having the highest density in the renal pelvis and being activated by an increase in wall tension like in the acute distension of the collecting system. Pain radiates in a dermatomal pattern covering the anterior abdominal wall and flanks as it happens during renal colics [39, 40].

## 1.12 Pyelocaliceal System of the Kidney

Minor renal calyces range from 5 to 14, being 8 on average, and enclose the pyramids (sometimes compound, enclosing 2 or 3 papillae together); they open into the major calyces, two or more, opening in turn into the renal pelvis, which can be intrarenal or extrarenal, with different degrees of accessibility and extent of urine drainage [1].

Pelvicalyceal system (PCS) anatomy might vary (Fig. 1.2), being the Brödel's kidney type (short and medially directed anterior calyx, longer and laterally directed posterior calyx) present in 69% of the right kidneys and the Hodson's one (longer anterior calyx close to the lateral border of the kidney, shorter and more medial posterior calyx) in 79% of left kidneys. Sampaio further classified into types A and B, with two subtypes each [55–57].

### 1.12.1 Clinical Implications for PCNL

Relevant anatomic parameters might be the infundibular width (better >5 mm) and length (better <3 cm), and the lower pole

**Table 1.1** Clinical implications of anatomical features

| Features of the kidney | Main relevance | Clinical implications |
|---|---|---|
| Number | Solitary (supernumerary) kidney | Related risk evaluation |
| Position | Ectopic kidney | Orthotopic kidney: influence of position and respiration |
| Morphology | Abnormal renal masses | Rule out tumors and abscesses |
| Renal orientation | Abnormal renal masses | Influence of position, BMI, gender, respiration, outcomes of previous surgeries |
| Size | Hypoplastic/hypotrophic kidney | Functional correlation |
| Relationships | Retrorenal colon, hepatomegaly, splenomegaly | Reference lines! Avoid surrounding organs during renal puncture |
| Arteries | Papillary puncture, Brödel's line | Prevent bleeding, know the consequences of angioembolization |
| Veins | Avoid traction/torqueing | Prevent bleeding |
| Nerves | Nociception by distension | Correlation with renal colic/insufficient ureteral drainage |
| Perirenal fat | Skin to stone distance | Additional metabolic role, renal compression |
| Collecting system | Adaptation of endoscopes and accessories | Static vs. dynamic anatomy, to avoid damage of the collecting system |

infundibulopelvic angle (better >45°). Such details may be obtained by contrast CT scan, identifying the so-called static anatomy of the PCS, and foreseeing the success rate of any treatment of urolithiasis. Intraoperative irrigation and contrast injection may provide additional data on the elasticity of the PCS, the so-called dynamic anatomy, relevant in order to adapt nephroscopes and accessories (mainly dilators and Amplatz sheath) to the PCS features rather than forcing a stiff infundibulum or calyx and causing its damage with bleeding [1, 11, 12, 58–60].

## 1.13 Conclusions

The knowledge of the gross, surgical, and radiological anatomy of the kidney is fundamental in the preoperative planning of PCNL, essential in the tailoring of the procedure on the patient, the urolithiasis, and the anatomy of the collecting system containing the stones, relevant for the optimization of PCNL success and the minimization of PCNL complications (Table 1.1).

## References


1. Cracco CM, Vercelli AV. Anatomy for PNL. In: Scoffone CM, Hoznek A, Cracco CM, editors. Supine percutaneous nephrolithotomy and ECIRS. Paris: Springer; 2014. p. 41–55.
2. Sampaio FJ, Mandarim-de-Lacerda CA. The kidney collecting system in man: systematization and morphometry based on 100 polyester resin casts. Bull AssocAnat (Nancy). 1985;69(207):297–304.
3. Özcan S, Huri E, Tatar I, et al. Impact of cadaveric surgical anatomy training on urology residents' knowledge: a preliminary report. Turk J Urol. 2015;41(2):83–7.
4. Veys R, Verpoort P, Van Haute C, et al. Thiel-embalmed cadavers as a novel training model for ultrasound-guided supine endoscopic combined intrarenal surgery. BJU Int. 2020;125(4):579–85.
5. Bork F, Stratmann L, Enssle S, et al. The benefits of an augmented reality magic mirror system for integrated radiology teaching in gross anatomy. SciEduc. 2019;12:585–98.
6. Patel U, Walkden RM, Ghani KR, Anson K. Three-dimensional CT pyelography for planning of percutaneous nephrostolithotomy: accuracy of stone measurement, stone depiction and pelvicalyceal reconstruction. EurRadiol. 2009;19(5):1280–8.
7. Koo K, Matlaga BR. New imaging techniques in the management of stone disease. UrolClin North Am. 2019;46(2):257–63.
8. Tatar I, Huri E, Selçuk I, et al. Review of the effect of 3D medical printing and virtual reality on urology training with 'MedTRain3Modsim' Erasmus + European Union Project. Turk J Med Sci. 2019;49:1257–70.
9. Wake N, Rosenkrantz AB, Huang R, et al. Patient-specific 3D printed and augmented reality kidney and prostate cancer models: impact on patient education. 3D Print Med. 2019;5(1):4.
10. Rassweiler J, Rassweiler MC, Klein J. New technology in ureteroscopy and percutaneous nephrolithotomy. Curr Opin Urol. 2016;26(1):95–106.
11. Scoffone CM, Cracco CM. Invited review: the tale of ECIRS (Endoscopic Combined IntraRenalSurgery)

in the Galdakao-modified supine Valdivia position. Urolithiasis. 2018;46(1):115–23.
12. Cracco CM, Scoffone CM. Endoscopic combined intrarenal surgery (ECIRS)—Tips and tricks to improve outcomes: a systematic review. Turk J Urolin Press. 2020; https://doi.org/10.5152/tud.2020.20282.
13. Cochat P, Febvev O, Bacchetta J, et al. Towards adulthood with a solitary kidney. Pediatr Nephrol. 2019;34(11):2311–23.
14. Parmar K, Manoharan V, Kumar S, et al. Supernumerary kidney with stone: successfully managed with semirigid ureteroscopy and laser lithotripsy. J Endourol Case Rep. 2019;30(5):92–5.
15. Shi X, Peng Y, Li X, et al. Propensity score-matched analysis comparing retrograde intrarenal surgery with percutaneous nephrolithotomy for large stones in patients with a solitary kidney. J Endourol. 2018;32(3):198–204.
16. Shi X, Peng Y, Li X, et al. Renal function changes after percutaneous nephrolithotomy in patients with renal calculi with a solitary kidney compared to bilateral kidneys. BJU Int. 2018;122(4):633–8.
17. Pietropaolo A, Reeves T, Aboumarzuk O, et al. Endourologic management (PCNL, URS, SWL) of stones in solitary kidney: a systematic review from European Association of Urologists Young Academic Urologists and Uro-Technology groups. J Endourol. 2020;34(1):7–17.
18. Duty B, Waingankar N, Okhunov Z, et al. Anatomical variations between the prone, supine, and supine oblique positions on computed tomography: implications for percutaneous nephrolithotomy access. Urology. 2012;79(1):67–71.
19. Marchini GS, Berto FC, Vicentini FC, et al. Preoperative planning with noncontrast computed tomography in the prone and supine position for percutaneous nephrolithotomy: a practical overview. J Endourol. 2015;29(1):6–12.
20. Karavaş E, Gürel S, Kıyan A, et al. Effect of prone and supine positioning on computed tomography urography examination. UrolInt. 2018;101(2):167–74.
21. Yamashita H, Yamashita M, Futaguchi M, et al. Individually wide range of renal motion evaluated by four-dimensional computed tomography. Springerplus. 2014;3:131.
22. Lezrek M, Bazine K, Asseban M, et al. Technique to overcome renal mobility during percutaneous tract dilation: bi-prong forceps renal parenchymal dissection. BJU Int. 2013;112:697–702.
23. Xiaofeng G, Zivu F, Chaoyue L, et al. Management of staghorn stones in special situations. Asian J Urol. 2020;7(2):130–8.
24. Salvi M, Muto G, Tuccio A, et al. Active treatment of renal stones in pelvic ectopic kidney: systematic review of the literature. Minerva Urol Nefrolin. 2020; https://doi.org/10.23736/S0393-2249.20.03792-3.
25. Li X, Li B, Meng Y, et al. Treatment of recurrent renal transplant lithiasis: analysis of our experience and review of the relevant literature. BMC Nephrol. 2020;21(1):238.
26. Vicentini FC, Mazzucchi E, Gökçe MI, et al. Percutaneous nephrolithotomy in horseshoe kidneys: results of a multicentric study. J Endourol. 2020; https://doi.org/10.1089/end.2020.0128.
27. Rana AM, Bhojwani JP. Percutaneous nephrolithotomy in renal anomalies of fusion, ectopia, rotation, hypoplasia, and pelvicalyceal aberration: uniformity in heterogeneity. J Endourol. 2009;23(4):609–14.
28. Aminsharifi A, Haghpanah R, Haghpanah S. Predictors of excessive renal displacement during access in percutaneous nephrolithotomy: a randomized clinical trial. Urolithiasis. 2014;42:61–5.
29. Lama DJ, Safiullah S, Yang A, et al. Three-dimensional evaluation of perirenal fat volume in patients with nephrolithiasis. Urolithiasis. 2018;46(6):535–41.
30. Geraci G, Zammuto MM, Mattina A, et al. Para-perirenal distribution of body fat is associated with reduced glomerular filtration rate regardless of other indices of adiposity in hypertensive patients. J ClinHypertens. 2018;20:1438–46.
31. Gadzhiev N, Oibilatov U, Kolotilov L, et al. Reducing kidney motion: optimizing anesthesia combining respiratory support for retrograde intrarenal surgery: a pilot study. BMC Urol. 2019;19(1):61.
32. Ezeofor SN, Anyanwu GE, Obikili EN (2020) Reference indices for evaluating kidney dimensions in children using anthropometric measurements. SA J Radiol 24(1):1882.
33. Assaf E, Chalhoub K, Lteif E, et al. A dynamic anatomical description of the parietal pleura setting safety limits for intercostal percutaneous access. J Endourol. 2018;32(10):919–22.
34. Aron M, Goel R, Keserwani PK, et al. Upper pole access for complex lower pole renal calculi. BJU Int. 2004;94(6):849–52.
35. Netto NR Jr, Ikonomidis J, Ikari O, Claro JA. Comparative study of percutaneous access for staghorn calculi. Urology. 2005;65(4):659–62.
36. Özturk H. Gastrointestinal system complications in percutaneous nephrolithotomy: a systematic review. J Endourol. 2014;28(11):1256–67.
37. Dahril OH, Mustafa A. Duodenal perforation and a broken guidewire fragment inside the duodenum during supine percutaneous nephrolithotomy (PCNL) without adequate prior imaging: a case report. Urol Case Rep. 2018;22:25–7.
38. Hopper KD, Sherman JL, Luethke JM, Ghaed N. Theretro renal colon in the supine and prone patient. Radiology. 1987;162(2):443–6.
39. Tuttle DN, Yeh BM, Meng MV, et al. Risk of injury to adjacent organs with lower-pole fluoroscopically guided percutaneous nephrostomy: evaluation with prone, supine, and multiplanar reformatted CT. J Vasc Interv Radiol. 2005;16:1489–92.
40. DiBona GF, Kopp UC. Neural control of renal function. Physiol Rev. 2007;77(1):75–197.
41. Kirkpatrick JJ, Foutz S, Leslie SW. Anatomy, abdomen and pelvis, kidney nerves. Treasure Island (FL): StatPearls Publishing; 2020.

42. Tokas T, Herrmann TRW, Skolarikos A, et al. Pressure matters: intrarenal pressures during normal and pathological conditions, and impact of increased values to renal physiology. Word J Urol. 2019;37(1):125–31.
43. Aminsharifi A, Alavi M, Sadeghi G, et al. Renal parenchymal damage after percutaneous nephrolithotomy with one-stage tract dilation technique: a randomized clinical trial. J Endourol. 2011;25(6):927–31.
44. Ferraro PM, D'Addessi A, Gambaro G. Randall's plaques, plugs and the clinical workup of the renal stone patient. Urolithiasis. 2015;43(Suppl 1):59–61.
45. Macchi V, Crestani A, Porzionato A, et al. Anatomical study of renal arterial vasculature and its potential impact on partial nephrectomy. BJU Int. 2017;120(1):83–91.
46. Klatte T, Ficarra V, Gratzke C, et al. A literature review of renal surgical anatomy and surgical strategies for partial nephrectomy. Eur Urol. 2015;68(6):980–92.
47. Macchi V, Picardi E, Inferrera A, et al. Anatomic and radiologic study of renal avascular plane (Broedel's line) and its potential relevance on percutaneous and surgical approaches to the kidney. J Endourol. 2018;32(2):154–9.
48. Pearle MS. Puncture for percutaneous surgery: is the papillary puncture a dogma? No! CurrOpinUrol. 2019;29(4):472–3.
49. Kallidonis P, Liatsikos E. Puncture for percutaneous surgery: is papillary puncture a dogma? Yes! CurrOpinUrol. 2019;29(4):470–1.
50. Xu C, Feng S, Lin C, Zheng Y. Reducing postoperative morbidity of mini-invasive percutaneous nephrolithotomy. Would it help if blood vessels are left unharmed during puncture? A CONSORT-prospective randomized trial. Medicine. 2018;97(47):e13314.
51. Chen C, Wang X, Xin F, et al. Large calcified renal artery aneurysm in the renal sinus misdiagnosed as an intrapelvic calculus followed by mistakenly performed PCNL: a case report. BMC Nephrol. 2020;21(1):335.
52. Liao X, Xu H, Liu F, et al. Value of angioembolization in the treatment of iatrogenic renal vascular injury assisted by 3-dimensional digital subtraction angiography. Med Sci Monit. 2020;26:e927208.
53. Mahmood SN, Toffeq HM. Renal vein injury during percutaneous nephrolithotomy procedure. J Endourol Case Rep. 2016;2(1):148–51.
54. Thrasher JB, Snyder JA. Post-nephrolithotomychyluria. J Urol. 1990;143:578–9.
55. Kaye KW. Renal anatomy for endourologic stone removal. J Urol. 1983;130:647–8.
56. Sampaio FJB. Surgical anatomy of the kidney. In: Smith AD, Badlani GH, Bagley DH, et al., editors. Smith's textbook of endourology (part II: percutaneous surgery) chapter 6. St Louis (USA): Quality Medical Publishing; 1996.
57. Sampaio FJB, D'Anunciacao AL, Silva ECH. Comparative follow up of patients with acute and obtuse infundibulum-pelvic angle submitted to extracorporeal shockwave lithotripsy for lower caliceal stones: preliminary report and proposed design study. Urology. 2007;79:61–6.
58. Binbay M, Akman T, Ozgor F, et al. Does pelvicaliceal system anatomy affect success of percutaneous nephrolithotomy? Urology. 2011;78:733–8.
59. Sengupta S, Donnellan S, Vincent JM, Webb DR. CT analysis of caliceal anatomy in the supine and prone positions. J Endourol. 2000;14(7):555–7.
60. Sampaio FJB. Renal collecting system anatomy: its possible role in the effectiveness of renal stone treatment. Curr Opin Urol. 2001;11:359–66.

# 2 Evolution and Classification of Minimally Invasive PCNL

Mehmet Ferhat and Kemal Sarıca

## 2.1 History

Currently, percutaneous nephrolithotomy is the procedure of choice for the minimally invasive management of large stones (>20 mm) both in adults and in children. Related to the evolution of the procedure, percutaneous procedures to the renal collecting system for different indications have been performed for a long time. In 1871, Simon G. was the first physician who mentioned the trocar puncture of hydro or pyonephrotic kidneys [1]. In other words, trocar puncturing the dilated kidneys for the drainage of the collecting system for the first time paved the way for renal puncture to do other intrarenal endoscopic procedures. Based on this evolved concept, an "**antegrade pyelography**" was done by CaseyWC and Goodwin WE in 1953 following an accidental entry into the renal collecting system during a needle biopsy of a "nonfunctioning" kidney [2–4]. They punctured the kidney and drained some urine and pus which thereafter let Goodwin WE and his colleagues describe "**percutaneous pyelostomy**" as the next logical step after percutaneous pyelography [5]. However, despite the establishment of renal puncture with this aim, it took another 10 years until this procedure was suggested and performed again for percutaneous stone removal (PNL) [6].

Related to the application of percutaneous renal access, initially, radiologists were the physicians performing the procedure and despite the widespread use of X-ray (fluoroscopy) to get an access to the kidney, combined sonography and fluoroscopy were first used by Pedersen JF with this aim [7]. Alken P and his co-workers initiated renal access to the collecting system under sonographic guidance on an X-ray table in 1978 and with this experience urologists began to perform the whole PNL procedure after this new approach in puncturing the kidney [8, 9].

Regarding the dilation of the percutaneous access tract, the use of malleable conical dilators and plastic sheaths were originally introduced by Seldinger SI in 1953 based on the accumulated experience from his angiographic radiological procedures [10]. Subsequently, Fernström I, a radiologist, used Couvelaire catheters up to 24 F and tapered plastic dilators for tract dilation at the beginning of this procedure [11, 12]. Another radiologist Rusnak B. et al. described the gradual dilation technique by using polyurethane dilators enlarging up to 30 F in 1982 where he used a 34 F sleeve remaining in place as the Amplatz sheath [13]. Balloon dilatation was described by Clayman R. et al. [14], which was also primarily used in radiological angioplasty procedures [15]. Last but not least, in 1980 by

M. Ferhat (✉)
Department of Urology, Bahcelievler Medicana Hospital, Istanbul, Turkey

K. Sarıca
Department of Urology, Medical School, Biruni University, Istanbul, Turkey


M. S. Agrawal et al. (eds.), *Minimally Invasive Percutaneous Nephrolithotomy*,
https://doi.org/10.1007/978-981-16-6001-6_2

Alken P. et al. described the principle of the metallic telescope dilators, a technique which enabled the urologists to perform a safe dilation process in one step [16, 17].

Although large bore tubes and dilators have been used in the beginning, in an attempt to limit the degree of invasiveness and the risk of serious complications small size tracts were popularized in recent years. By using a 12.5 F ureteroscope, while Wu W. et al. performed Mini-PNL procedures in staghorn stones since 1988 in China [18], an 11/13 F sheath and a 7.7 F pediatric cystoscope were used by Jackman SV et al. in their "mini-perc" series in 1998. All these procedures were done after one-step dilation [19]. A similar procedure in pediatric PNL was published by Helal M et al. [20] again with a single-step dilation technique and this approach became even more popular [21] with smaller tracts [22].

Regarding the first successful stone removal from the punctured kidney, Fernström I. et al. performed the first percutaneous procedure under radiological control during which they extracted kidney stones through percutaneously established tracts first in 1974 and published three successful cases together with the urologist Johansson in 1976 [11].

Regarding the intracorporeal stone disintegration, electrohydraulic lithotripsy was the first modality applied in operatively established tracts in 1969 [23], which was associated with the highest risk to tissue and instruments [24]. Later on ultrasound lithotripsy was introduced [25–27] and the use of this modality along with the development of new accessory instruments (i.e., continuous flow nephroscope), PNL began to be applied more commonly by different groups. Following its clinical introduction, this new procedure replaced 50% of our surgical procedures for large stones in a successful manner [24, 28, 29]. Although it was not necessary to leave a nephrostomy tube following the extraction of stones after an uneventful procedure (by leaving the tract to close on its own), Bellman et al. reported the first concept of planned no-nephrostomy strategy with successful outcomes [30]. This "tubeless PNL" concept was performed by inserting a double-J stent instead of a nephrostomy tube in the beginning and as a result of increasing experience "totally tubeless PNL" concept has evolved in uncomplicated cases (with no bleeding, perforation, and residual fragments left) by leaving no tube and/or stent after the procedure.

## 2.2 In Summary

- Fernström and Johansson published the first percutaneous access under radiologically controlled percutaneous renal stone extraction [11].
- Kurth et al. first removed a staghorn stone by using ultrasound lithotripsy [31].
- Rolf Günther, Gerd Hutschenreiter, and Peter Alken developed endoscopically controlled percutaneous renal stone removal in 1976 [32].

## 2.3 Evolution of Minimally Invasive Percutaneous Nephrolithotomy (PNL)

### 2.3.1 Miniaturization in PNL: A New but Rapidly Evolving Concept

With an increasing incidence both in adults and in children in all parts of the world, stone disease requires an appropriate treatment to prevent possible functional and morphologic changes in the affected kidneys. Management mainly aims at a completely stone-free status with minimal or no risk of complications. Currently available contemporary management options of urinary stones include extracorporeal shock wave lithotripsy (ESWL), retrograde intrarenal surgery (RIRS), and percutaneous nephrolithotomy (PNL). With the efficient and judicious use of these techniques, open and laparoscopic surgeries are being performed rarely (1–2%) in selected complex cases with relatively larger stones.

Of these available options, PNL was first described by Fernstrom I. and Johansson S. in 1976 [11], since then this modality has been accepted and applied as the treatment of choice in the minimal invasive removal of renal calculi sizing >2 cm [33]. Despite its relatively more invasive nature which may be associated with certain severe complications (bleeding, perforation, and infection), PNL enables the endourologists to render the patients stone free in a single session when compared to other treatment modalities associated with relatively lower stone-free and higher re-treatment rates [34]. It is clear that with the clinical introduction of PNL, the morbidity and mortality associated with open renal surgery were significantly reduced. On the other hand again, although the role of ESWL and RIRS has considerably increased as a result of the developments in endoscopic instruments and techniques, PNL still has certain indications with many advantages over ESWL and RIRS in patients with large and complex stones. Excellent stone-free rates (SFR) ranging from 76% to 98% have been reported following PNL [35].

As mentioned above although PNL is the most efficient method with respect to the stone-free rates, complications such as extravasation, blood transfusion, fever, septicemia, colonic injury, and pleural injury may be encountered during and after the procedure. In addition to postoperative sepsis (2%), fever (10–16%) and adjacent organ perforation (0.4%); blood transfusion (3–6%) and significant bleeding (8%) could be encountered during and/or after the procedure. Based on the data reported by the British Association of Urological Surgeons (BAUS) [36] and Clinical Research Office of the Endourological Society (CROES) [37], risks associated with PCNL include postoperative sepsis (2%), fever (10%–16%), and perforation of adjacent organs (0.4%). In particular, blood transfusion (3%–6%) and significant bleeding (8%) are not uncommon complications after PCNL, with potentially devastating consequences.

Taking the evident invasive nature and higher risk of complications associated with standard PNL into account, endourologists aimed to lower the invasiveness and decrease the risk of severe complications (mainly bleeding) by using smaller tract sizes to limit the trauma induced in the renal parenchyma. As a result of the continuous efforts on this aspect, the concept of "miniaturization" has evolved and relatively smaller-sized instruments began to be used in recent years. As the cornerstone of this new era, Jackman SV et al. [38] have first developed a specifically designed minimally invasive PNL (mini-PCNL) device for children in 1998. Following this advancement, a specially designed miniaturized nephroscope for mini-PCNL in adults was first designed and used by Lahme S. et al. [39] in Germany in 2001.

**Since then, the "miniaturized-PCNL" technique has developed rapidly with the introduction of other techniques** designed by using other types of specially designed miniaturized systems (Ultra-mini-PNL, Micro-PNL, and Super-Mini-PNL) became increasingly popular worldwide.

Although limited, published data in recent years demonstrated that these newer miniaturized techniques using relatively smaller size tracts and instruments seemed to reduce the morbidity rates, increase the efficacy of PNL, and also increase the range of its indications. Current European Association of Urology (EAU) guidelines recommend standard PNL as the first treatment alternative for large renal calculi sizing >20 mm and also for moderate-sized lower calyceal stones (10–20 mm) when unfavorable factors for ESWL exist [40].

## 2.4 Currently Available Miniaturized PCNL Techniques

With the clinical introduction of "miniaturization" concept, endourologists began to use the smaller instruments through smaller diameter sheaths in an attempt to reduce the extent of injury induced in the renal parenchyma with similar success rates and reduced complications. With this aim, a variety of endoscopes with different sizes have been used for stone disintegration and removal, by using the access sheaths sizing from11 to 20 Fr. However, over the past 20 years different surgical techniques have been defined and this situation brought the terminology of mini-PNL into a more complex position necessitating further clarification for the term of "mini-PNL" where many studies used the same terminology for the different sized sheaths (14–22 F sheaths).

### 2.4.1 Mini-PCNL

Based on these observations to decrease the morbidity associated with larger tracts, reduction of the tract size with the use of smaller instruments have been proposed. As a result of these efforts, the new technique using a small caliber working sheath was defined as "mini-PNL" or "miniperc." This technique was originally developed for the management of large renal stones in pediatric patients. However, as stated above the term "mini-perc" has been used in the literature, for varying sized sheaths between 11 and 20 Fr [19, 41, 42]. Related to this issue, Helal et al. [20] were the first group reporting miniaturized PNL for a 2-year-old pediatric patient with renal stones by using a 15-Fr peel-away vascular sheath. Following the definition and first application of this technique, Jackman SV et al. [19] performed mini-PNL by using an 11-Fr access sheath. The stone-free rate was significantly high (89%) in this first series without any procedure-related complications.

### 2.4.2 Minimally Invasive PCNL

Within the concept of miniaturization which aims to use smaller instruments and reduced tract sizes, Minimally Invasive PCNL (MIP) approach was first described by Nagele U. et al. in 2007 [41]. Regarding the instrumentation, this system was found to use a 12 Fr nephroscope with a 6.7 Fr working channel, single-stage dilators and corresponding operating sheaths. Stones are being disintegrated by using a ballistic lithotripter and the fragments formed are evacuated due to the difference of the intrarenal pressure and the pressure outside the apparatus, a phenomenon described as the "vacuum cleaning effect" of the system [43].

### 2.4.3 Ultra-Mini-PCNL

In an attempt to decrease the size of the PNL instruments further; "Ultramini-PNL" (UMP) concept has been brought into the agenda of endourologists by Desai J. et al. This new technique used a specially designed 7.5 Fr nephroscope enabling the surgeon to carry out PNL through 11 to 13 Fr sheaths [44]. As the most important characteristic advantage of this technique, this special design of the working sheath allows stone fragment retrieval without the use of baskets or graspers with a minimal complication rate, a high SFR and very limited need for auxiliary procedures [45, 46].

### 2.4.4 Micro-PCNL

This technique is carried out using a 4.85 Fr "all-seeing needle" [47], which aims to perform the renal access and PCNL procedure in one single step under direct visualization. The main aim of the "all-seeing needle" was to establish a perfect initial tract under direct vision, to limit the risk of tract-related morbidity. The microoptics of the needle was planned to help in the confirmation of a correct papilla, to puncture and avoid to injure and viscera on the way to renal parenchyma.

### 2.4.5 Super-Mini-PCNL and Authors' Experience

Related to the ongoing miniaturization process, some drawbacks such as lack of or limited continuous irrigation flow, relatively poorer endoscopic visualization, difficulty in stone extraction, and more importantly the theoretical risk of persistent intraoperative elevation of renal pelvic pressure have led the urologists to look for new techniques to overcome such important disadvantages, which closely affect the final outcome of the procedures. As a result of these efforts, G. Zeng et al. developed the Super-mini-PCNL (SMP) system in 2016 [48]. The basic components of the original SMP system were a 7 Fr miniature nephroscope with enhanced irrigation capability and a modified nephrostomy access sheath, which allows a continuous negative pressure aspiration. The nephroscope has a 3.3 Fr working and irrigation channel which allows the use of both a 0.8-mm pneumatic lithotripter probe, a laser fiber up to 365 mm, and also a 2.5 Fr stone basket.

In conclusion, following the first description of miniaturized PCNL technique nearly two decades ago, all those different smaller-sized systems have not gained a widespread acceptance so far, and their exact roles within the armamentarium of renal stone surgery remain to be defined. Accumulated experience so far has clearly demonstrated that the miniaturized PCNL technique appears to be a reasonable alternative for adult patients with small-to-medium-sized stones and particularly in pediatric ones which allow the application of the procedure in a "totally tubeless" manner. However, further well-designed, randomized controlled studies are certainly needed to outline the specific role of these systems better in a comparative manner with the currently available standard PCNL technique.

*# We are grateful and thankful to Prof. Peter ALKEN for having his published paper on History of PNL as the only available main source for the preparation of our chapter.*

## 2.5 Classification

Following its first clinical introduction nearly 40 years ago, although the indications and applications of PNL have been well assessed and performed with well-established guidelines. However, based on the well-known severe complications (i.e., bleeding and infection) a trend of equipment miniaturization has been emerged to reduce the tract related above mentioned morbidity with the currently available relatively large sized tracts [49]. With this aim and strong desire, endourologists began to use smaller caliber instruments.

However, although the idea and subsequent use of smaller tracts merit certain attention, the clinical introduction of the "miniaturization concept in PNL" has been accompanied by confusion in the terminology, as there is no established consensus among the clinicians. The investigators introducing different techniques have suggested a variety of terms for their newly proposed techniques. On the other hand, practicing endourologists began to look for a unified, commonly accepted terminology based on the size of the access sheaths used [19, 45, 49–53].

This search basically originated from the use of several new PNL terms, like mini-PNL (<22 Fr) [19], MIP [52], ultra-mini-PNL [44], super-mini-PNL [48], and micro-PNL [54], by different investigator groups and confusion regarding the appropriate use of terminology for PNL applications increased substantially. Based on this confusion arising from the "personal author definitions" in the published literature, endourologists realized the importance of a single, widely accepted reporting nomenclature, which will definitely ease the documentation and comparison of currently available techniques.

Related to this issue evaluation of the published data has shown that majority of the proposed miniaturized systems have been put into the concept of "Mini-PNL procedure." However, as one cannot put a 24F sheath and 10F sheath into the same concept, once again to avoid confusion with regard to various names used in PCNL although limited some authors tried to propose a uniform nomenclature based on sheath size used [49] (Table 2.1).

Accumulated experience on this aspect so far has clearly indicated that PNL techniques using access sheath size smaller than 24 Fr could be considered miniaturized approaches. Concerning the formation of a new nomenclature for clinical use, Schilling et al. [49] proposed a categorization of PNL based on the diameter of the outer sheath. Any diameter > 25 Fr was considered to be XL size, 20–24 Fr as L size, 15–19 Fr as M size, 10–14 as S size, 5–9 Fr as XS size, and finally <5 Fr XXS size. Similarly, Tepeler et al. [51] proposed labeling based on the size of the access tract. PNL techniques were categorized as PNL + 30, PNL + 20, and PNL + 12 (Table 2.1). We believe that once established and commonly used, the further acceptance of these techniques

**Table 2.1** Comparative evaluation of the nomenclature used for the currently available PCNL techniques based on the instrument and stone characteristics

| Procedure | Sheath outer diameter | Scope size | Stone size |
|---|---|---|---|
| Standard PCNL [56, 67] | 24–30 Fr | | >2 cm |
| Mini-PCNL [19] | < 22 Fr | 12–14 Fr | <1.5–2 cm |
| The minimally invasive PCNL (MIP) [45] | 18F | 12 Fr | <1.5 cm |
| Ultra-mini-PCNL [44, 52] | 11–13 Fr | 3.5–6 Fr | <1.5 cm |
| Süper-Mini-PCNL [48] | 10–14 | 7 Fr | <1.5 cm |
| Superperc-PCNL)[68] | 10–12 | 4.5/6F | |
| Micro-PCNL [50, 54] | 4.85 Fr–8 Fr | 0.9 mm fiber telescope | <1.5 cm, diverticula and pediatric stone |
| Mini-Micro-PCNL [53] | 8F | | <1.5 cm, diverticula and pediatric stone |

will eventually result in an expert consensus that would clarify the issue of terminology.

Although the main concept for the use of smaller instrumentation was to induce less stress on the kidney, which may result in less bleeding compared with standard 30F instruments; however, to date, most studies comparing minimally invasive PNL with standard PNL have failed to demonstrate considerable differences in outcomes [48, 50, 54–66].

## References


1. Simon G.: Chirurgie der Nieren. Enke Erlangen 1871. https://archive.org/details/chirurgiedernier00simo. Accessed 21 June 2019.
2. Casey WC, Goodwin WE. Percutaneous antegrade pyelography and hydronephrosis. J Urol. 1955;74(1):164–73.
3. Kapandji EM. Ponction de Bassinet et Radiomanometrie Meato-uretreo-pyelocalicielle. Rev C Par. 1949;68:270–90. (Abstracted in. Internat. Abstr. Surg. 1950 June; 90: 577–578)
4. Wickbom I. Pyelography after direct puncture of the renal pelvis. Acta Radiol. 1954;41(6):505–12.
5. Goodwin WE, Casey WC, Woolf W. Percutaneous trocar (needle) nephrostomy in hydronephrosis. JAMA. 1955;157:891–4.
6. Valdivia Uría JG, Lachares Santamaría E, Villarroya Rodríguez S, Taberner Llop J, Abril Baquero G, Aranda Lassa JM. Percutaneous nephrolithectomy: simplified technic (preliminary report). Arch Esp Urol. 1987;40(3):177–80.
7. Pedersen JF. Percutaneous nephrostomy guided by ultrasound. J Urol. 1974;112(2):157–9.
8. Hutschenreiter G, Alken P, Klippel KF. Percutaneous nephrostomy under ultrasound guidance. Urologe A. 1979;18(3):157–63.
9. Thüroff JW, Hutschenreiter G. Fallbericht: Perkutane Nephrostomie und instrumentelle Steinentfernung in Lokalanästhesie. Urol Int. 1980;35:375–80.
10. Seldinger SI. Catheter replacement of the needle in percutaneous arteriography: a new technique. Acta Radiol. 1953;39(5):368–76.
11. Fernström I, Johannsson B. Percutaneous pyelolithotomy: a new extraction technique. Scand J Urol Nephrol. 1976;10:257–9.
12. Fernström I, Johansson B. Percutaneous extraction or renal calculi. Front Eur Radiol. 1982;1:1–24.
13. Rusnak B, Castaneda-Zuniga W, Kotula F, Herrera M, Amplatz K. An improved dilator system for percutaneous nephrostomies. Radiology. 1982;144(1):174.
14. Clayman RV, Castaneda-Zuniga WR, Hunter DW, Miller RP, Lange PH, Amplatz K. Rapid balloon dilatation of the nephrostomy track for nephrostolithotomy. Radiology. 1983;147(3):884–5.
15. Olbert F, Hanecka L. Transluminale Gefässdilatation mit einem modifizierten Dilatationskatheter. Wien Klin Wochenschr. 1977;89:281–4.
16. Alken P. Teleskopbougierset zur perkutanen Nephrostomie. Aktuelle Urol. 1981;12:216–9.
17. Alken P, Gunther R, Thüroff J. Percutaneous nephrolithotomy—a routine procedure? BJU Special Suppl. 1983:1–5.
18. Wu KJ, et al. Secondary minimally invasive PCNL followed by nephrostomy for staghorn stones. Acad J Guangzhou Med Coll. 1993;2:13–6.
19. Jackman SV, Docimo SG, Cadeddu JA, Bishoff JT, Kavoussi LR, Jarrett TW. The "mini-perc" technique: a less invasive alternative to percutaneous nephrolithotomy. World J Urol. 1998;16(6):371–4.
20. Helal M, Black T, Lockhart J, Figueroa TE. The Hickman peel-away sheath: alternative for pediatric percutaneous nephrolithotomy. J Endourol. 1997;11(3):171–2.
21. Frattini A, Barbieri A, Salsi P, Sebastio N, Ferretti S, Bergamaschi E, Cortellini P. One shot: a novel method to dilate the nephrostomy access for percutaneous lithotripsy. J Endourol. 2001;15(9):919–23.
22. Alken P. Dilation of the nephrostomy tract. In: Smith A, Preminger G, Kavoussi L, Badlani G, editors.

Smith's textbook of endourology. 4th ed. Hoboken: Wiley; 2019.

23. Sachse H. Erfahrungen mit der Elektrolithotripsie. Verh Deutsche Ges Urol. 1970;23:171–3. 1 History of PNL 12
24. Alken P. Intracorporeal lithotripsy. Urolithiasis. 2018;46(1):19–29.
25. Lutzeyer W, Pohlman R, Terhorst B, Cichos M. Die Zerstörung von Harnsteinen durch Ultraschall. I. Experimentelle Untersuchungen. Urol Int. 1970;25:47–63.
26. Terhorst B, Lutzeyer W, Cichos M, Pohlman R. Destruction of urinary calculi by ultrasound. II. Ultrasound lithotripsy of bladder calculi. Urol Int. 1972;27(6):458–69.
27. Gasteyer KH. A new method of bladder calculi fragmentation: ultrasonic lithotripsy. Urologe. 1971;10(1):30–2.
28. Marberger M, Stackl W, Hruby W. Percutaneous litholapaxy of renal calculi with ultrasound. Eur Urol. 1982;8(4):236–42.
29. Segura JW, Patterson DE, LeRoy AJ, McGough PF, Barrett DM. Percutaneous removal of kidney stones. Preliminary report. Mayo Clin Proc. 1982;57(10):615–9.
30. Bellman GC, Davidoff R, Candela J, Gerspach J, Kurtz S, Stout L. Tubeless percutaneous renal surgery. J Urol. 1997;157(5):1578–82.
31. Kurth KH, Hohenfellner R, Altwein JE. Ultrasound litholapaxy of a staghorn calculus. J Urol. 1977;117:242–3.
32. Alken P: History of PNL. In: Zeng G, Sarica K, ediors. Percutaneous nephrolithotomy. https://doi.org/10.1007/978-981-15-0575-1_1.
33. Xue W, Pacik D, Boellaard W, Breda A, Botoca M, Rassweiler J, et al. Management of single large nonstaghorn renal stones in the CROES PCNL global study. J Urol. 2012;187:1293e7.
34. Zhu W, Liu Y, Liu L, Lei M, Yuan J, Wan SP, et al. Minimally invasive versus standard percutaneous nephrolithotomy: a meta-analysis. Urolithiasis. 2015;43:563e70.
35. Michel MS, Trojan L, Rassweiler JJ. Complications in percutaneous nephrolithotomy. Eur Urol. 2007;51:899–906.
36. Armitage JN, Irving SO, Burgess NA. British Association of Urological Surgeons Section of endourology. Percutaneous nephrolithotomy in the United Kingdom: results of a prospective data registry. Eur Urol. 2012;61:1188e93.
37. De la Rosette J, Assimos D, Desai M, Gutierrez J, Lingeman J, Scarpa R, et al. The clinical research Office of the Endourological Society percutaneous nephrolithotomy global study: indications, complications, and outcomes in 5803 patients. J Endourol. 2011;25:11e7.
38. Jackman SV, Hedican SP, Peters CA, Docimo SG. Percutaneous nephrolithotomy in infants and preschool age children: experience with a new technique. Urology. 1998;52:697–701.
39. Lahme S, Bichler KH, Strohmaier WL, Gotz T. Minimally invasive PCNL in patients with renal pelvic and calyceal stones. Eur Urol. 2001;40:619–24.
40. Türk C, Knoll T, Petrik A, Sarica K, Skolarikos A, Straub M, et al. Guidelines on Urolithiasis. Arnhem (The Netherlands): European Association of Urology (EAU); 2013.
41. Nagele U, Horstmann M, Sievert K-D, Kuczyk MA, Walcher U, Hennenlotter J, et al. A newly designed amplatz sheath decreases intrapelvic irrigation pressure during mini percutaneous nephrolitholapaxy: an in-vitro pressure-measurement and microscopic study. J Endourol. 2007;21:1113e6.
42. Li X, He Z, Wu K, Li SK, Zeng G, Yuan J, et al. Chinese minimally invasive percutaneous nephrolithotomy: the Guangzhou experience. J Endourol. 2009;23:1693e7.
43. Mager R, Balzereit C, Gust K, Husch T, Herrmann T, Nagele U, et al. The hydrodynamic basis of the vacuum cleaner effect in continuous-flow PCNL instruments: an empiric approach and mathematical model. World J Urol. 2016;34:717e24.
44. Desai J, Solanki R. Ultra-mini percutaneous nephrolithotomy (UMP): one more armamentarium: ultramini PCNL. BJU Int. 2013;112:1046e9.
45. Desai J, Zeng G, Zhao Z, Zhong W, Chen W, Wu W. A novel technique of ultra-mini-percutaneous nephrolithotomy: introduction and an initial experience for treatment of upper urinary calculi less than 2 cm. Biomed Res Int. 2013;2013 https://doi.org/10.1155/2013/490793.
46. Agrawal MS, Agarwal K, Jindal T, Sharma M. Ultra-minipercutaneous nephrolithotomy: a minimally-invasive option for percutaneous stone removal. Indian J Urol IJU J Urol Soc India. 2016;32:132e6.
47. Desai M, Mishra S. "Microperc" micro percutaneous nephrolithotomy: evidence to practice. Curr Opin Urol. 2012;22:134e8.
48. Zeng G, Wan S, Zhao Z, Zhu J, Tuerxun A, Song C, et al. Supermini percutaneous nephrolithotomy (SMP): a new concept in technique and instrumentation. BJU Int. 2016;117:655e61.
49. Schilling D, Hüsch T, Bader M, Herrmann TR, Nagele U. Nomenclature in PCNL or the tower of babel: a proposal for a uniform terminology. World J Urol. 2015;33:1905e1907. https://doi.org/10.1007/s00345-015-1506-7.
50. Desai MR, Sharma R, Mishra S, Sabnis RB, Stief C, Bader M. Single step percutaneous nephrolithotomy (microperc): the initial clinical report. J Urol. 2011;186:140–5.
51. Tepeler A, Sarica K. Standard, mini, ultra-mini, and micro percutaneous nephrolithotomy: what is next? A novel labeling system for percutaneous nephrolithotomy according to the size of the access sheath used during procedure. Urolithiasis. 2013;41:367–8.
52. Nagele U, Schilling D, Anastasiadis AG, Walcher U, Sievert KD, Merseburger AS, Kuczyk M, Stenzl

A. Minimally invasive percutaneous nephrolitholapaxy (MIP). Der Urologe Aug A. 2008;47(9):1068–73. https://doi.org/10.1007/s00120-008-1814-2.
53. Sabnis RB, Ganesamoni R, Ganpule AP, Mishra S, Vyas J, Jagtap J, Desai M. Current role of microperc in the management of small renal calculi. Ind J Urol Soc India. 2013;29(3):214–8. https://doi.org/10.4103/0970-1591.117282.
54. Bader MJ, Gratzke C, Seitz M, Sharma R, Stief CG, Desai M. The "allseeing needle": initial results of an optical puncture system confirming access in percutaneous nephrolithotomy. Eur Urol. 2011;59:1054–9.
55. Cheng F, Yu W, Zhang X, Yang S, Xia Y, Ruan Y. Minimally invasive tract in percutaneous nephrolithotomy for renal stones. J Endourol. 2010;24:1579–82.
56. Knoll T, Wezel F, Michel MS, Honeck P, Wendt-Nordahl G. Do patients benefit from miniaturized tubeless percutaneous nephrolithotomy? A comparative prospective study. J Endourol. 2010;24:1075–9.
57. Giusti G, Piccinelli A, Taverna G, et al. Miniperc? No, thank you! Eur Urol. 2007;51:810–5. discussion 815
58. Abdelhafez MF, Bedke J, Amend B, et al. Minimally invasive percutaneous nephrolitholapaxy (PCNL) as an effective and safe procedure for large renal stones. BJU Int. 2012;110:E1022–6.
59. Mishra S, Sharma R, Garg C, Kurien A, Sabnis R, Desai M. Prospective comparative study of miniperc and standard PNL for treatment of 1 to 2 cm size renal stone. BJU Int. 2011;108:896–9. discussion 899–900
60. Sabnis RB, Jagtap J, Mishra S, Desai M. Treating renal calculi 1–2 cm in diameter with minipercutaneous or retrograde intrarenal surgery: a prospective comparative study. BJU Int. 2012;110:E346–9.
61. Zeng G, Zhu W, Li J, et al. The comparison of minimally invasive percutaneous nephrolithotomy and retrograde intrarenal surgery for stones larger than 2 cm in patients with a solitary kidney: a matched-pair analysis. World J Urol. 2015;33:1159–64.
62. Kirac M, Bozkurt OF, Tunc L, Guneri C, Unsal A, Biri H. Comparison of retrograde intrarenal surgery and mini-percutaneous nephrolithotomy in management of lower-pole renal stones with a diameter of smaller than 15 mm. Urolithiasis. 2013;41:241–6.
63. Pan J, Chen Q, Xue W, et al. RIRS versus mPCNL for single renal stone of 2–3 cm: clinical outcome and cost-effective analysis in Chinese medical setting. Urolithiasis. 2013;41:73–8.
64. Kruck S, Anastasiadis AG, Herrmann TR, et al. Minimally invasive percutaneous nephrolithotomy: an alternative to retrograde 394 EUROPEAN UROLOGY 70 (2016) 382–396 intrarenal surgery and shockwave lithotripsy. World J Urol. 2013;31:1555–61.
65. Sabnis RB, Ganesamoni R, Doshi A, Ganpule AP, Jagtap J, Desai MR. Micropercutaneous nephrolithotomy (microperc) vs retrograde intrarenal surgery for the management of small renal calculi: a randomized controlled trial. BJU Int. 2013;112:355–61.
66. Hatipoglu NK, Tepeler A, Buldu I, et al. Initial experience of micropercutaneous nephrolithotomy in the treatment of renal calculi in 140 renal units. Urolithiasis. 2014;42:159–64.
67. Kamal W, Kallidonis P, Kyriazis I, Liatsikos E. Minituriazed percutaneous nephrolithotomy: what does it mean? Urolithiasis. 2016;44:195–201.
68. Shah K, Agrawal MS, Mishra DK. Superperc: a new technique in minimally-invasive percutaneous nephrolithotomy. Indian J Urol. 2017;33:48–52.

# 3 Diagnostic Imaging for Mini Percutaneous Nephrolithotomy

Susanne Sloth Osther and Palle Jörn Sloth Osther

## 3.1 Introduction

Traditionally, percutaneous nephrolithotomy (PCNL) has been advocated for the treatment of patients with large and/or complex renal calculi. During recent years miniaturizing the access in PCNL (mini PCNL) has widened the indications for PCNL, and continuing evolutions in access and intracorporeal lithotripsy technology have increased the possibilities of a true Personalized Stone Approach (PSA), taking into consideration best available evidence, patients' preferences, and expectations as well as surgeons' clinical expertise (Fig. 3.1) [1]. In this perspective, imaging is an essential tool for patient selection, access planning, as well as for complication and outcome evaluation.

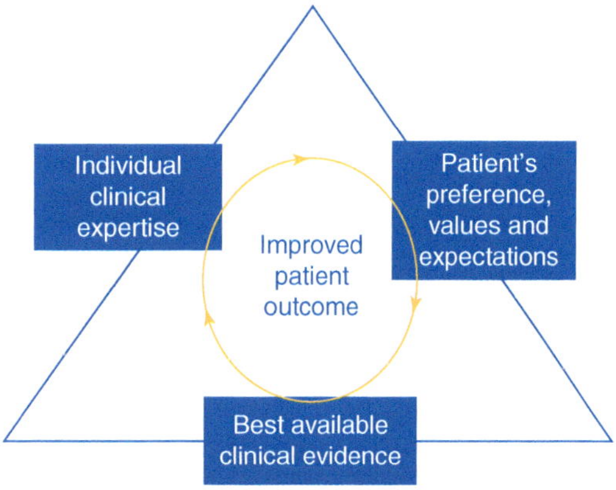


**Fig. 3.1** PSA in an EBM perspective. (PSA = Personalized Stone Approach; EBM = Evidence Based Medicine; [Adapted from Axelsson et al. World J Urol [1]])

## 3.2 Introducing the RALARA Principle and Imaging in Nephrolithiasis

Nephrolithiasis is often recurrent, and patients with kidney stones are at risk of high radiation exposure [2]. To reduce ionized radiation in stone patients it is of upmost importance to apply the ALARA principle. ALARA stands for "as low as reasonably achievable", which should be an integral part of all activities that involve the use of ionized radiation to prevent unnecessary exposure as well as overexposure. Further details regarding the ALARA principle will be outlined in the next chapter.


S. S. Osther (✉) · P. J. S. Osther
Department of Urology, Urological Research Center, Vejle Hospital—A Part of Hospital Littlebelt, University Hospital of Southern Denmark, Vejle, Denmark
e-mail: susanne.sloth.osther@rsyd.dk; Palle.Joern.Osther@rsyd.dk





M. S. Agrawal et al. (eds.), *Minimally Invasive Percutaneous Nephrolithotomy*, https://doi.org/10.1007/978-981-16-6001-6_3

In patients undergoing PCNL there are several additional factors contributing to high radiation exposure, including high body mass index (BMI), multiple tract access, complex renal anatomy, and increased stone burden [3]. Therefore, the concept of ALARA is of special importance in this group of patients. On the other hand, we need sufficient and reliable diagnostic imaging to define indication for treatment, for performing safe surgery, and for evaluation of outcome. In this respect, we introduce the concept of **RALARA**, "risk as low as reasonably achievable", taking into consideration both 1) risk of performing the imaging procedure (radiation risk) and 2) risk of not performing the imaging procedure, potentially resulting in insufficient information for treatment decisions. Therefore, imaging strategy needs to be personalized (Fig. 3.2).

### 3.2.1 Paediatric Nephrolithiasis

Since mini PCNL plays a particular role in management of paediatric urolithiasis, special attention should be on imaging modalities for paediatric upper urinary tract stone disease. Ideally radiation free imaging should be used; however, for planning PCNL procedures this may not be sufficient. Ultrasonography (US) is the preferred initial diagnostic examination in children with the advantages of being easily available and with no radiation exposure [4] (Fig. 3.3). However, US for diagnosis of urolithiasis and characterization of renal anatomy do have limitations. US accuracy is very operator dependent, and sensitivity and specificity for detection of renal stones have been reported to be 61–93% and 95–100%, respectively [4, 5]. Additionally, US often does not present renal and perirenal anatomy and details of stone burden accurately. Therefore, additional imaging is often necessary for treatment planning, especially if PCNL is considered. The other radiation free alternative, Magnetic Resonance Urography (MRU), is seldomly used [6]. Although Gadolinium-enhanced-excretory MRU has shown up to 90–100% sensitivity for urolithiasis diagnosis and is excellent for presenting anatomical details and severity of obstruction, the examination has considerable limitations, including longer procedure duration, need for general anaesthesia, motion artefacts, and high costs [4, 6]. Combining US and plain abdominal radiography (Kidney-Ureter-Bladder = KUB) with retrograde pyelography at surgery may be enough for PCNL surgical strategy; however, since ultra-low dose CT (ULD-CT) protocols with radiation

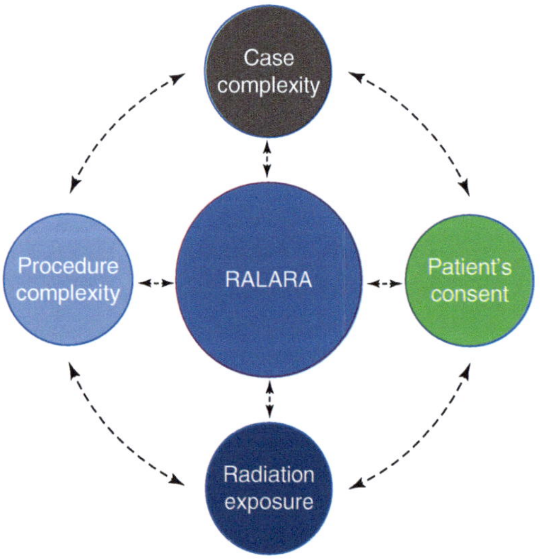


**Fig. 3.2** RALARA—Risk as Low as Reasonably Achievable. (Risk of performing imaging [ionized radiation hazards] should be weighed up against risk of not performing sufficient and reliable diagnostic imaging, in order to be able to select the right treatment for the right patient. In this clinical decision-making scenario, the concept of RALARA interacts dynamically with case and procedure complexity, patient's consent and potential radiation risks for the individual patient)

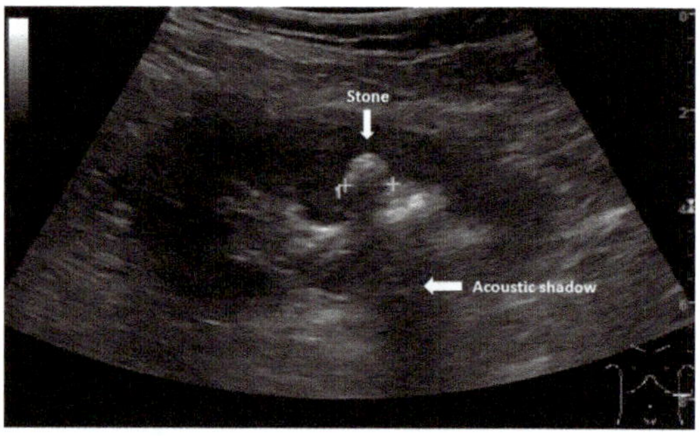


**Fig. 3.3** Ultrasonography [ULS] of kidney with a stone in the middle calyx. (The stone strongly reflect ultrasonic waves and appears as a bright echogenic structure with an acoustic shadow behind, due to the fact that that the ultrasonic waves are unable to penetrate through the stone)

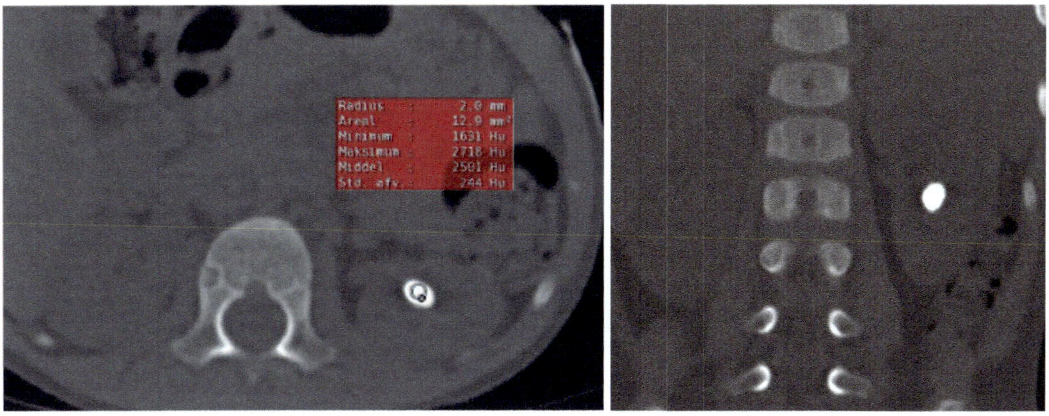


Axia plane

Coronal plane

**Fig. 3.4** Ultralow dose computerized tomography [ULD-CT]. (ULD-CT in a 3-year-old boy with a very dense stone [mean HU 2501]. The examination could be designed with a radiation dose of 0.36 mSv, which is comparable or even less than a KUB. The boy was treated by mini-PCNL and Thulium fiber laser lithotripsy, since this very hard stone probably would have been Shock Wave Lithotripsy [SWL] resistant. In this way the imaging modality helped choosing the right treatment up front, thereby enabling a personalized stone approach [PSA])

doses close to KUB (0.5 mSv) and without limiting image quality in the paediatric population, ULD-CT has been suggested as standard prior to PCNL in children [7] (Fig. 3.4). Again, due to the extreme diversity of stone disease, especially in the population needing PCNL, a PSA imaging strategy in children should be applied, taking into consideration the concept of RALARA.

Overall diagnostic imaging considerations concerning mini PCNL will be discussed in the following.

## 3.3 Preoperative Diagnostic Imaging

Preoperative imaging is considered the major tool for individualizing stone management; thereby enabling PSA [1]. Ideally imaging should characterize the stone, present renal and perirenal anatomy as well as estimate kidney function [8].

### 3.3.1 Stone Characteristics and Renal Anatomy

Previously, Intravenous Urography (IVU) (Fig. 3.5) was considered the gold standard for diagnosis and treatment planning of urolithiasis; however, nowadays CT has almost completely taken over the stone imaging scenario. For assessment of acute flank pain, Non-contrast CT (NCCT) with sensitivities and specificities for evaluating renal and ureteral calculi approaching 100% performs significantly better than IVU (evidence level 1a) [9–12]. Regarding treatment strategies in PCNL, CT examinations are of particular value for (1) assessment of stone characteristics (composition and volume) and (2) for defining renal anatomy, in order to choose optimal access size and site, which both are paramount in mini PCNL.

#### 3.3.1.1 Stone Characteristics

CT-attenuation values, expressed as Hounsfield Units (HU), are widely used to estimate stone composition and hardness [13]. This may be of importance, when selecting endoscopic procedures (RIRS, mini PCNL) instead of SWL, since higher HU values (above 900–1200 HU) have been found to be independent predictors of SWL failure [13, 14]. It has been shown, however, that the correlation between HU and SWL failure is not linear despite identical stone composition, suggesting a multitude of factors involved (15). By using high-resolution detection of internal structure of renal calculi with helical CT, it was found that internal structure rather than HU of

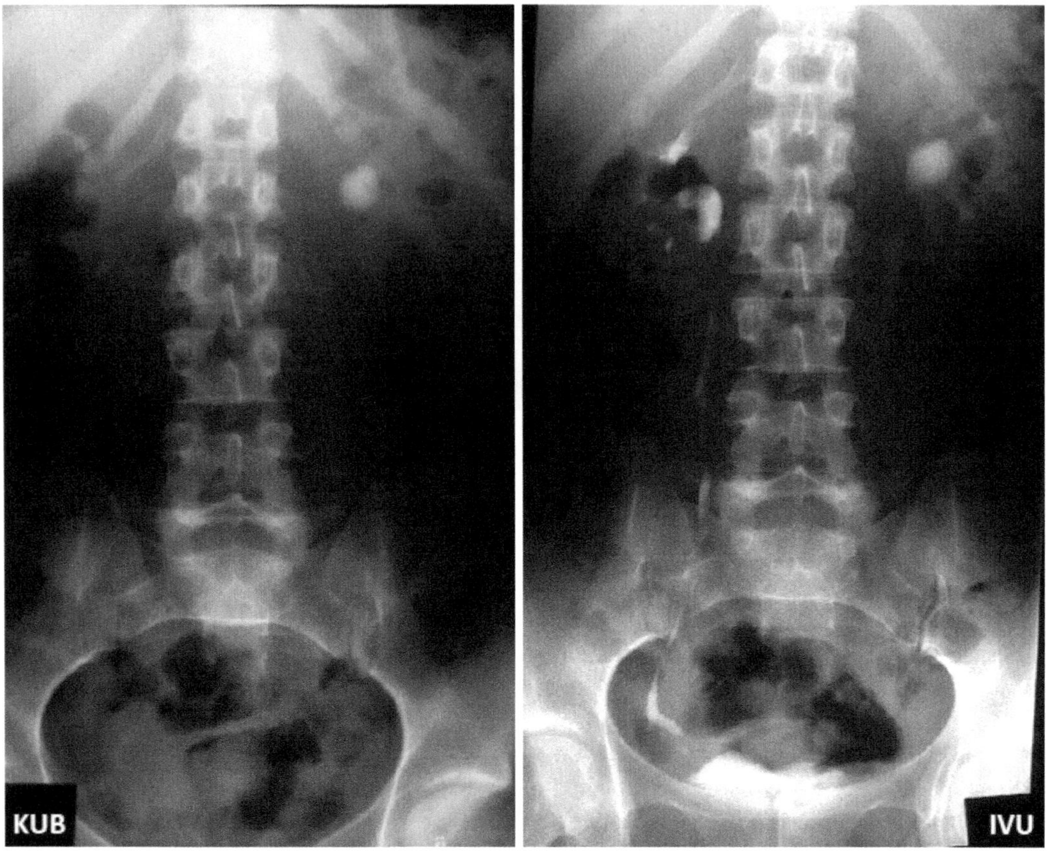


**Fig. 3.5** Plain abdominal radiography [KUB] and intravenous urography [IVU]. (KUB [left] showing large radiopaque stone in the left kidney. IVU [right] demonstrating that the stone is located in the renal pelvis with a slight degree of obstruction, resulting in dilatation of calyces)

calcium oxalate monohydrate (COM) [15] and cystine stones [16] predicted lithotripsy fragility in vitro. COM and cystine stones of homogeneous structure required almost twice as many Shock Waves (SWs) to comminute than stones of similar mineral composition that exhibit internal structural features (void regions) that were visible by CT (Fig. 3.6). Hounsfield unit values of COM as well as cystine stones did not correlate with stone fragility. Thus, it seems that it is stone morphology, rather than X-ray attenuation, which correlates with fragility to SWs in COM and cystine stones, and these stone characteristics may be used for selection of patients to primary SWL or primary endoscopic treatment, such as mini PCNL, increasing efficacy of both (Fig. 3.7).

Traditionally, stone diameters have been used to characterize stone burden. This is a routine that stems from the era of plain abdominal radiography (KUB) and IVU; however, with use of CT technology exact volume of stone burden is achievable, and volume seems to correlate better to treatment outcome and should be used in clinical as well as research settings [17, 18].

Whether a KUB should be added to the NCCT before stone treatment is a matter of debate [19]. KUB envisions radiopaque stones; including calcium stones, cystine and struvite stones, whereas uric acid stones are radiolucent (Fig. 3.8). This may be useful information during access as well as during endoscopy when evaluating residual fragments with fluoroscopy. This

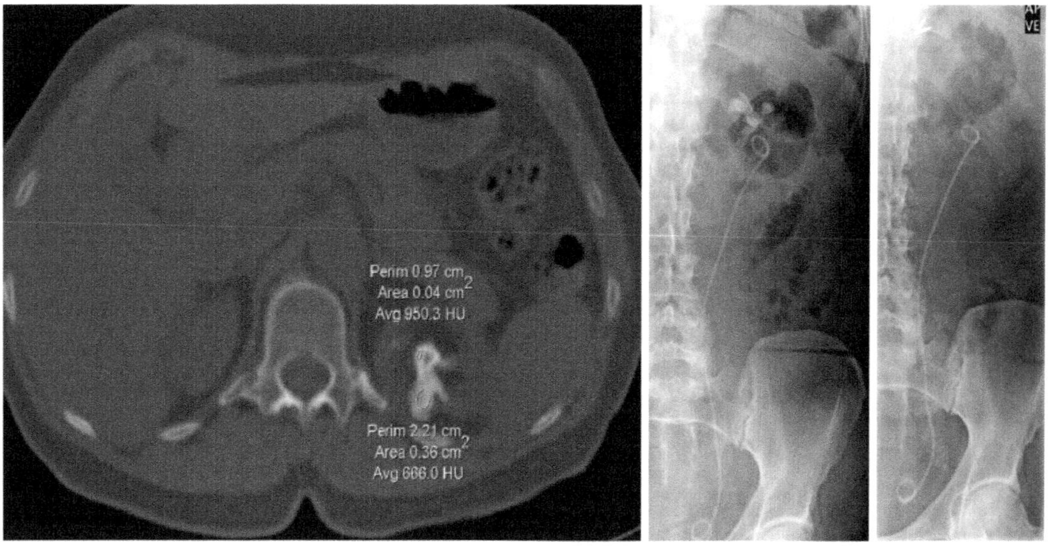


**Fig. 3.6** Non-contrast CT[NCCT] in bone window. (NCCT [left] demonstrating a branched stone in the upper pole of the left kidney that has a close relation to the spleen, which potentially would be a problem in an upper pole access. In the bone window it appears that the stone is heterogenous with void regions, which makes the stone easier fragmentable with SWL. Therefore, SWL was preferred, and after one SWL session the patient was almost stone free with only minor fragments left in the lower pole demonstrated on KUB [right]. Prior to SWL the patient had a JJ inserted to prevent adverse events of a Steinstrasse. In this way imaging helped personalizing treatment, focusing on both efficacy and safety)

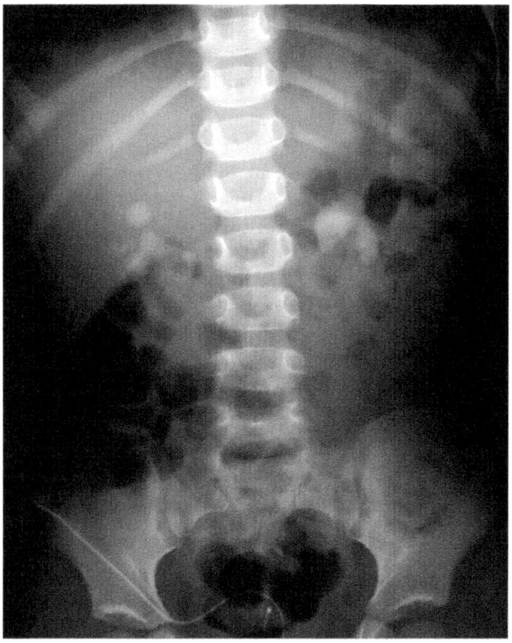

**Fig. 3.7** Plain abdominal radiography [KUB] of cystine stones. (KUB demonstrating weak radiopaque staghorn stones in both kidneys of a 3-year-old boy with cystinuria)

information may also be achieved using the CT planning image (CTI, Scout, Topogram, etc.), since it has been shown that kidney stones visible on CTI are also visible on KUB/fluoroscopy (positive predictive value 100%) [20]. Thus, adding a KUB seems to be unnecessary exposure of ionized radiation, if a CTI is available.

#### 3.3.1.2 Renal Anatomy

Regarding anatomical information, NCCT has been considered less suitable than IVU, and patients with complex stones or anatomy scheduled for PCNL may need additional imaging [13]. This can be done by a retrograde contrast study during surgery, which often is enough for a safe puncture. Additionally, this gives an impression of the dynamic anatomy of the collecting system, which may define need for a miniaturized access (narrow calyceal neck, diverticulum stones. Etc.). This also may be achieved by a contrast enhanced CT, which according to the Guidelines of European Association of Urology (EAU) should be done if renal stone removal is planned and the

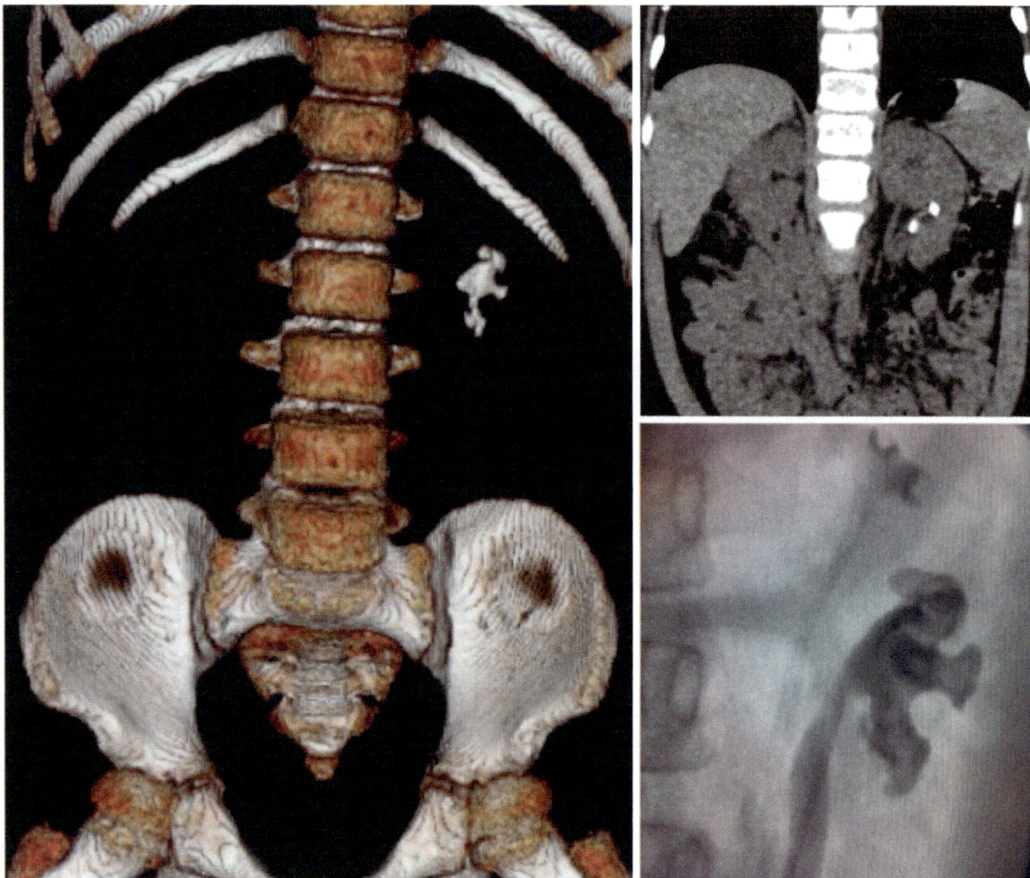

**Fig. 3.8** Low-dose 3-D CT. (In this 9-year-old boy initial ultrasonography gave the suspicion of a large stone in the lower part of the left kidney. For treatment planning a low-dose CT [1.7 mSv] was performed, and this examination gave the suspicion of a dual system [upper right], which was confirmed by a retrograde pyelography during surgery [lower right]. 3-D reformatting [left] helped deciding proper calyx for access in mini PCNL. Thus, the slightly higher radiation dose was justified by the additional information achieved, securing efficacious and safe surgery)

anatomy of the renal collecting system needs to be assessed [13, 21, 22]. Excretory contrast studies (ECT) may mask stones [8, 23]; however, viewing the images in the bone window most often will give valuable information regarding stone and calyceal system interrelations. In complex cases where access difficulties are anticipated, 3-D CT pyelography may be beneficial for detailed evaluation of stone burden and anatomy as well as for perirenal organ mapping, thereby helping to choose the right plane of access and at the same time avoiding injury to adjacent organs (Fig. 3.9). This may be of especial importance in patients with abnormal body habitus (Fig. 3.10). Three-dimensional CT pyelography demonstrates calculi in parallel calyces, calyceal orientation, and size of calyceal necks as well as presence of a calyceal diverticulum and other anatomical abnormalities, which may be highly valuable when deciding the best route of access, access size, and when performing combined endoscopic intrarenal surgery (ECIRS) (Fig. 3.11) [21, 24, 25]. In this way the advantages of a miniaturized access often become evident.

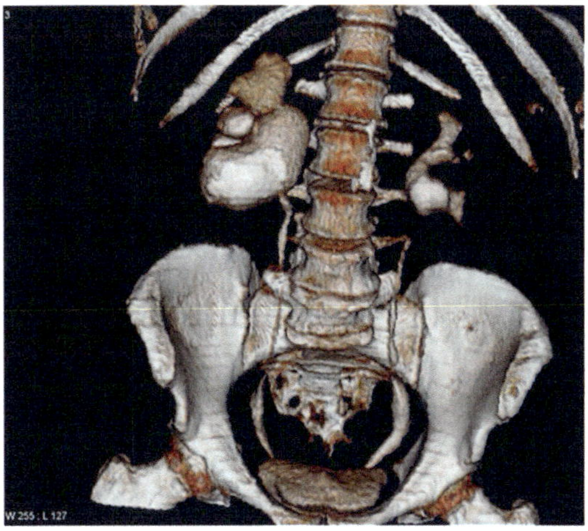

**Fig. 3.9** 3-D CT in renal anomaly. (3-D CT reconstruction in a patient with bilateral UPJ stenosis, showing the large stone burdens and the upper urinary tract in rich 3-D format that may be rotated to visualize the system from all directions, in order to plan optimal access)

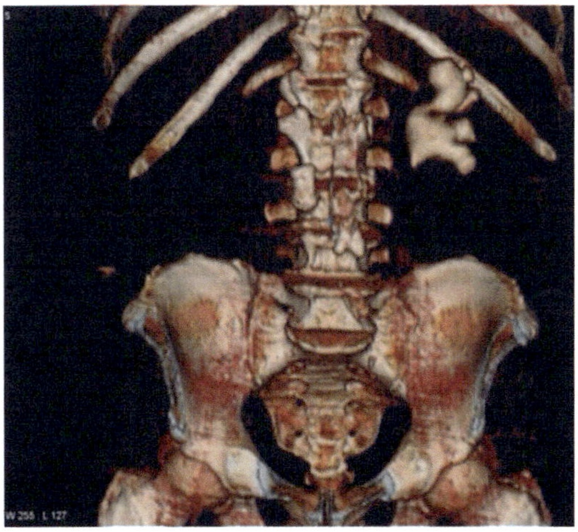

**Fig. 3.10** 3-D CT in complex stone scenario. (CT with 3-D reconstruction of large calcium oxalate monohydrate staghorn stone. 3-D reformatting helped deciding best route of access in an endoscopic intrarenal surgical [ECIRS] procedure)

## 3.3.2 Perirenal Organ Mapping

Preoperative imaging should provide information regarding interpositioned organs (colon, spleen, liver, pleura and lung) within the planned percutaneous access route, thereby reducing risk of organ injury during PCNL [23]. In a study comparing CTs in supine and prone position, it was shown that colon is more often positioned behind the colon (retrorenal) in prone (10%) compared to the supine position (1.9%) [26], which may suggest a lower risk of colon injury in supine PCNL. Another study has demonstrated that colon is more often retrorenal on the left side, especially in women [27] (Fig. 3.12). This information may be used when planning patient positioning and access route. Theoretically, preoperative CT for PCNL planning should be performed with the patient in the same position in which surgery is planned [28]. In our practice we perform all CTs in supine position, and when the colon position is considered a problem, multiplanar reformatted images (3-D CT) are provided, since these often gives a more reliable estimate of risk of colon injury compared to evaluation of axial CT images [29].

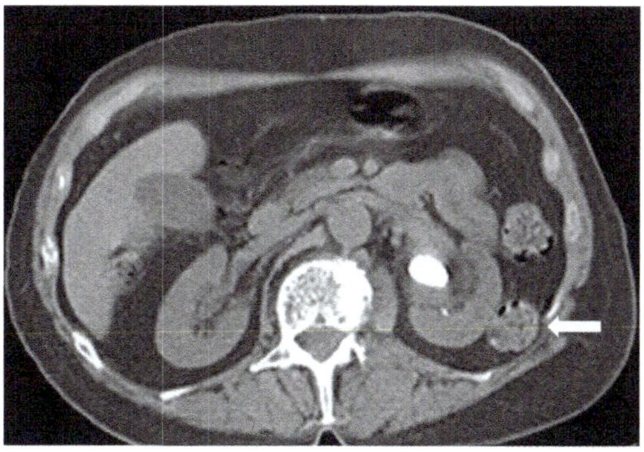

**Fig. 3.11** NCCT and perirenal organ mapping. (Non-contrast CT [NCCT] in a female with solitary stone in the left kidney. Examination revealed a retrorenal colon [arrow], which one must be aware, when access is planned)

If a supracostal puncture is planned, the relation of the access tract to the pleura and the lung must be considered. 3-DCT in both inspiratory and expiratory phases may be helpful in showing the relationships between the kidney and pleura/diaphragm/ribs [30]. It is generally recommended to do percutaneous puncture while the patient is in expiration [8].

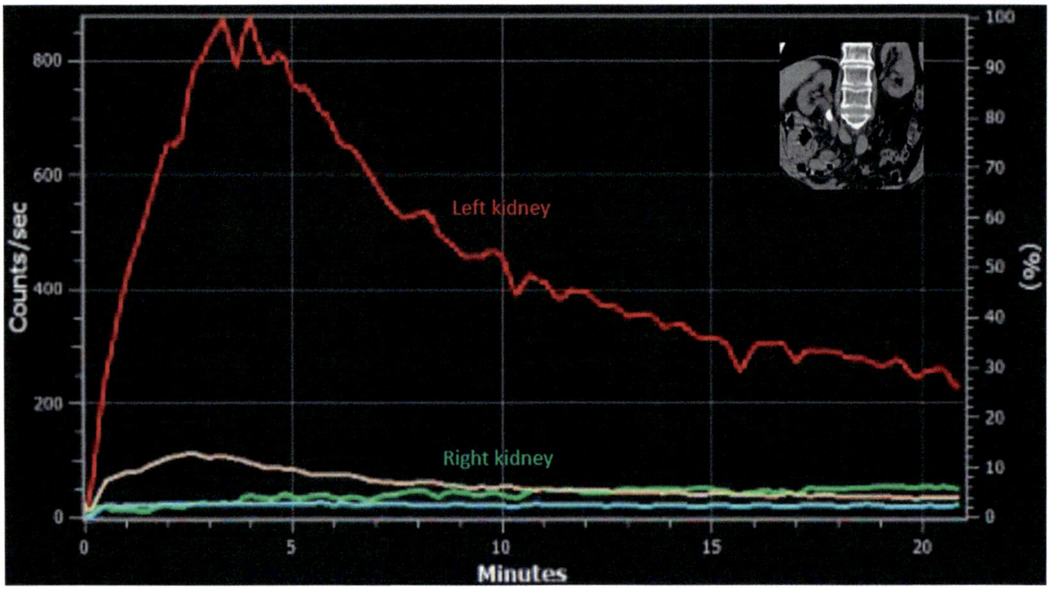


**Fig. 3.12** Renogram for deciding best approach. (Female admitted with right sided flank pain. NCCT showing large stone just below the UPJ of a right nephropathic kidney [right corner]. Renogram unveiled a non-functioning right kidney. Patient was treated by laparoscopic nephrectomy)

### 3.3.3 Estimation of Renal Function

If the kidney function of the stone-bearing kidney is suspected to be severely decreased (reduced parenchymal thickness), a renogram/scintigraphy is considered mandatory for exact evaluation of the renal split function. The threshold deciding whether the patient should be offered PCNL or nephrectomy is depending on the total combined renal function, which must be evaluated by a clearance estimate (Fig. 3.13).

## 3.4 Postoperative Imaging

### 3.4.1 Evaluation of Complications

Although, miniaturized PCNL seems to have a lower complication rate, suspicion of procedure related complications postoperatively should prompt immediate imaging according to the specific clinical symptoms to limit serious sequelae.

Access above the ribs is associated with a higher risk of pleural injury [8]. In supra 12th and supra 11th accesses, hydro- or pneumothorax have been reported in up to 12% and 35%, respectively [8]. Chest fluoroscopy during surgery can be used to detect pleural complications, and this allows immediate drainage [8, 31]. If the patient develops symptoms indicative of pleural injury postoperatively, a chest X-ray or CT should be performed (Fig. 3.14).

If the patient develops postoperative diarrhoea/haematochezia, signs of peritonitis, or passage of gas or faeces through the nephrostomy tract, a colonic perforation should be suspected, and such findings should prompt an abdominal CT, possibly with injection of contrast medium through the nephrostomy tube, if this has been placed [32]. Since colonic injuries are most often retroperitoneal, most of these can be managed conservatively.

Bleeding during and after PCNL is most often venous and usually self-limiting. Severe postprocedural haemorrhage is rarely seen in mini PCNL. However, if it happens, an arteriovenous fistula or a pseudoaneurysm must be suspected, and the patient should undergo immediate angiography with the possibility of performing superselective embolization, which is both a lifesaving and a nephron-sparing intervention [33]. Using B-mode with colour Doppler ultrasound for access guidance may avoid injury to the renal blood vessels during PCNL [34].

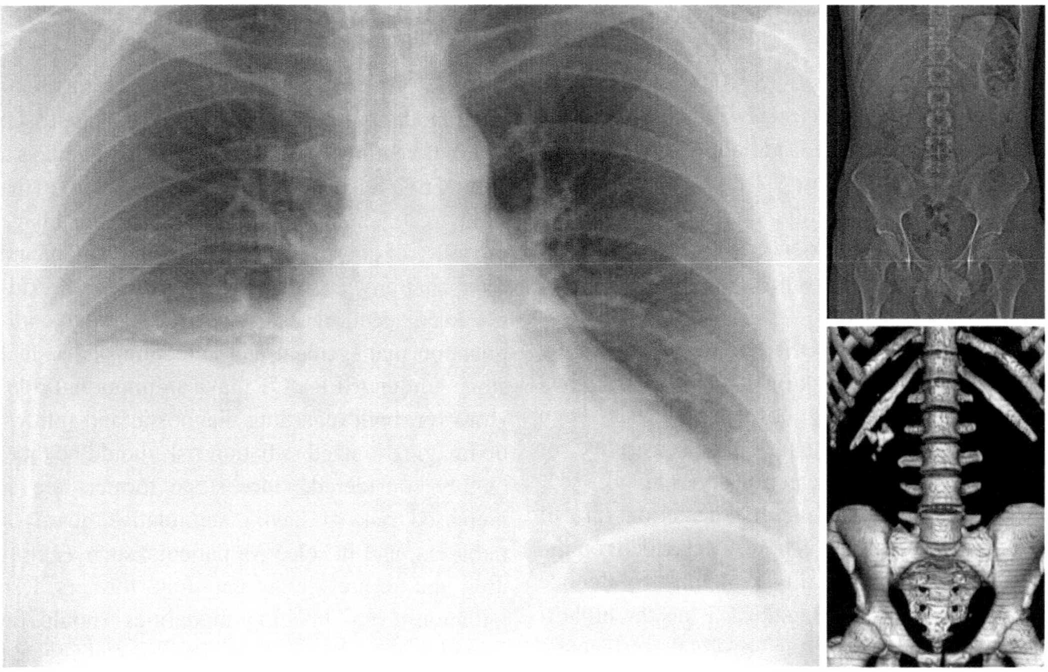

**Fig. 3.13** Plain chest X-ray. (PCNL was performed through an upper pole access for a right-sided partial staghorn stone [right]. Upper calyx was dilated and accessed just above costa 12. Surgery was uneventful, and patient was rendered stone free. Postoperatively, patient developed dyspnoea and pain at deep inspiration. Patient was hemodynamic stable with no haemoglobin drop. Plain chest X-ray showed pleural fluid accumulation on the right side. The pleural cavity was drained for clear fluid with an 8.3 Fr pigtail drain that could be removed two days postoperatively)

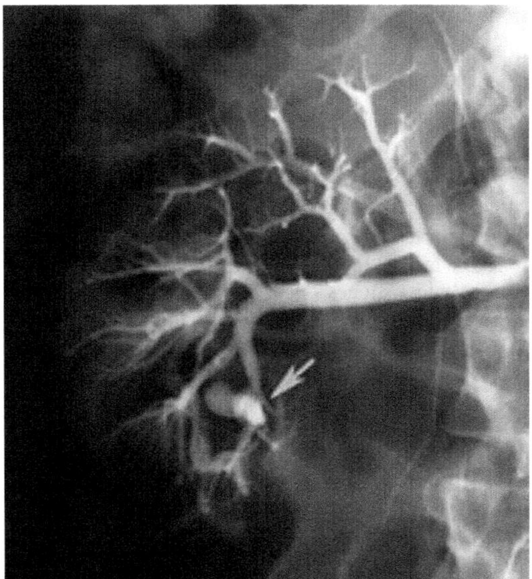

**Fig. 3.14** Angiography with transarterial superselective embolization. (The patient presented with intermittent haemorrhage through the nephrostomy drain and haemoglobin drop 18 hours post-PCNL. Transarterial angiography was performed, showing an intrarenal pseudoaneurism that was treated by superselective embolization)

### 3.4.2 Evaluation of Residual Stones

*Intraoperative imaging.* Fluoroscopy during the PCNL procedure is used for nephroscopy guidance to detect residual stones. High magnification rotational fluoroscopy as an adjunct to aggressive nephroscopy has been shown to increase detection rate of residual calculi, and thereby may increase stone free rate (SFR) [35].

*Postoperative imaging.* Postoperative imaging for residuals helps deciding whether the patient needs additional treatment (repeat nephroscopy, SWL, ureteroscopy, etc.). Also, postoperative imaging is used for selecting patients that are candidates for metaphylaxis. Need of sensitive image studies is highlighted by the fact that patients with residual fragments are at higher risk for recurrence compared with patients rendered stone free [36]. In this perspective, KUB and nephrotomograms have been challenged, since these imaging modalities seem to overestimate SFR by 35% and 17% [8], respectively. In prospective series of patients undergoing PCNL for large and staghorn calculi, NCCT has been shown to be superior to KUB with regard to detecting residuals (NCCT sensitivity 100% compared to KUB sensitivity 46%) [8, 37–39]. The downside to conventional NCCT is radiation dose, and subsequently ultra-low dose CT protocols have been developed with radiation doses close to KUB [40], and in our experience such protocols may be equally good for postprocedural evaluation of SFR.

Ultrasonography (US) may be an appealing modality without radiation concerns for residual fragment evaluation; however, it has been documented that US has a poor sensitivity for residual fragment detection post-PCNL [41, 42]. Thus, it is evident that detection rate of residual stone burden is highly dependent on the applied imaging modality, which may influence clinical decision making. NCCT has the highest sensitivity for detecting residual fragments; however, less than half of patients with residual fragments on NCCT seem to experience a subsequent stone-related event [43], and thus early CT evaluation may lead to overtreatment. Taking into account the potential hazards of ionized radiation, this calls for a selective, personalized approach, in which the highly sensitive CT evaluation should be restricted to those patients, who have a high risk of residuals, and in whom residual calculi mandate aggressive treatment, for instance, infection and cystine stones. Timing of follow-up imaging has been a matter of debate. On the one hand, an early follow-up within the first days postoperatively may diagnose dust or residual fragments that will pass spontaneously without causing any adverse events, and as a consequence of this the EAU Guidelines propose imaging at four weeks to be most appropriate for evaluating stone free rate (SFR) [22, 44, 45]. On the other hand, early diagnosis of significant residual stone fragments will enable second-look nephroscopy in case a nephrostomy tube was placed. Thus, due to the diversity of stone disease follow-up timing of course also will have to be personalized, and according to above considerations a selective approach seems advisable [46].

## 3.5 Summary

Mini PCNL has evolved as an important treatment modality to enable a personalized approach to stone treatment (PSA). In this, imaging plays a crucial role for selection of the right patient to the right treatment. CT has emerged as the image modality of choice for defining stone burden and renal anatomy, as well as relationship of the kidney to adjacent organs. Also, with regard to complication management and detection of residual stone burden (SFR), CT plays an important role. However, both regarding diagnostic and follow-up imaging ionized radiation risk should be thoroughly considered, since stone formers are at increased risk of having cumulative doses of radiation, and in selective patients, such as children and severely recurrent stone formers, less radiation-heavy imaging modalities should be considered. In other words, the risks of ionized radiation should outweigh the risks of overlooking stone characteristics, anatomical details, and residual fragments (RALARA). Uroradiologists and urologists should work in close collaboration to design selective imaging protocols in such a way that the amount of ionized radiation is stratified and justified according to the clinical question.

## References

1. Axelsson T, Cracco C, Desai M, Hasan MN, Knoll T, Montanari E, Pérez-Fentes D, Starub M, Thomas K, Williams JC Jr, Brehmer M, Osther PJS. Consultation on kidney stones, Copenhagen 2019: lithotripsy in percutaneous nephrolithotomy. World J Urol. 2020 Jul 29; https://doi.org/10.1017/s00345-020-03383-w.
2. Miller DT, Semins MJ. Minimizing radiation dose in management of stone disease: how to achieve 'ALARA'. Curr Opin Urol, 2020 dec 31. Publish ahead of print. https://doi.org/10.1097/MOU.0000000000000845. Online ahead of print PMID: 33394609.
3. Lipkin ME, Preminger GM. Risk reduction strategy for radiation exposure during percutaneous nephrolithotomy. Curr Opin Urol. 2012;22(2):139–43. https://doi.org/10.1097/MOU.0b013e32834fc36a.
4. Grivas N, Thomas K, Drake T, Donaldson J, Neisius A, Petrik A, Ruhayel Y, Seitz C, Türk C, Skolarikos A. Imaging modalities and treatment of paediatric

upper tract urolithiasis: a systematic review and update on behalf of the EAU uroliothiasis guidelines panel. J Ped Urology. 2010:612–24.
5. Robertson NP, Dillman JR, O'Hara SM, DeFoor WR Jr, Reddy PP, Giordano RM, et al. Comparison of ultrasound versus computed tomography for the detection of kidney stones in the pediatric population: a clinical effectiveness study. Pediatr Radiol. 2018;48:962–72.
6. Routh JC, Graham DA, Nelson CP. Trends in imaging and surgical management of pediatric urolithiasis at American pediatric hospitals. J Urol. 2010;184(4 suppl):1816–22.
7. Gedik A, Tutus A, Kayan D, Yilmaz Y, Bircan K. Percutaneous nephrolithotomy in pediatric patients: is computerized tomography a must? Urol Res. 2011;39:45–9.
8. Park S, Pearle MS. Imaging for percutaneous renal access and management of renal calculi. Urol Clin N Am. 2006:353–64.
9. Chen TT, Wang C, Ferrandino MN, Scales CD, Yoshizumi TT, Preminger GM, Lipkin ME. Radiation exposure during the evaluation and management of nephrolithiasis. J Urol. 2015;194:878–85.
10. Miller OF, Rineer SK, Reichard SR, Buckley RG, Donovan SM, Graham IR, Goff WB, Kane CJ. Prospective comparison of unenhanced spiral computed tomography and intravenous urogram in the evaluation of acute flank pain. Urology. 1998;52:982–7.
11. Pfister SA, Deckhart A, Laschke S, Dellas S, Otto U, Buitrago C, Roth J, Wiesner W, Bontgartz G, Gasser TC. Unenhanced helical computed tomography vs intervenous urography in patients with acute flank pain: accuracy and economic impact in a randomized prospective trial. Eur Radiol. 2003;13:2513–20.
12. Shine S. Urinary calculus IVU vs. CT renal stone? A critical appraised topic. Comput Biol Med. 2008;33:41–3.
13. Villa L, Giusti G, Knoll T, Traxer O. Imaging for urinary stones: update in 2015. Eur Urol Focus. 2016;2:122–9.
14. Ouzaid I, Al-qahtani S, Dominique S, et al. A 970 Hounsfield units (HU) threshold of kidney stone density on non-contrast computed tomography (NCCT) improves patients' selection for extracorporeal shockwave lithotripsy (ESWL): evidence from a prospective study. BJU Int. 2012;110:E438–42.
15. Williams JC Jr, Saw KC, Paterson RF, Hatt EK, McAteer JA, Lingeman JE. Variability of renal stone fragility in shock wave lithotripsy. Urology. 2003;61:1092–6.
16. Zarse CA, Hameed TA, Jackson ME, Pischalnikov YA, Lingemen JE, JA MA, Williams JC Jr. CT visible internal stone structure, but not Hounsfield unit value, of calcium oxalate monohydrate (COM) calculi predicts lithotripsy fragility in vitro. Urol Res. 2007;35:201–6.
17. Kim SC, Burns EK, Lingeman JE, Paterson RF, McAteer JA, Williams JC Jr. Cystine calculi: correlation of CT-visible structure, CT number, and stone morphology with fragmentation by shock wave lithotripsy. Urol Res. 2007;35:319–24.
18. Panthier F, Doizi S, Illoul L, Berthe L, Traxer O. Developing free three-dimensional software for surgical planning for kidney stones: volume is better than diameter. Eur Urol Focus 2020; 23: S2405–4569(20)30161–9. https://doi.org/10.1016/j.euf.2020.06.003.
19. Brehmer M, Beckman MO, Magnusson A. Three-dimensional computed tomography planning improves percutaneous surgery. Scand J Urol. 2014;48(3):316–23.
20. Bariol SV, Tolley DA. What is the best imaging for stone management? BJU Int. 2005;95(1):4–5.
21. Graumann O, Osther SS, Spasojevic D, Osther PJ. Can the CT planning image determine whether a kidney stone is radiopaque on a plain KUB? Urol Res. 2012;40(4):333–7.
22. Patel U, Walkden RM, Ghani KR, Anson K. Three-dimensional CT pyelography for planning of percutaneous nephrolithotomy: accuracy of stone measurement, stone detection and pelvicalyceal reconstruction. Eur Radiol. 2009;19:1280–8.
23. European Association of Urology (EAU) guidelines on Urolithiasis. ISBN 978-94-92671-04-2. https://uroweb.org/guideline/urolithiasis/#note_42-44. Accessed 17 Jan 2021.
24. Nolte-Emsting C, Cowan N. Understanding multislice CT urography techniques: many roads lead to Rome. Eur Radiol. 2006;16:2670–86.
25. Thiruchelvam N, Mostafid H, Ubhayakar G. Planning percutaneous nephrolithotomy using multidetector computed tomography urography, multiplanar reconstruction and three-dimensional reformatting. BJU Int. 2005;95:1280–4.
26. Heyns CF, van Geldern WF. 3-dimensional imaging of the pelviocalyceal system by computerized tomographic reconstruction. J Urol. 1990;144:1335–8.
27. Hopper KD, Sherman JL, Lurthke JM, Ghaed N. The retrorenal colon in the supine and prone patient. Radiology. 1987;162:443–50.
28. Azhar RA, Szymanski KM, Lemercier E, Valenti D, Andonian S, Anidjar M. Visceral organ-to-percutaneous tract distance is shorter when patients are placed in the prone position on bolsters compared with the supine position. J Endourol. 2011;25:687–90.
29. Chalasani V, Bissoon D, Bhuvanagir AK, Mizzi A, Dunn IB. Should PCNL patients have a CT in the prone position preoperatively? Can J Urol. 2010;17:5082–6.
30. Traxer O. Management of injury to the bowel during percutaneous stone removal. J Endourol. 2009;23:1777–80.
31. Tuttle DN, Yeh BM, Meng MV, Breiman RS, Stoller ML, Coakley FV. Risk of injury to adjacent organs with lower-pole fluoroscopically guided percutaneous nephrostomy: evaluation with prone, supine, and

multiplanar reformatted CT. J Vasc Interv Radiol. 2005;16:1489–92.
32. Ogan K, Corwin SC, Smith T, Watumull LM, Mullican MA, Cadeddu JA, Pearle MS. Sensitivity of chest fluoroscopy compared with chest CT and chest radiography for diagnosing hydropneumothorax in association with percutaneous nephrolithotomy. Urology. 2003;62:988–92.
33. Valdivia JG, Scarpa RM, Duvdevani M, Gross AJ, Nadler RB, Nutahare K, de la Rosette JJ. Supine versus prone position during percutaneous nephrolithotomy: a report from the clinical research Office of the Endourological Society Percutaneous Nephrolithotomy Global Study. J Endourol. 2011;25:1619–25.
34. Jain V, Ganpule A, Vyas J, Muthu V, Sabnis MRB, Rajapurkar MM, Desai MR. Management of non-neoplastic renal hemorrhage by transarterial embolization. Urology. 2009;74:522–7.
35. Lu M-H, Pu X-Y, Gao X, Zhou X-F, Qiu J-G, Si-Tu J. A comparative study of clinical value of single B-mode ultrasound guidance and B-mode combined with color doppler ultrasound guidance in mini-invasive percutaneous nephrolithotomy to decrease hemorrhagic complications. Urology. 2010;76:815–20.
36. Portis AJ, Laliberte MA, Drake S, Holtz C, Rosenberg MS, Bretzke CA. Intraoperative fragment detection during percutaneous nephrolithotomy: evaluation of high magnification rotational fluoroscopy combined with aggressive nephroscopy. J Urol. 2006;175:162–6.
37. Gettman MT, Pearle MS. Evaluation of residual stones following percutaneous nephrolithotomy. Braz J Urol. 2000;26:579–83.
38. Pearle MS, Watamull LM, Mullican MA. Sensitivity of noncontrast helical computerized tomography and plain film radiography compared to flexible nephroscopy for detecting residual fragments after percutaneous nephrolithotomy. J Urol. 1999;162:23–6.
39. Park J, Hong B, Park T, Park HK. Effectiveness of noncontrast computed tomography in evaluation of residual stones after percutaneous nephrolithotomy. J Endourol. 2007;21:684–7.
40. Osman Y, El-Tabey N, Rafai H, Elnahas A, Shoma A, Eraky I, Kenwy M, El-Kapany H. Detection of residual stones after percutaneous nephrolithotomy: role of nonenhanced spiral computerized tomography. J Urol. 2008;179:198–200.
41. Hyams ES, Shah O. Evaluation and follow-up of patients with urinary lithiasis: minimizing radiation exposure. Curr Urol Rep. 2010;11:80–6.
42. Fowler KAB, Locken JA, Duchesne JH, Williamson MR. US for detecting renal calculi with nonenhanced CT as a reference standard. Radiology. 2002;222:109–33.
43. Ulusan S, Koc Z, Tokmak N. Accuracy of sonography for detecting renal stone: comparison with CT. J Clin Ultrasound. 2007;35(5):256–61.
44. Gokce MI, Ozden E, Suer E, Gulpinar B, Gulpinar O, Tangal S. Comparison of imaging modalities for detection of residual fragments and prediction of stone related events following percutaneous nephrolithotomy. Int Braz J Urol. 2015;41(1):86–90.
45. Olvera-Posada D, Ali SN, Dion M, Alenezi H, Denstedt J, Razvi H. Natural history of residual fragments after percutaneous nephrolithotomy: evaluation of factors related to clinical events and intervention. Urology. 2016;97:46–50.
46. Tokas T, Habicher M, Junker D, Herrmann T, Jessen JP, Knoll T, Nagele U. Uncovering the real outcomes of active renal stone treatment by utilizing non-contrast computer tomography: a systematic review of the current literature. World J Urol. 2017;35(6):897–905.

# 4 ALARA: How to Reduce Radiation Exposure

B. M. Zeeshan Hameed, Milap Shah, and Bhaskar Somani

## 4.1 Introduction

### 4.1.1 Radiation Exposure Amongst Patients

Recent published literature has shown an exponential rise in the incidence of renal calculus disease [1, 2]. Ionizing radiation is an integral part of diagnosis, pre-operative planning, and post-operative follow-up in urology. So, residents and practicing urologists should have awareness and knowledge regarding practices of radiation safety and strategies to mitigate radiation exposure (RE). United Nation Scientific Committee on The Effects of Atomic Radiation (UNSCEAR) [3] defined the risk to the public in terms of "collective dose." The definition of the collective dose is "the product of the number of exposed individuals and their average effective dose." In the USA annually, almost 400 million diagnostic medical X-ray examinations are performed. The annual individual and collective effective doses have been estimated as 0.5 mSv and 130,000 mSv, respectively [4]. A study from India suggested that in 2010, the annual collective dose received from diagnostic radiology was 47.3 mSv (1.23 mSv/patient) [5]. The guidelines regarding the annual limit of RE for occupational exposure for individuals in healthcare have been issued by International Commission on Radiological Protection (ICRP). No guidelines are issued for patient-related RE. As per literature, very few single center studies have assessed the patient radiation exposure [6–9].

### 4.1.2 Radiation Exposure Amongst Healthcare Professionals

As per guidelines laid by ICRP, 20 mSv is the annual safe limit for healthcare personnel for the maximum duration of 5 years. Therefore, a total of 100 mSv over the 5-year period is considered within acceptable limits [10]. Literature suggests that urologists are protected by shields and receive less than 1% of the total scattered dose [11].

### 4.1.3 Radiation Exposure Amongst Urologists

A substantial source of radiation dose taken by the operator is the radiation from the patient [12]. Sahin et al. observed that radiation exposure to urologist's hand, feet, head, and neck area were 0.021 mSv, 0.003 mSv and less than 0.1 mSv, respectively [12]. Majidpour et al. reported the

B. M. Zeeshan Hameed (✉) · M. Shah
Department of Urology, Kasturba Medical College, Manipal, Karnataka, India

B. Somani
Professor and Consultant Urological Surgeon, University Hospital Southampton, Hampshire, UK


M. S. Agrawal et al. (eds.), *Minimally Invasive Percutaneous Nephrolithotomy*,
https://doi.org/10.1007/978-981-16-6001-6_4

radiation exposures of urologist in order for head, eye, hand, and foot were 0.47 μGy, 0.04 μGy, 0.21 μGy and 4.1 μGy (1 microgray = 0.001 millisievert) [13]. The mean fluoroscopy time in these studies ranged from 2.5 min to 12 min. Overall, it was observed that radiation exposure decreased with fluoroscopy time [12, 13]. In another German study, the authors reported mean values of RE as recorded by forehead and ring dosimeter during various procedures. The results from the forehead dosimeter showed mean RE of 0.04 mSv, 0.03 mSv, 0.18 mSv and 0.1 mSv during ureteral stent change (USC) and ureteral stent placement (USP), percutaneous stent change (PCS), percutaneous nephrolithotomy (PCNL) and ureteroscopy (URS), respectively. While the ring dosimeter showed mean values of 0.1 mSv, 0.2 mSv, 0.2 mSv, 0.1 mSv, and 4.3 mSv during USC, USP, PSC, URS, and PCNL, respectively [14]. Even for an average screening time of 10 min for an annual workload of 50 such cases, the surgeon would receive less than 2% (10 mGy) of the annual dose limit. Assuming a high error of estimation of 100%, it is unlikely that radiation exposure would increase to greater than 4% of the annual dose limit. Therefore, the annual dose received is well below the threshold dose for deterministic effects of ionizing radiation. Doses to surgeons and staff assisting in such procedures involving radiation are therefore low and should never approach the regulatory dose limits [15].

### 4.1.4 Awareness of ALARA and Radiation Exposure Amongst Urologists

Due to lack of awareness and knowledge with respect to principles of ALARAthere is an element of risk of increased RE amongst residents and practicing urologists [16]. Simple practice such as keeping the image intensifier closer to the patient and maximizing the distance between the X-ray tube and the patient can considerably reduce the radiation exposure (Fig. 4.1) and use of collimation to avoid the scattering of the X-ray beam (Fig. 4.2). Arslanoglu et al. showed that nearly 70% to 97% of urologists undervalue the

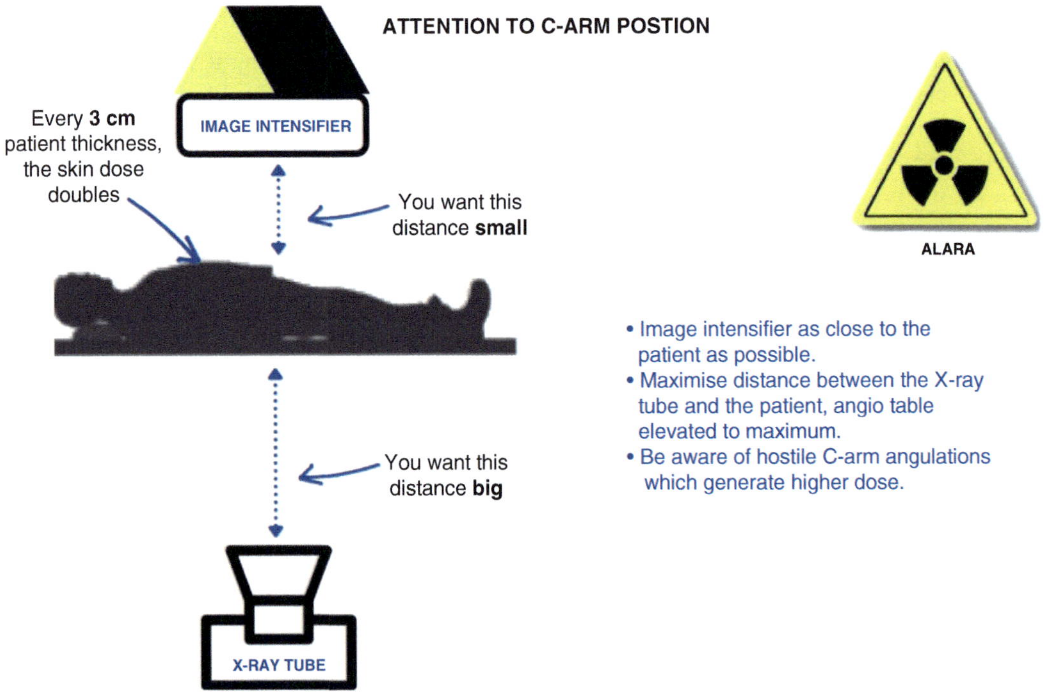


**Fig. 4.1** Showing the ideal spacing of the image intensifier and the distance between the X-ray tube and the patient to reduce the radiation exposure

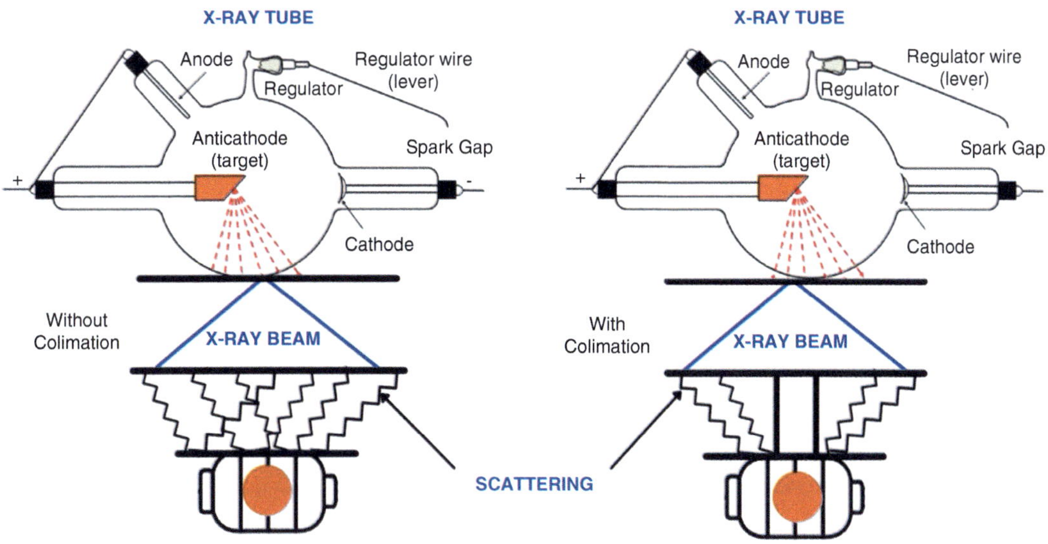


**Fig. 4.2** Use of collimation to avoid the scattering of X-ray beam

RE of patients during diagnostic procedures [17]. Friedman et al. demonstrated the lacunae of knowledge of radiation safety among trainees through an online survey. The survey showed that the ALARA principle was adequately practiced by 88% of trainees, but more than two-third did not use dosimeters, and only just above 50% had received proper radiation safety training [16]. The results of this survey threw light on the fact that there was still room for improvement in terms of educating urology residents regarding radiation safety [16].

## 4.2 Applications of Radiation in Urology and its Effective Dose

The prime priority is the need for accurate, accessible, and cost-effective radiological imaging modalities which can aid in the diagnosis of renal calculus, planning of treatment and monitoring response [18]. One of the major concerns is the cumulative dose exposure amongst recurrent stone formers. With this in mind, various newer and alternative modalities have been implemented as the first line of imaging [19]. The effective radiation doses of various diagnostic and interventional imaging modalities are as mentioned in Table 4.1 [20].

**Table 4.1** Effective dose of diagnostic and interventional modalities

| Diagnostic imaging modalities | | Mean effective dose (mSv) |
|---|---|---|
| X-ray KUB | | 0.7–1.1 |
| IVU | | 1.5–3.5 |
| CT abdomen and pelvis | Standard dose | 5–10 |
| | Low dose | 2.0–3.5 |
| | Ultra-low dose | 0.5–1.5 |
| CT Urogram | | 10–31 |
| Interventional modalities (fluoroscopy) | | |
| SWL | | 1–8 |
| Ureteroscopy | | 1–7 |
| PCNL | | 3–18 |

### 4.2.1 Diagnostic Modalities

**X-Ray KUB**

Earlier, the first imaging modality of choice for patients with suspected renal calculus was plain X-ray KUB. The sensitivity and specificity of X-ray KUB are 59% and 71%, respectively [21]. Part from low sensitivity, other drawbacks of plain radiography were inability to detect radiolucent stones and poor quality images due to shadows of overlying bowel gas [21]. The only advantages include easy availability, low cost and lowRE as compared to other modalities (effective radiation dose of 0.2–0.7 mSv) [22].

**Intravenous Urography (IVU)**

The added advantages of IVU over KUB are the ability to delineate the anatomy as well as give an idea regarding the functioning of the kidney. The effective radiation dose is higher as compared to plain radiography (0.7–3.7 mSv). It also depends on the number of films taken [23]. The limitations of IVU are that it can be more time consuming and needs trained personnel technicians to perform it. The risk of contrast-induced nephropathy and allergic reactions due to contrast material also persist.

**Computed Tomography (CT)**

CT is useful in the diagnosis of stones as well as pre-operative planning. As per the American Urologic Association and Endourological Society Guideline for the Surgical Management of Stones, non-contrast CT (NCCT) should be done before performing PCNL in children and adults [24]. It also recommendsNCCT to help in deciding the interventional procedure between ESWL and URS [25]. Various stone scoring systems which assesses the complexity of PCNL procedure also require NCCT as a pre-operative imaging modality [26, 27]. One major disadvantage is the increased radiation exposure and cost of the procedure [23]. Low dose (LDCT) or ultra-low dose CT (ULDCT) is an appropriate alternative to standard CT in order to overcome the drawback of increased RE. Studies have shown that the dose can be reduced by 56%, and yet the sensitivity and specificity of LDCT remains the same with minimal intra- and inter-observer difference [28, 29]. Hence, it is now the first choice of imaging for the diagnosis of urolithiasis. It is also the first choice for follow-up cases, especially in patients with recurrent nephrolithiasis [30].

### 4.2.2 Interventional Modalities

**Fluoroscopy**

Fluoroscopy is an integral part of various interventional procedures used in the treatment of urolithiasis such as URS, SWL, and PCNL. There are various techniques to achieve a perfect puncture during PCNL, and the most common one is the Bulls eye technique which needs the C-arm to be positioned at 0° and 30° position during the puncture (Fig. 4.3). A validated model is used to quantify RE in patients undergoing URS and PCNL [31, 32]. The mean effective dose exposure in URS, SWL, and PCNL is mentioned in Table 4.1 [20]. Details regarding the methods to reduce radiation exposure during these procedures are discussed later in the chapter.

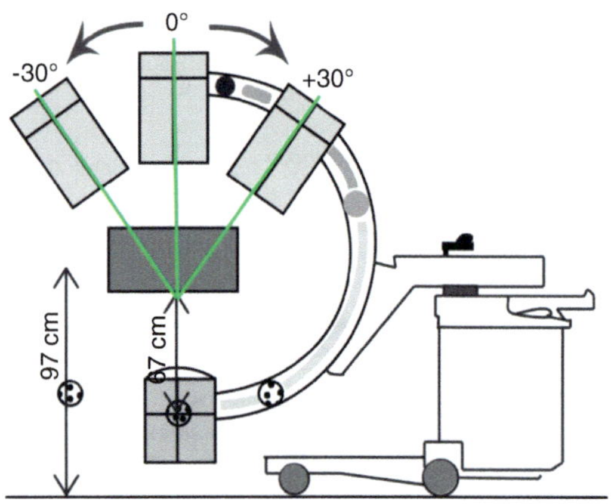


**Fig. 4.3** The C-arm position at 0° and 30° during the PCNL procedure to aid the Bull's Eye technique of PCNL puncture

### 4.2.3 Newer Technology

**Digital Tomosynthesis (DT)**

It is the reconstruction of X-ray images by removing overlying bowel gas shadows. This improves the overall image quality [30]. Various studies have suggested that the dose of radiation exposure in IVP decreases when combined with DT as the time taken to complete the procedure is less. Also, when compared to low dose CT, the radiation exposure in DT is lower [33, 34].

## 4.3 Occupational Limits of Radiation Exposure Set by National Organization

ICRP has given organ-specific permissible limits for radiation exposure. These values can only be used in those specific organs when exposed to radiation rather than the whole body, these dose

**Table 4.2** Dose limitation recommendations as per ICRP-2007 [6]

| Part of the body | Occupational exposure | Public exposure |
|---|---|---|
| Whole body (effective dose) | 20 mSv/year averaged over 5 consecutive years;<br>30 mSv in any single year | 1 mSv/y |
| Lens of eyes (equivalent dose) | 150 mSv in a year | 15 mSv/y |
| Skin (equivalent dose) | 500 mSv in a year | 50 mSv/y |
| Extremities: Hands and feet (equivalent dose) | 500 mSv in a year | – |

Note: For pregnant radiation workers, after declaration of pregnancy 1 mSv on the embryo/fetus should not exceed

limits are summarized in Table 4.2 [6]. Atomic Energy Regulatory Board of India (AERB) has also laid down radiation exposure dose limitations which are in line with ICRP recommendations. As per AERB "No practice or source within a practice should be authorized unless the practice produces sufficient benefit to the exposed individuals or to society to offset the radiation harm that it might cause; that is: unless the practice is justified, taking into account social, economic, and other relevant factors" [35].

## 4.4 Effects of Increased Radiation Exposure

### 4.4.1 Deterministic Effects

Deterministic effects occur as a result of cell killing. Cataract formation is an exception to this rule [36]. These effects occur only when a certain dose threshold has been crossed. No effect is observed below this dose limit while the severity increases as the dose increases above the threshold. The mode of delivery of the dose also plays an important role. Large dose single exposure is more harmful than smaller dose exposure over an extended period. At doses of approximately 2 Gy, radiation sickness occurs while bone marrow suppression occurs at dose range 1–10 Gy [37, 38]. Risk of cataract formation increases after a single exposure of 2 Gy or more than 10 Gy if radiation exposure is infractions. At 5–20 Gy small intestinal cells are affected, and an acute dose of more than 10 Gy may cause internal bleeding due to damage of the GI tract. CNS is affected at dose of 20–50 Gy, and cerebrovascular syndrome occurs at100 Gy. Radiation severity can be assessed by noting the reduction in lymphocyte count. Lymphocyte count can be used as a biological radiation dosimeter [37].

### 4.4.2 Stochastic Effects

Cancer induction is one of the most prominent stochastic effects resulting from RE. Unlike deterministic effects, there is no threshold limit in this case, and the severity is independent of the dose [39]. Stochastic effects can also be seen in the form of stroke, respiratory, heart, and GI tract disease at dose levels above 1 Sv [39].

## 4.5 Factors Affecting Increased Radiation Exposure Amongst Urologists

Multiple factors such as obesity, stone number, size, location, Hounsfield units (HU) and operative factors such as the side of procedure, access technique, multiple tracts and operative time have been studied to assess their influence on the radiation exposure (RE) amongst urologists. Balaji et al. [40] showed that the multiple tracts, large stone size, low stone density, use of fluoroscopy to gain PCS access and larger sheath size resulted in increased RE. Factors that had no impact on RE were operative time, stone number and location, BMI and age of the patient [40]. In obese patients, it is logical that more fluoroscopy time (FT) will be required for better visualization of images [41]. Ritter et al. [42] reported that experienced surgeons (> 2 years-experience) could easily reduce the FT up to 55% in comparison to novice surgeons (< 2 years-experience) during relatively easier endourological interventions. This leads to lesser RE of patients as well as OT personnel.

**Table 4.3** RE measurements based on Sheath size/type of PCNL and stone location [40]

| Type of PCNL | Sheath size (Fr), mean (SD) | RE (mSv), mean (SD) |
|---|---|---|
| RE based on type of PCNL/sheath size | | |
| Standard PCNL | 26.5 (1.6) | 0.29 (0.12) |
| Miniperc | 21.2 (1.7) | 0.18 (0.1) |
| MIP-M | 15.7 (0.8) | 0.21 (0.08) |
| MIP-S | 10.7 (0.6) | 0.16 (0.08) |
| RE based on stone location | | |
| Pelvis | 79 (37.3) | 0.2 (0.06) |
| Lower calyx | 45 (21.2) | 0.17 (0.1) |
| Middle calyx | 14 (6.6) | 0.18 (0.08) |
| Upper calyx | 12 (5.7) | 0.21 (0.09) |
| Proximal ureter | 9 (4.2) | 0.17 (0.1) |
| Multiple (different calyx) | 53 (25) | 0.25 (0.12) |

Lipkin et al. [43] reported that for a right and left PCNL, the expected dose rate (EDR) was a mean 0.014 and 0.021 mSv/s, respectively. But no such variation was noted in the study by Balaji et al. [40]. The latter also mentioned the mean RE measurements based on the type of PCNL (sheath size) and stone location which is described in Table 4.3 [40].

## 4.6 Measures to Reduce Radiation Exposure

### 4.6.1 ALARA Principles

The principles of ALARA or "as low as reasonably achievable" has three lines of defense:

time (minimum), distance (maximum) and shielding (protective gear).

Such strategies should be cost-effective, avoid delay in the procedure, should not affect the outcomes of the procedure.

Strategies to follow ALARA principles are as mentioned in Table 4.4.

**Time (Minimizing Time)**

Decreasing radiation time to as minimum as possible is an effective strategy to reduce RE. Strategies to achieve this are mentioned in Table 4.4 [44–48].

**Table 4.4** Principles and strategies to achieve ALARA

| Time (minimize) | Distance (maximize) | Shielding (use shields) |
|---|---|---|
| 1. Substitute fluoroscopy with other imaging modalities such as US-guided PCNL puncture | 1. Avoid being in the room during the procedure, whenever possible (IVP, CT) | 1. Lead-impregnated eyeglasses, gloves, thyroid shields, chest and pelvic aprons, and ceiling-mounted shields. |
| 2. Use digital fluoroscopy | 2. Lens-mounted video cameras decreases the distance of the surgeon and radiation source | |
| 3. Use "last-image-hold" technique | | |
| 4. Pulsed fluoroscopy with still frames should be used | | |
| 5. Track FT and keep reminders or alarms if it exceeds a certain limit | | |
| 6. Cumulative dose history should be documented if patient has underwent multiple procedures | | |

**Distance (Maximizing Distance)**

Maximizing distance is a cost-effective strategy to minimize RE. RE follows the inverse square law. When the distance is doubled, the RE decreases to one-quarter, and at a distance of 3meters, the radiation dose becomes similar to background levels [48, 49].

**Shielding (Protective Gear)**

This is important for personnel who will be within the radiation field. The most common heavy metal used for shielding is lead which is capable of attenuating radiation, but 100% protection is not provided by lead shields. So shielding should not be considered as a substitute for other principles [49–51].

### 4.6.2 Use of Protective Shields/Gear for Reducing RE

#### 4.6.2.1 Effect of Shielding on Imaging

Shielding (using protective shields) is one of the key principles of ALARA [52]. The results regarding the effect of shields on image noise are controversial and contradictory [53–58]. If shields are placed over the area of interest, it is known as "in-plane" shielding. If placed over areas outside of the area of interest, it is called "out-of-plane" shielding. The former increases the image noise and hence can result in poor image quality [55]. Improper application of in-plane shielding can result in loss of protective effect of the shield. Due to these limitations, Iball and Brettle strongly recommend the use of "out-of-plane" shielding [54].

#### 4.6.2.2 Protective Gear Equipment

Shields can be ceiling-mounted, lead-based gloves, eyeglasses, thyroid shields, pelvic, and chest aprons. The thickness of lead aprons is variable. 0.5 mm Lead thickness can attenuate radiation by more than 95%. Annual inspection of these aprons is necessary to check for cracks. Thyroid shields also attenuate the RE by almost 23 times (reduce from 46 mSv to 0.02 mSv). This is almost equivalent to background radiation levels [51]. One major limitation of the chest and pelvic shields is the weight of the aprons. In literature, survey results have shown urologists complaint of orthopedic problems in the form of back pain, neck, hip, and knee and even hand problems [59]. The compliance associated with wearing chest and pelvic aprons was high and reported to be 97%. While the results showed poor compliance with the use of thyroid shields, dosimeters, eyeglasses, and gloves [59].

### 4.6.3 Techniques to Reduce Radiation during Pre-Operative Imaging and Evaluation

Radiation exposure in a patient with nephrolithiasis is increasing owing to the increase in the use of CT for diagnosis as well as for follow-ups. Various studies have reported that increased use of CT does not alter the rate of re-admissions [60, 61]. Alternatives such as X-ray and US have lower cost and RE, but the sensitivity is also low when compared with standard CT [62]. As per the American Urological Association guidelines regarding appropriate imaging Selection for the evaluation of ureteral calculi "low dose" NCCT should be the initial imaging modality for a patient with flank pain and a suspected ureteral stone if the body mass index is less than 30 kg/m$^2$ and a standard dose NCCT if the patient is obese [Table 4.5]. They recommend a KUB concurrently with the NCCT if the stone is not seen on the scout image. For follow-up of radio-opaque

**Table 4.5** Tips to reduce radiation exposure during pre-operative evaluation, intraoperative procedure, and post-operative follow-up

| Pre-operative | Intraoperative | Post-operative |
|---|---|---|
| 1. X-ray KUB/ US should be performed first. If the stone is not visible on scout film or US, then perform NCCT | 1. Pulsed fluoroscopy | 1. For radio-opaque stones: X ray or US can be preferred |
| 2. LDCT should be preferred | 2. Air pyelography | 2. For radiolucent stones: • USG can be done initially • NCCT can be done if stone not visualized on USG |
| 3. ULDCT can also be considered for stones >4 mm | 3. Endoscopic-guided puncture | |
| | 4. US-guided access | |
| | 5. Use of protective gear | |
| | 6. Improve surgical training regarding US and endoscopic-guided access | |
| | 7. Optimize positioning and magnification | |

stones, they recommend ultrasound along with KUB. In cases of radiolucent stones, they recommend follow-up imaging with NCCT. From results of meta-analysis, the pooled sensitivity and specificity of Low Dose CT (LDCT) was 96% and 95% respectively [63]. The estimated radiation doses for the various modalities have been mentioned earlier. ULDCT is defined as CT protocol, which is comparable to X-ray KUB and emits an effective dose of less than 1 mSv. The specificity and sensitivity of ULDCT were reported to be as high as 96% and 92%, respectively, for stones more than 4 mm in size. But when generalized to all stone sizes, the sensitivity dropped to 72% [64]. Increase in BMI of the patient also reduces the sensitivity of ULDCT [65]. So in order to reduce RE of patient, US can be deployed as the first line of imaging followed by LDCT if required for pre-operative planning. Following this protocol can reduce RE from 17.2 mSv to 1.4 to 2.0 mSv [22]. Another alternative is Digital Tomosynthesis (DT) having ERD of 0.8 mSv which is lower than LDCT [33].

### 4.6.4 Methods to Reduce Radiation during PCNL

The RE during NCCT of the abdomen and PCNL has been reported to be similar [30]. PCNL has the highest radiation exposure when compared with other interventional endourological procedures [49, 66–68]. We have already highlighted the factors which add to the increase in radiation exposure during PCNL. There are several strategies for reducing radiation exposure during PCNL. [Table 4.5]

1. Pulsed Fluoroscopy: Using this strategy at 4 frames per second resulted in the decrease of FT by 65% [47]. This value was further reduced to 80% when pulsed fluoroscopy was done at 1 frame per second by an experienced technician in conjugation with the use of a laser-guided C-arm with fixed lower current and kVp [69].
2. Air pyelography reduced the ERD by almost 40–50% [32].
3. Endoscopic-guided PCS access using retrograde flexible ureterorenoscopy and ultrasound-guided puncture has been associated with fewer access tracts, less operative time and decreased transfusion rates [70–73]. It also reduced fluoroscopy time (FT) and RE during PCNL with comparable outcomes [74–78].
4. Blind Access: This technique can be performed without the use of fluoroscopy. Very few studies have reported the outcomes of the blind access technique. It resulted in increased operative time and low stone free rates. This strategy can be adopted in the absence of ultrasound. This technique should be performed only by experts in selected cases [79].

### 4.6.5 Radiation Exposure in Pediatric Age Group and Measures to Reduce the Exposure

PURSE (Pediatric Urology Radiation Safety Evaluation) study was one of the first to clearly show that radiation exposure during pediatric endourological procedures was not insignificant [80].

**Strategies to Reduce RE in Pediatric Age Group [81, 82]**

1. Position optimization: The skin entry dose can be reduced by keeping the fluoroscopy table away from the source. The image capture can be maximized by keeping it near to image intensifiers (II). The position of II should be focused over the area of interest before fluoroscopy is started rather than adjusting during fluoroscopy.
2. Reduce Radiation Scatter: This can be achieved by installing a lead drape around the II. Lead covers should be avoided around the patient as it leads to an increase in radiation scatter. Bismuth impregnated drapes can be used [16].
3. Pulse fluoroscopy during the interventional procedure and still images for reviewing the findings can be used.

4. Perform non-magnified fluoroscopy whenever possible.
5. Avoid angulating beam over radiosensitive areas (eyes, thyroid, breast, gonads).
6. Experienced technicians help in avoiding inadvertent fluoroscopy and thereby reduce overall FT.
7. Alarm bells or live intraoperative read outs can be used when fluoroscopy time extends beyond a certain limit.
8. Ultrasound can be used as the primary modality for diagnosis, pre-operative planning, intraoperative setting, and follow-up whenever feasible.
9. Proper Documentation: Cumulative dose history should be documented in cases where multiple procedures are done in children.
10. Equipment modification can be done by integrating dose-measurement and dose reduction devices.

### 4.6.6 Radiation Exposure in Pregnant Women

RE reducing strategies are of prime importance in this set of populations. It poses a challenge for the urologists in diagnosis, pre-operative planning and decision making [83]. The most adopted strategy is to ensure the safety of the fetus. The safe cumulative dose limit set by various organizations is not more than 50 mGy.Level more than 10–20 mGy doubles the risk of leukemia over a background rate of 1 in 3000 [84–86]. One thing to be kept in mind while considering the risks of radiation in the management of urolithiasis is balanced against the risk of a negative ureteroscopy (URS). This may be due to ambiguity in the diagnosis of stones. One trial reported negative URS of 4.2% only when both US and NCCT were used in diagnosis in comparison to more than 20% negative URS when either US or MRI was used alone [87]. ESWL is an absolute contraindication in pregnancy due to the increased risk of fetal death and malformations observed in animal studies [88, 89]. PCNL is considered a contraindication in pregnancy due to the need for general anesthesia, difficulty in patient positioning, and need for fluoroscopy [90]. There are case reports of PCNL being performed safely in all three trimesters, but there is not enough literature to recommend PCNL outside of an experimental setting [90–92].

### 4.6.7 Ultrasound and Virtual Reality Simulator Training Models

#### 4.6.7.1 Ultrasound-Guided Access and Training

Certain studies have reported higher fluoroscopy time required for fluoroscopy-guided access (FGA) in PCNL, which directly results in more radiation exposure [93–95]. As per a Meta-analysis by Wang et al., the X-ray exposure was 2.6 min longer for FGA compared to the USG guided access (USGA) group [95]. The use of ultrasound in endourological procedures is not just a safe and efficient alternative for adult and pediatric populations but also in lines with the principles of ALARA [96]. Ultrasound-guided access training will become one of the key components in mitigating RE during PCNL. Various training models are proposed for US guided punctures for trainees [97]. Veys et al. proposed a Thiel-embalmed cadavers training model for ultrasound-guided supine endoscopic combined intrarenal surgery (ECIRS) [97]. US-guided renal puncture reduces radiation exposure in obese patients, and it reduces costs compared to fluoroscopy [98, 99]. Complete US-guided procedures can be safely performed in the absence of fluoroscopic guidance and are considered to be as effective, feasible, and secure as conventional fluoroscopic PCNL with the advantage of zero radiation exposure [100, 101]. Surgical skill development on training models can help in reducing the trainees' learning curve.

#### 4.6.7.2 Virtual Reality Simulator Training

Competency and proficiency in PCNL can be achieved only after an average of 36–45 and 105–115 cases, respectively [101]. Studies have shown that urology residents with previous training in PCNL perform the procedure with reduced

FT. This was confirmed with the decrease in RE when virtual reality simulators (VRS) were used for training residents in achieving percutaneous access. Therefore, VRS can be incorporated in the early phase of training, which can lead to a decrease in radiation exposure to urologists and patients [102–104].

### 4.6.8 Clinical Governance and Radiation Safety Culture [105]

#### 4.6.8.1 Clinical Governance [105]

The four key components of clinical governance are:

- Clinical effectiveness.
- Clinical audit.
- Risk management strategies.
- Education, training, and continuing professional development.

Radiation safety is an integral part of all four components [105].

#### 4.6.8.2 Strategies to Improve Radiation Safety Culture [105]

1. Education and creating awareness.
2. Standardize the norms and guidelines.
3. Proper training and feedback.
4. Quality improvement based on feedback.

## References


1. Scales CD Jr, Smith AC, Hanley JM, et al. Urologic diseases in America P. Prevalence of kidney stones in the United States. Eur Urol. 2012;62(1):160–5.
2. Turney BW, Reynard JM. The cost of stone surgery. Eur Urol. 2014;66(4):730–1.
3. United Nations Scientific Committee on the Effects of Atomic Radiation (UNSCEAR) sources and effects of ionizing radiation. UNSCEAR 2000 Report Vol. I to the General Assembly, with scientific annexes.
4. National Academy of Sciences. Health risks from exposure to low levels of ionizing radiation, Board on Radiation Effects Research, Division on Earth and Life Studies, 2006.
5. Durga Prasada Rao A, Dellie ST. Radiation exposure of patients undergoing common diagnostic X-ray examinations in some major hospitals in Visakhapatnam, India. J Med Diagn Meth. 2012;1:101. https://doi.org/10.4172/2168-9784.1000101.
6. International Commission on Radiological Protection (ICRP). The 2007 recommendations of the International Commission on Radiological Protection. ICRP publication 103. Ann ICRP. 2007;37:1–332.
7. Hanna L, Walmsley BH, Devenish S, Rogers A, Keoghane SR. Limiting radiation exposure during percutaneous nephrolithotomy. J Endourol. 2015;29:526–30.
8. Jamal JE, Armenakas NA, Sosa RE, Fracchia JA. Perioperative patient radiation exposure in the endoscopic removal of upper urinary tract calculi. J Endourol. 2011;25:1747–51.
9. Martin J, Hennessey DB, Young M, Pahuja A. Radiographer delivered fluoroscopy reduces radiation exposure during endoscopic urological procedures. Ulster Med J. 2016;85:8–12.
10. ICRP Publication 60. Recommendations of the International Commission on Radiological Protection, 60. Ann ICRP. 1990;1991(21):1–3.
11. Christodoulou EG, Goodsitt MM, Larson SC, Darner KL, Satti J, Chan HP. Evaluation of the transmitted exposure through lead equivalent aprons used in a radiology department, including the contribution from backscatter. Med Phys. 2003;30:1033–8.
12. Şahin E, Kara C, Reşorlu B, Sönmez MG, Ünsal A. Radiation exposure during percutaneous nephrolithotomy; is there a risk of the patient and the operating team? Int J Radiat Res. 2018;16(1):133–8.
13. Majidpour HS. Risk of radiation exposure during PCNL. Urol J. 2010;7(2):87–9.
14. Ritter M, Krombach P, Martinschek A, et al. Radiation exposure during endourologic procedures using over-the-table fluoroscopy sources. J Endourol. 2012;26:47–51.
15. Hellawell G, Mutch S, Thevendran G, Wells E, Morgan R. Radiation exposure and the urologist: what are the risks? J Urol. 2005;174(3):948–52.
16. Friedman A, Ghani K, Peabody J, Jackson A, Trinh Q, Elder J. Radiation safety knowledge and practices among urology residents and fellows: results of a nationwide survey. J Surg Educ. 2013;70(2):224–31.
17. Arslanoğlu A, Bilgin S, Kubah Z, et al. Doctors' and intern doctors' knowledge about patients' ionizing radiation exposure doses during common radiological examinations. Diagn Interv Radiol. 2007;13:53–5.
18. Matlaga BR. The need for better decision tools in managing stone disease. J Urol. 2012;188(3):698–9.
19. Yecies T, Averch TD, Semins MJ. Identifying and managing the risks of medical ionizing radiation in endourology. Can J Urol. 2018;25(1):9154–60.

20. Yasser A, Noureldi SA. Radiation safety during diagnosis and treatment. In: Smiths textbook of endourology, vol. 1. 4th ed. Chichester: Wiley-Blackwell; 2019. p. 14–37.
21. Levine JA, Neitlich J, Verga M, et al. Ureteral calculi in patients with flank pain: correlation of plain radiography with unenhanced helical CT. Radiology. 1997;204:27–31.
22. IAEA. Radiation protection of patients (RPOP) (Urology). https://www.iaea.org/resources/rpop/Health-professionals/other-specialities-and-imaging-modalities/urology/patients.
23. Mettler FA Jr, Thomadsen BR, Bhargavan M, et al. Medical radiation exposure in the U.S. in 2006: preliminary results. Health Phys. 2008;95:502–7.
24. Assimos D, Krambeck A, Miller NL, et al. Surgical management of stones: American Urological Association/Endourological Society guideline, PART I. J Urol. 2016;196(4):1153–60.
25. Fulgham PF, Assimos DG, Pearle MS, et al. Clinical effectiveness protocols for imaging in the management of ureteral calculous disease: AUA technology assessment. J Urol. 2013;189(4):1203–13.
26. Okhunov Z, Friedlander JI, George AK, et al. S.T.O.N.E. nephrolithometry: novel surgical classification system for kidney calculi. Urology. 2013;81(6):1154–9.
27. Jeong CW, Jung JW, Cha WH, et al. Seoul National University renal stone complexity score for predicting stone-free rate after percutaneous nephrolithotomy. PLoS One. 2013;8(6):e65888.
28. Zilberman DE, Tsivian M, Lipkin ME, et al. Low dose computerized tomography for detection of urolithiasis—its effectiveness in the setting of the urology clinic. J Urol. 2011;185(3):910–4.
29. White WM, Zite NB, Gash J, et al. Low-dose computed tomography for the evaluation of flank pain in the pregnant population. J Endourol. 2007;21(11):1255–60.
30. Lipkin M, Preminger G. Imaging techniques for stone disease and methods for reducing radiation exposure. Urol Clin N Am. 2013;40(1):47–57.
31. Lipkin ME, Mancini JG, Toncheva G, et al. Organ specific radiation dose rates and effective dose rates during percutaneous nephrolithotomy. J Endourol. 2012;26(5):439–43.
32. Lipkin ME, Wang AJ, Toncheva G, et al. Determination of patient radiation dose during ureteroscopic treatment of urolithiasis using a validated model. J Urol. 2012;187(3):920–4.
33. Wang AJ, Nguyen G, Toncheva G, et al. Radiation exposure from non-contrast CT, digital tomosynthesis, and standard KUB and tomograms. J Endourol. 2011;25(S1):A304–5.
34. Mermuys K, De Geeter F, Bacher K, et al. Digital tomosynthesis in the detection of urolithiasis: diagnostic performance and dosimetry compared with digital radiography with MDCT as the reference standard. AJR Am J Roentgenol. 2010;195(1):161–7.
35. Principles R, Public B. Radiation protection principle [Internet]. Aerb.gov.in. 2020. Available from: https://www.aerb.gov.in/english/radiation-protection-principle.
36. Fry M. Deterministic effects. Health Phys. 2001;80:338–43.
37. Hall E, Giaccia A. Radiobiology for the radiologist. Philadelphia: Lippincott Williams &Wilkins; 2005.
38. Thomas O, Mahe M, Campion L, Bourdin S, Milpied N, Brunet G, Lisbona A, Le MA, Moreau P, Harousseau J, Cuilliere J. Long-term complications of total body irradiation in adults. Int J Radiat Oncol Biol Phys. 2001;49:125–31.
39. Pierce DA, Shimizu Y, Preston DL, Vaeth M, Mabuchi K. Studies of the mortality of atomic bomb survivors. Report 12, Part I. Cancer: 1950–1990. Radiat Res. 1996;146:1–27.
40. Balaji S, Vijayakumar M, Singh A, Ganpule A, Sabnis R, Desai M. Analysis of factors affecting radiation exposure during percutaneous nephrolithotomy procedures. BJU Int. 2019;124(3):514–21.
41. Hsi R, Zamora D, Kanal K, Harper J. Severe obesity is associated with 3-fold higher radiation dose rate during ureteroscopy. Urology. 2013;82(4):780–5.
42. Ritter M, Siegel F, Krombach P, et al. Influence of surgeon's experience on fluoroscopy time during endourological interventions. World J Urol. 2013;31:183–7. https://doi.org/10.1007/s00345-012-0923-0.
43. Lipkin ME, Wang AJ, Toncheva G, Ferrandino MN, Yoshizumi TT, Preminger GM. Determination of patient radiation dose during ureteroscopic treatment of urolithiasis using a validated model. J Urol. 2012;187:920–4.
44. Mooney RB, McKinstry J. Paediatric dose reduction with the introduction of digital fluorography. Radiat Prot Dosimetry. 2001;94:117–20.
45. Persliden J, Helmrot E, Hjort P, et al. Dose and image quality in the comparison of analogue and digital techniques in paediatric urology examinations. Eur Radiol. 2004;14:638–44.
46. Ngo TC, Macleod LC, Rosenstein DI, et al. Tracking intraoperative fluoroscopy utilization reduces radiation exposure during ureteroscopy. J Endourol. 2011;25(5):763–7.
47. Elkoushy MA, Shahrour W, Andonian S. Pulsed fluoroscopy in ureteroscopy and percutaneous nephrolithotomy. Urology. 2012;79(6):1230–5.
48. Elkoushy MA, Alkhayal A, Andonian S. Radiation safety for urologists. J Endourol B Videourol. 2014; https://doi.org/10.1089/vid.2013.0067.
49. Andonian S, Atalla MA. Radiation safety in urology. AUA update series, volume 28, lesson 26, 2009;228–247.
50. National Council for Radiation and Measurement. Structural shielding design and evaluation for medical use of x-rays and gamma rays of energies up to 10 MeV. Report No. 49. Bethesda, MD: National Council on Radiation Protection; 1976.

51. Tse V, Lising J, Khadra M, et al. Radiation exposure during fluoroscopy: should we be protecting our thyroids? Aust N Z J Surg. 1999;69:847–8.
52. McCollough CH, Wang J, Gould RG, Orton CG. Point/counterpoint: the use of bismuth breast shields for CT should be discouraged. Med Phys. 2012;39:2321–4.
53. Ciarmatori A, Nocetti L, Mistretta G, Zambelli G, Costi T. Reducing absorbed dose to eye lenses in head Ct examinations: the effect of bismuth shielding. Australas Phys Eng Sci Med. 2016;39:583–9.
54. Iball GR, Brettle DS. Organ and effective dose reduction in adult chest CT using abdominal lead shielding. Br J Radiol. 2011;84:1020–6.
55. Alonso TC, Mourão AP, Santana PC, da Silva TA. Assessment of breast absorbed doses during thoracic computed tomography scan to evaluate the effectiveness of bismuth shielding. Appl Radiat Isot. 2016; https://doi.org/10.1016/j.apradiso.2016.03.018.
56. Kim YK, Sung YM, Choi JH, Kim EY, Kim HS. Reduced radiation exposure of the female breast during low-dose chest CT using organ-based tube current modulation and a bismuth shield: comparison of image quality and radiation dose. Am J Roentgenol. 2013;200:537–44.
57. Einstein AJ, Elliston CD, Groves DW, et al. Effect of bismuth breast shielding on radiation dose and image quality in coronary CT angiography. J Nucl Cardiol. 2012;19:100–8.
58. Goren A, Prins R, Dauer L, et al. Effect of leaded glasses and thyroid shielding on cone beam CT radiation dose in an adult female phantom. Dentomaxillofac Radiol. 2013;42:20120260.
59. Elkoushy MA, Andonian S. Prevalence of orthopedic complaints among endourologists and their compliance with radiation safety measures. J Endourol. 2011;25(10):1609–13.
60. Westphalen AC, Hsia RY, Maselli JH, et al. Radiological imaging of patients with suspected urinary tract stones: national trends, diagnoses, and predictors. Acad Emerg Med. 2011;18(7):699–707.
61. Kirpalani A, Khalili K, Lee S, et al. Renal colic: comparison of use and outcomes of unenhanced helical CT for emergency investigation in 1998 and 2002. Radiology. 2005;236(2):554–8.
62. Brisbane W, Bailey MR, Sorensen MD. An overview of kidney stone imaging techniques. Nat Rev Urol. 2016;13(11):654–62.
63. Niemann T, Kollmann T, Bongartz G. Diagnostic performance of low-dose CT for the detection of urolithiasis: a meta-analysis AJR. Am J Roentgenol. 2008;191:396.
64. Pooler BD, Lubner MG, Kim DH, et al. Prospective trial of the detection of urolithiasis on ultralow dose (sub mSv) noncontrast computerized tomography: direct comparison against routine low dose reference standard. J Urol. 2014;192:1433.
65. Poletti PA, Platon A, Rutschmann OT, et al. Low-dose versus standard-dose CT protocol in patients with clinically suspected renal colic. AJR Am J Roentgenol. 2007;188:927.
66. Hellawell GO, Mutch SJ, Thevendran G, et al. Radiation exposure and the urologist: what are the risks? J Urol. 2005;174(3):948–52.
67. Hristova-Popova J, Saltirov I, Vassileva J. Exposure to patient during interventional endourological procedures. Radiat Prot Dosimetry. 2011;147(1–2):114–7.
68. Jindal T. The risk of radiation exposure to assisting staff in urological procedures: a literature review. Urol Nurs. 2013;33:136–9.
69. Blair B, Huang G, Arnold D, et al. Reduced fluoroscopy protocol for percutaneous nephrostolithotomy: feasibility, outcomes and effects on fluoroscopy time. J Urol. 2013;190(6):2112–6.
70. Grasso M, Lang G, Taylor FC. Flexible ureteroscopically assisted percutaneous renal access. Tech Urol. 1995;1:39–43.
71. Sountoulides PG, Kaufmann OG, Louie MK, et al. Endoscopy-guided percutaneous nephrostolithotomy: benefits of ureteroscopic access and therapy. J Endourol. 2009;23:16491654.
72. Khan F, Borin JF, Pearle MS, et al. Endoscopically guided percutaneous renal access: "seeing is believing". J Endourol. 2006;20:451–5.
73. Isac W, Rizkala E, Liu X, et al. Endoscopic-guided versus fluoroscopic-guided renal access for percutaneous nephrolithotomy: a comparative analysis. Urology. 2013;81:251–6.
74. Andonian S, Scoffone CM, Louie MK, et al. Does imaging modality used for percutaneous renal access make a difference? A matched case analysis. J Endourol. 2013;27(1):24–8.
75. Basiri A, Ziaee AM, Kianian HR, et al. Ultrasonographic versus fluoroscopic access for percutaneous nephrolithotomy: a randomized clinical trial. J Endourol. 2008;22:281–4.
76. Falahatkar S, Neiroomand H, Enshaei A, et al. Totally ultrasound versus fluoroscopically guided complete supine percutaneous nephrolithotripsy: a first report. J Endourol. 2010;24(9):1421–6.
77. Zhou T, Chen G, Gao X, et al. 'X-ray'-free balloon dilation for totally ultrasound-guided percutaneous nephrolithotomy. Urolithiasis. 2015;43(2):189–95.
78. Jagtap J, Mishra S, Bhattu A, et al. Which is the preferred modality of renal access for a trainee urologist: ultrasonography or fluoroscopy? Results of a prospective randomized trial. J Endourol. 2014;28(12):1464–9.
79. Basiri A, Mehrabi S, Kianian H, et al. Blind puncture in comparison with fluoroscopic guidance in percutaneous nephrolithotomy: a randomized controlled trial. Urol J. 2007;4:79–83.
80. Dudley AG, Dwyer ME, Fox JA, et al. Prospective assessment of radiation in pediatric urology: the

pediatric urology radiation safety evaluation study. J Urol. 2016;196:202.
81. Connolly B, Racadio J, Towbin R. Practice of ALARA in the pediatric interventional suite. Pediatr Radiol. 2006;36(S2):163–7.
82. Kameda T, Taniguchi N. Overview of point-of care abdominal ultrasound in emergency and critical care. J Intensive Care. 2016;4:53.
83. Yecies T, Bandari J, Fam M, et al. Risk of radiation from computerized tomography urography in the evaluation of asymptomatic microscopic hematuria. J Urol. 2018;200:967–72.
84. Anon. Committee opinion no. 723: guidelines for diagnostic imaging during pregnancy and lactation: correction. Obstet Gynecol. 2018;132:786.
85. Anon. ACR-SPR practice parameter for imaging pregnant or potentially pregnant adolescents and women with ionizing radiation. Am Coll Radiol. 2018. Resolution 39
86. Streffer C, Shore R, Konermann G, et al. Biological effects after prenatal irradiation (embryo and fetus). A report of the International Commission on Radiological Protection. Ann ICRP. 2003;33:5–206.
87. White WM, Johnson EB, Zite NB, et al. Predictive value of current imaging modalities for the detection of urolithiasis during pregnancy: a multicenter, longitudinal study. J Urol. 2013;189:931–4.
88. Streem SB. Contemporary clinical practice of shock wave lithotripsy: a reevaluation of contraindications. J Urol. 1997;157:1197–203.
89. Smith DP, Graham JB, Prystowsky JB, et al. The effects of ultrasound-guided shock waves during early pregnancy in Sprague-Dawley rats. J Urol. 1992;147:231–4.
90. Somani B, Dellis A, Liatsikos E, et al. Review on diagnosis and management of urolithiasis in pregnancy: an ESUT practical guide for urologists. World J Urol. 2017;35:1637–49.
91. Shah A, Chandak P, Tiptaft R, et al. Percutaneous nephrolithotomy in early pregnancy. Int J Clin Pract. 2004;58:809–10.
92. Holman E, Toth CS, Khan MA. Percutaneous nephrolithotomy in late pregnancy. J Endourol. 1992;6:421–4.
93. Agarwal M, Agrawal MS, Jaiswal A, Kumar D, Yadav H, Lavania P. Safety and efficacy of ultrasonography as an adjunct to fluoroscopy for renal access in percutaneous nephrolithotomy (PCNL). BJU Int. 2011;108(8):1346–9.
94. Jagtap J, Mishra S, Bhattu A, Ganpule A, Sabnis R, Desai MR. Which is the preferred modality of renal access for a trainee urologist: ultrasonography or fluoroscopy? Results of a prospective randomized trial. J Endourol. 2014 Dec 1;28(12):1464–9.
95. Wang K, Zhang P, Xu X, Fan M. Ultrasonographic versus fluoroscopic access for percutaneous Nephrolithotomy: a meta-analysis. Urol Int. 2015;95(1):15–25.
96. Emiliani E, Kanashiro A, Chi T, Pérez-Fentes DA, Manzo BO, Angerri O, et al. Fluoroless endourological surgery for stone disease: a review of the literature—tips and tricks. Vol. 21, Current Urology Reports. Springer; 2020.
97. Veys R, Verpoort P, Van Haute C, Wang Z, Chi T, Tailly T. Thiel-embalmed cadavers as a novel training model for ultrasound-guided supine endoscopic combined intrarenal surgery. BJU Int. 2019;125(4):579–85.
98. Usawachintachit M, Masic S, Chang HC, Allen IE, Chi T. Ultrasound guidance to assist percutaneous nephrolithotomy reduces radiation exposure in obese patients. Urology. 2016;98:32–8.
99. Hudnall M, Usawachintachit M, Metzler I, et al. Ultrasound guidance reduces percutaneous nephrolithotomy cost compared to fluoroscopy. Urology. 2017;103:52–8.
100. El-Shaer W, Kandeel W, Abdel-Lateef S, Torky A, Elshaer A. Complete ultrasound-guided percutaneous nephrolithotomy in prone and supine positions: a randomized controlled study. Urology. 2019;128:31–7.
101. Armas-Phan M, Tzou DT, Bayne DB, Wiener SV, Stoller ML, Chi T. Ultrasound guidance can be used safely for renal tract dilatation during percutaneous nephrolithotomy. BJU Int. 2019; https://doi.org/10.1111/bju.14737.
102. Noureldin YA, Elkoushy MA, Andonian S. Assessment of percutaneous renal access skills during urology objective structured clinical examinations (OSCE). Can Urol Assoc J. 2015;9(3–4):E104–8.
103. Noureldin YA, Fahmy N, Anidjar M, et al. Is there a place for virtual reality simulators in assessment of competency in percutaneous renal access? World J Urol. 2016;34(5):733–9.
104. Papatsoris AG, Shaikh T, Patel D, et al. Use of a virtual reality simulator to improve percutaneous renal access skills: a prospective study in urology trainees. Urol Int. 2012;89(2):185–90.
105. World Health Organization. (2016). Communicating radiation risks in paediatric imaging: information to support health care discussions about benefit and risk.

# Part II

# Armamentarium for Mini-PCNL

# Instrumentation for Mini-PCNL (Access Sheaths, Endoscopes, and Accessories)

5

Ajay Bhandarkar, Dipen Patel, and Manasi Parikh

## 5.1 Introduction

Various minimally invasive techniques like Percutaneous Nephrolithotomy (PCNL), Extracorporeal ShockWave Lithotripsy (ESWL), flexible ureteroscopy (fURS)/Retrograde IntraRenal surgery (RIRS) have dominated upper urinary tract calculi management in the last several decades. Even though Rupel and Brown [1] removed renal calculi from pre-existing nephrostomy tract in1941, formal credit goes to Fernstromand Johansson [2] for reporting the first PCNL in three patients in 1976. Since then, several people have contributed to make PCNL a safe and popular treatment modality [3–5]. As per EAU and AUA guidelines, PCNL is the preferred treatment modality for renal stones greater than 2 cm in size [6, 7]. In 1980s, ESWL appeared to be a more promising modality due to its minimally invasive appeal. However, stone-free rates were consistently poor, especially if the stone size was found to be greater than 20 mm, and it was lower calyceal calculi. Stone-free rates of PCNL procedures are higher than ESWL and RIRS [8]. Till the late 1990s, conventional PCNL with tract size 24–30 F had complications like bleeding, postoperative pain, and prolonged hospitalization [9]. Even though the incidence of bleeding was not very high, it was the most feared adverse event [10]. As preference for ESWL, especially in larger calculi (greater than 15 mm), gradually faded in the last two decades, RIRS emerged as a promising modality [11]. Advancements in technology have led to better quality of flexible endoscopes over the years. Nevertheless, the attractive feature of RIRS is that renal parenchymal transgression can be avoided and there is a minimal chance of bleeding due to injury to segmental renal vessels. Stone-free rates in RIRS for smaller calculi (less than 15 mm) in lower calyces were comparable to PCNL [12].

To avoid hemorrhagic complications of conventional PCNL (cPCNL), an attempt was made to reduce the size of the tract, and smaller endoscopes were used to break stones. The term coined for this procedure was Mini-PCNL or Mini-Perc. Helal et al. [13] were the first to attempt a small size tract in a pediatric patient. Additionally, Jackman et al. [14] published the possibility of using a smaller tract in adults with a peel-away sheath and ureteroscope. Both the studies showed 89% stone-free rates. Monga [15] and many others [16, 17] also published their experiences with a miniaturized tract for PCNL. The idea of a miniaturized tract was not well accepted initially, as stone-free rates were

A. Bhandarkar (✉) · D. Patel
Sujay Urological Hospital, Vadodara, Gujarat, India

M. Parikh
Boston University, Boston, MA, USA
e-mail: manasib@bu.edu


M. S. Agrawal et al. (eds.), *Minimally Invasive Percutaneous Nephrolithotomy*,
https://doi.org/10.1007/978-981-16-6001-6_5

less compared to cPCNL and operative time was more with Mini-PCNL [18]. However, Lahme [19] and Udo Nagele [20] with their teams as well as several centers from China [21, 22], persisted with improvised techniques to enable better outcomes in Mini-PCNL. Sasha C. Druskin et al. [23] in 2016 accepted the fact that stone-free rates of MPCNL were comparable to standard PCNL, however, the lower morbidity claim of MPCNL may need well-designed multicentric studies.

In this chapter, we shall look into various sheath and instrument options available for Mini-PCNL.

## 5.2 Innovative Sheaths and Mini Endoscopes

Helal et al. in 1997, used a 15 F Hickman catheter introduction kit in a 2-year-old girl with left renal calculus. The sheath was peeled away to accommodate a 10 F pediatric cystoscope to use graspers and remove the calculus. His experience of manipulation with a small endoscope was easy and there was no bleeding [13]. Stephen W Jackman [14] published his experience of using 11 F Vascular access sheaths in 7 pediatric patients in October, 1998 [24] and 13 F Ureteroscopy sheaths in 9 adults in December, 1998 [14]. During his study, he found that 6 children out of 7 and 8 adult patients out of 9 were stone free at 3–6 weeks follow-up. Chan and Jarrett [25] from the same John Hopkins Institute modified Jackman's technique in prone split-leg position and attempted flexible ureteroscopic access to lower calyceal calculus. If flexible ureteroscopy failed, they punctured lower calyx and proceeded with dilatation up to 16 F using fascial dilators. Ureteroscopy sheath with 13 F size was used for access and 10 F peditric cystoscope as nephroscope. Excess sheath was trimmed if necessary. At 1 month follow-up, 16 out of 17 patients in their cohort series were stone free. Occasionally, poor visualization and grasper-related issues were noted as primary limitations in their miniaturized PCNL.

Generally, Mini-PCNL term is used when access sheath size is between 11 and 20 F and in conventional PCNL access sheath size is 26–30 F. Monga et al. in 2000 [15], used Cook balloon dilator with 20F Amplatz Sheath and used 8 F/9.5 F Richard wolf uretero-renoscope with Laser/Ultrasonic lithotrite for stone fragmentation. Their study achieved a single procedure stone-free rate of 90%.

M I Feng et al. [26] published their prospective randomized study of 30 patients with Standard PCNL (sheath size 34 F) and labelled Mini-PCN (sheath size 24 F) in 2001. They observed no significant advantage for Mini-PCN versus Standard technique. Lipsky et al. in 2013 [27] reported the use of 24 F Amplatz sheath after balloon dilatation of the tract and used conventional 26 F Storz made nephroscope without its outer sheath. They could use conventional energy sources and graspers through this scope. By using this technique, they could avoid limitations of Mini-PCNL like poor visualization or irrigation issues, using specialized miniaturized instruments and telescopes. This strategy helped in better irrigation and ability to remove larger fragments with minimal post-procedural morbidity. They termed this as the Modified Technique of PCNL with modified instruments.

Desai et al. designed an innovative 13 F metallic outer sheath with a 6 F inner sheath, a small tube of 3 F welded to the inner wall, and finally connected to a port outside for injecting saline. An ultrathin 3 F telescope in a newly designed 7.5 F nephroscope was used for this procedure, which was labelled as "UltraMini PCNL." [28] This technique is described in Sect. 5.6 of this book.

Song et al. in 2011 [29] published their study of using a patented sheath with Lithotripsy and suctioning/clearance system to address high incidence of residual stones after Chinese Mini-PCNL. They designed a 16 F metallic sheath with a side port for attaching suction device. They used a specially designed small 12 F nephroscope and holmium laser for lithotripsy.

Shah et al. [30] also mentioned in their study a similar device −10/12 metallic sheath (Shah sheath) used with a small pediatric ureteroscope 4.5/6 F (Richard Wolf) as nephroscope. This technique termed "Superperc" is also described in Sect. 5.6.

Bader et al. [31] in 2011 used a 0.9-mm diameter micro-optical needle connected to a light source to perform an optical puncture into the targeted calyx in 15 patients undergoing PCNL. This was further developed so that the entire PCNL procedure was done through a 4.85F tract using the optical needle as camera without dilatation. There were several limitations of using a 4.8 F sheath, as it was extremely fragile to manipulate. To overcome the limitations of micro-PCNL, an additional technical modification on micro-PCNL was proposed [32]. A bigger 8 F metallic sheath has been proven to restrict the bending of the sheath in the collecting system and also makes it possible to accommodate a 1.6-mm ultrasonic lithotripter probe. This technique of "Microperc" is described in detail in Sect. 5.6.

## 5.3 "Peel Away" Sheath

The concept of Mini-PCNL originated at the John Hopkins Institute, USA. However, it was made more popular by Urologists in Germany and China. Sung Y M [17] and his colleagues in the year 2006 published their study involving the largest patient cohort group at the time. Seventy-two patients were included from 1999 to 2002, with 3 years follow-up. They used 14 F Peel away sheath and 8/9.5 F ureteroscope for Mini-PCNL. They observed 95.7% stone-free rates in cumulative stone burden less than 6 $cm^2$, but 52% in stone burden more than 6 $cm^2$.

Guohua Zeng et al. [33] and Xun Li [34] from the Guongzhou, China has the record of the largest number of Mini-PCNLs in a single center. They described the use of Ureteroscope through a mature nephrostomy tract as a part of staged PCNL from 1992 to 1998. They modified their technique from 1998 by using Peel Away Sheath 16–20 F size, with 8/9.5 F Ureteroscope and used Holmium laser or Pneumatic Lithotrity for stone fragmentation. Their center utilizes indigenously designed Pressure Pump for irrigation. Zeng et al. attributed their success of Chinese MPCNL to the selection of the middle calyx as puncture site as well as the use of a pressure pump to facilitate flushing of fragments [35]. Zhaohui He [36] from the same center also published their experience of Mini-PCNL for successful stone removal in 7 patients with transplant kidneys.

## 5.4 LahmeNephroscope and Sheath

In 2001, Sven Lahme [19] and his group from the Department of Urology, University of Tübingen, Germany, published their initial experience with a newly designed, dedicated 12 F Mini Nephroscope (Richard Wolf) and 15 F or 18 F metallic sheath with working length of 205 mm. The instrument is designed as a continuous-flow version. It allows irrigation via the nephroscope (12F) and outflow via the sheath. As an alternative, it is possible to work via an Amplatz sheath. The instrument has a straight 6 F working channel. The angle of the view is 12°. The light conductor consists of 50,000 pixels. Between January 2000 and February 2001, minimally invasive percutaneous nephrolitholapaxy (MPCNL) was performed in 19 patients. The mean stone size was 2.4 $cm^2$. All the patients were treated with ultrasound access and the average operative time was 99 min. Re-treatment rate was 0.7 and none required blood transfusion. They also promoted one-step dilatation. MPCNL of 12 F requires only 1/5 of the cross-sectional area compared with a conventional instrument caliber of 26 F. In 2011, V. Zimmermann [37], S. Lahme and his group expanded their experience with the same technique in 649 patients. On average re-treatment rate was 26.4%. The mean stone size was 4.1 $cm^2$. The average operating time was 65 min. The overall stone-free rate was 93.6%. Blood transfusions were needed in nine cases (1.4%).

## 5.5 Minimally Invasive PCNL

Udo Nagele and his group at the Department of Urology, University of Tübingen, Germany (same as Sven Lahme initiated Mini-PCNL) carried forward their research on improving outcomes of Mini-PCNL. Their new Gelatin Matrix Haemostatic Sealant (GMHS) for closing the tract of Mini-PCNL in a tubeless procedure was published in September, 2006 [38]. They retrospectively reviewed 11 patients in whom GMHS was used at the end of Mini-PCNL. They were the first to describe the use of indigenously designed 18 F metallic sheath. Proximally open-ended sheath and 12 F Lahme Mini Nephroscope were used for this study. Subsequently, in April 2007 [39] they published their experience with a new application device that can be used to close the renal-access tract with GMHS.

In September 2007, an experimental study was done by Udo Nagele et al. [20] in a fresh, perfused cadaveric porcine kidney model. The study tested a new 18 F nephroscope sheath specially designed to decrease intrapelvic pressure during Mini-PCNL. It was compared against conventional closed 18 F metal sheath (used with Lahme Mini-Nephroscope) with Luer-Lok. Intrarenal pressure peaks were measured with a urodynamic workstation. In 1999 [40], Roger Low first studied nephroscopy sheath characteristics. He postulated that intrarenal pressure generated during percutaneous nephroscopy is affected by the height of the irrigation fluid and the sheath characteristics. A shorter length and larger diameter may help in reducing intrarenal pressures. Udo Nagele et al [41]. concluded that by using a 12F nephroscope in connection with the new open 18 F access sheath, critical intrarenal pressure can be avoided, even if the inflow pressure is as high as 125 cm $H_2O$. In contrast, using a closed sheath of an equal diameter resulted in pressure peaks as high as 137 cm $H_2O$.

In August 2008 [42], Udo Nagele coined the term Minimally Invasive PCNL (MIP) for the procedure which was characterized not only by the diameter of the miniaturized 18 F Amplatz sheath that was adopted from the Mini-Perc, but also, by the following features: (1) Ultrasound-guided puncture of the kidney, (2) single-step dilatation of the access tract, (3) ballistic lithotripsy, (4) a low-pressure irrigation system together with stone retraction by irrigation with a specially designed nephroscope sheath, for the so-called vacuum cleaner effect, and (5) a sealed and tubeless access tract with primary closure of the channel independent of hemorrhage and without a second-look procedure. The results of the first 57 patients demonstrated primary stone-free rates of 92.9% with operating times averaging 62 (25–123) minutes. Severe complications, such as sepsis or bleeding requiring blood transfusion, did not occur. Their experience of treatment of lower calyceal calculi (0.8–1.5 cm size) with new MIP technique was published in September 2008 [43]. Stone disintegration was achieved by ballistic lithotripsy through a 12 F minis cope with a 6F working channel (modular miniature nephroscope system with automatic pressure control by Nagele, Karl Storz, Tuttlingen, Germany). Hydrodynamic effects of a specially designed sheath were used to evacuate fragmented stones without additional pressure or suction. When fragments adhered to the parenchyma, a 2.4F tipless nitinol basket was used for stone retrieval. Mean operative time was 54 min (range 32–94 min). The average postoperative hospital stay was 3.2 days. One patient received a flexible Ureteroscopy (URS) for the removal of residual stone fragments and was stone-free thereafter. Together with this secondary ureteroscopy procedure, a complete stone-free status could be achieved in all patients.

The MIP system is available in three different sizes, including the 15/18, 16.5/19.5, and 21/24 F sheaths (representing the inner and outer circumferences). There is an irrigation channel within the sheath as well as the working channel.

Hennessey et al. [41] highlighted several advantages of MIP over standard PCNL and RIRS, for example—flexible patient position, simple single-step dilatation, sleek but robust metallic sheath easy to manipulate during supracostal access and easy learning curve for an experienced surgeon doing standard PCNL. It is safe to learn this procedure for novice surgeons as well due to lower risk of trauma and bleeding.

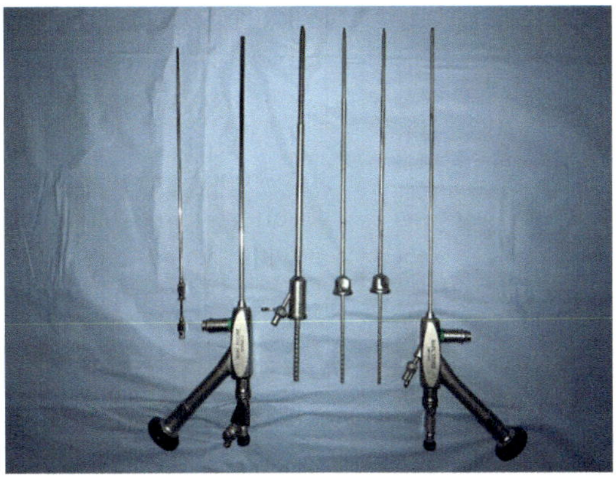

**Fig. 5.1** Sheath size 15 F, MIP S and XS with 7.5 F and 12 F telescope

Bergmann et al. [44] also observed that MIP can be safely and effectively implemented with a mentor-based approach.

The new MIP generation of nephroscope comes with more versions and even smaller diameters (MIP XS and S), and hence offers the chance for even less access trauma (Fig. 5.1). This upgraded concept of MIP is geared to serve as an alternative to retrograde intrarenal surgery while at the same time allowing for an increase in size (MIP M and MIP L systems), to select the best possible treatment option for the management of larger or multiple stones. Thus, this way full advantage of the specific features inherent to MIP is ensured.

## 5.6 Endoscopes and Accessories

The idea of miniaturization of instruments was to reduce the size of nephrostomy tract and use a smaller sheath (18 F instead of 30 F) to reduce renal parenchymal trauma. Any small endoscope with a proper working channel (greater than 5 F) for energy sources and irrigation, which could pass through a small sheath, was good enough to visualize and break the stone. Short Uretero-renoscopes or pediatric cystoscopes worked well in initial trials. First dedicated 12 F Mini-Nephroscope was designed by Sven Lahme in 2001. This was manufactured by Richard Wolf company. But, MIP system was designed by Udo Nagele team and it was manufactured by Karl Storz. Currently, the different endoscope options available for Mini-PCNL are described in Table 5.1. Special endoscopes for Ultramini PCNL and Microperc will be discussed in respective sections of this book. Invention of vacuum cleaner effect/hydrodynamic effects has led to a decline in the use of accessories in MIP [45, 46]. Various accessories for Mini-PCNL are described in Table 5.2.

## 5.7 Irrigation and Suction Pumps

One of the reasons for compromised vision during Mini-PCNL is the smaller working channel of the endoscopes. Proper flow of irrigation fluid is mandatory to wash away blood or debris during endoscopic surgery. If working channel is the same for irrigation flow and accessory instruments like forceps or lithotripsy probes, irrigation flow reduces further while using these instruments. Increasing the height of irrigation fluid bottle is one option, but, various centers use some sort of a pressure system to increase the flow of irrigation. Li et al. [34] described use of a specially designed irrigation pump (MMC Yiyong, Guangzhou, China) during Chinese PCNL. This pulsatile pump generates high pressure (>300 mm Hg) for 3 s followed by low pressure which helps in retrieval of fragments during withdrawal of the nephroscope without using forceps. Alternate high and low pressures created by this pump do not contribute to persistently high Renal Pelvic Pressures and avoid its detrimental effects. Udo Nagele et al. [43] described use of a suction irrigation pump (UROMAT E.A.S.I. SCB) where suction (100–1800 ml/minute) and pressure irrigation (20–200 mm of Hg) are regulated. They recommended use of a suction pump during MIP XS or S, where sheath size is small, and the suction is attached to ureteric catheter to reduce intrarenal pressure. Omar et al. [47] described use of the Thermedx Fluid Smart System™ for pressure irrigation, where, the irrigant temperature was maintained at 21C or higher.

**Table 5.1** Specifications of endoscopes and sheaths available for Mini-PCNL

| | | | | | Sheaths | |
|---|---|---|---|---|---|---|
| | Size (Fr) | Viewing angle (Deg) | Working length (cm) | Working channel (Fr) | Size (F) | Length (CM) |
| *Karl Storz*™ | | | | | | |
| A) Conventional | | | | | | |
| MIP XS/S | 7.5 | 6 | 24 | 2 | 8.5/9.5 | 15, 18 |
| | | | | | 11/12 | 15, 18 |
| MIP M | 12 | 12 | 22 | 6.7 | 15/16 | 15, 18 |
| | | | | | 16.5/17.5 | 15, 18 |
| | | | | | 21/22 | 15, 18 |
| MIP L | 19.5 | 12 | 22 | 12.4 | 23/24 | 15, 18 |
| | | | | | 25/26 | 15, 18 |
| B) Unconventional | | | | | | |
| PED URS (R) | 7.3 | 6 | 25 | 3.6 | | |
| URS (R) | 7 | 6 | 34 | 4.8 | | |
| URS (R) | 8 | 6 | 34 | 5 | | |
| URS (R) | 9.5 | 6 | 34 | 6 | | |
| *Richard wolf*™ | | | | | | |
| A) Conventional | | | | | | |
| Lahme | 12 | 12 | 22.5 | 6 | 15 | 20.5 |
| Nephroscope | | | | | 18 | 20.5 |
| B) Unconventional | | | | | | |
| Flexible cystoscope | 15 | 120 (150–210) | 40 | 7.5 | | |
| Olympus™ | | | | | | |
| A) Conventional | | | | | | |
| PED Nephroscope | 11 | 7 | 22 | 7.5 | 15.9 | 22 |
| B) Unconventional | | | | | | |
| Flexible cystoscope | 8.1 | 120 (130–220) | 38 | 6.6 | | |
| URS (R) | 7.8 | 7 | 33 | 4.2 | | |

**Table 5.2** Instruments and accessories used during Mini-PCNL

| | Size (F) | Length (cm) |
|---|---|---|
| *Storz* | | |
| Fenestrated forcep | | |
| MIP- L | 11.5 | 38 |
| | 10.5 | 38 |
| Triprong forcep | | |
| MIP- L | 10.5 | 38 |
| MIP- M | 5 | 36 |
| Stone grasper | | |
| Adult | 10.5 | 38 |
| | 5 | 40 |
| Pediatric | 3 | 28 |
| | 5 | 30 |
| Biopsy forceps | | |
| Adult | 5 | 40 |
| Pediatric | 3 | 28 |
| | 5 | 30 |
| Flexible instruments | | |
| Stone grasper | | |
| Biopsy forceps | 5 | 73 |
| Stone basket | 5 | 73 |
| | 5 | 60 |
| *Wolf* | | |
| Triprong forceps | 6 | 36.5 |
| Alligator forceps | 6 | 41 |
| Stone grasper | | |
| Rigid | 6 | 36.5 |
| Flexible | 5 | 55 |
| Biopsy forceps (Flexible) | 5 | 55 |
| *Olympus* | | |
| Stone grasper | | |
| Rigid | 5 | 34 |
| Flexible | 3 | 28 |
| Triprong forceps | 5 | 34 |
| Biopsy forceps | 5 | 34 |
| | 3 | 28 |

## 5.8 Sealants

"Tubeless" PCNL exit strategy is considered as one of the advanced techniques used in conventional PCNL. In MIP, tubeless exit and nephrostomy tract sealing is an essential step. A variety of materials are used for sealing the tract to effectively control tract bleeding, prevent urine leakage and thus reduce postoperative pain after PCNL [48]. Lee et al. [49] first described use of GMHS for tubeless PCNL in 2004. The major advantage of GMHS over other sealants is that it dissolves completely in the urine within 5 days. This prevents it from acting as a nidus for future stone formation. Udo Nagele et al. [42] published their study about sealant applicators for MIP. They concluded that this new applicator facilitated application of the GMHS sealant and prevented its migration into the pelvicalyceal system. However, no convincing evidence in the literature about the advantages of using any tissue sealants after tubeless PCNL. Well-controlled, prospective multicenter trials with proper randomization of large numbers of patients are needed for ascertaining further trend related to usage of these sealants [50, 51].

## 5.9 Conclusion

Idea of using miniaturized instruments for percutaneous stone removal has revolutionized the management of upper tract calculi over the last two decades. Especially, 10–20 mm lower calyceal calculi can be managed with high stone-free rates, reduced ancillary procedures and lower morbidity. Specially designed equipment like MIP sheaths and telescopes are worthy investments for all specialized centers managing upper urinary tract calculi. Alternatively, small Amplatz sheaths or Peel Away sheaths (14–20 F) are available which can be used with short Ureterorenoscopes as nephroscope for Mini-PCNL. With proper irrigation pressure and vacuum cleaner effect for stone fragment removal, use of accessory equipment can be minimized.

## References

1. Rupel E, Brown R. Nephroscopy with removal of stone following nephrostomy for obstructive calculous anuria. J Urol. 1941;46(2):177–82. https://doi.org/10.1016/S0022-5347(17)70906-8.
2. Fernström I, Johansson B. Percutaneous pyelolithotomy. A new extraction technique. Scand J Urol Nephrol. 1976;10(3):257–9. https://doi.org/10.1080/21681805.1976.11882084.
3. Wickham JEA, Kellett MJ, Miller RA. Elective percutaneous Nephrolithotomy in 50 patients:an analysis of the technique, Results and Complications. J

Urol. 1983;129(5):904–5. https://doi.org/10.1016/S0022-5347(17)52450-7.
4. Wilfrido R. Castaneda-Zuniga, Ralph Clayman, Arthur Smiths, Barry Rusnak, Marcos Herreral AND Kurt Amplatz “Nephrostolithotomy: percutaneous techniques for urinary calculus removal”. J Urol. 2002;167:849–53.
5. Alken P, Hutschenreiter G, Günther R, Marberger M. Percutaneous stone manipulation. J Urol. 1981;125(4):463–6. https://doi.org/10.1016/S0022-5347(17)55073-9.
6. Türk C, Petřík A, Sarica K, et al. EAU guidelines on diagnosis and conservative Management of Urolithiasis. Eur Urol. 2016;69(3):468–74. https://doi.org/10.1016/j.eururo.2015.07.040.
7. Assimos D, Krambeck A, Miller NL, et al. Surgical Management of Stones: American urological association/Endourological society guideline. PART I J Urol. 2016;196(4):1153–60. https://doi.org/10.1016/j.juro.2016.05.090.
8. Albala DM, Assimos DG, Clayman RV, et al. Lower pole I: a prospective randomized trial of extracorporeal shock wave lithotripsy and percutaneous nephrostolithotomy for lower pole nephrolithiasis-initial results. J Urol. 2001 Dec;166(6):2072–80.
9. Michel MS, Trojan L, Rassweiler JJ. Complications in percutaneous Nephrolithotomy. Eur Urol. 2007;51(4):899–906. https://doi.org/10.1016/j.eururo.2006.10.020.
10. Clayman RV, Surya V, Hunter D, et al. Renal vascular complications associated with the percutaneous removal of renal calculi. J Urol. 1984;132(2):228–30. https://doi.org/10.1016/S0022-5347(17)49573-5.
11. Geraghty RM, Jones P, Somani BK. Worldwide trends of urinary stone disease treatment over the last two decades: a systematic review. J Endourol. 2017;31(6):547–56. https://doi.org/10.1089/end.2016.0895.
12. Kumar A, Kumar N, Vasudeva P, Kumar Jha S, Kumar R, Singh H. A prospective, randomized comparison of shock wave lithotripsy, retrograde intrarenal surgery and Miniperc for treatment of 1 to 2 cm radiolucent lower Calyceal renal calculi: a single Center experience. J Urol. 2015;193(1):160–4. https://doi.org/10.1016/j.juro.2014.07.088.
13. Helal M, Black T, Lockhart J, Figueroa TE. The Hickman Peel-away sheath: alternative for Pediatric percutaneous Nephrolithotomy. J Endourol. 1997;11(3):171–2. https://doi.org/10.1089/end.1997.11.171.
14. Jackman SV, Docimo SG, Cadeddu JA, Bishoff JT, Kavoussi LR, Jarrett TW. The “mini-perc” technique: a less invasive alternative to percutaneous nephrolithotomy. World J Urol. 1998;16(6):371–4. https://doi.org/10.1007/s003450050083.
15. Monga M, Oglevie S. Minipercutaneous Nephrolithotomy. J Endourol. 2000;14(5):419–21. https://doi.org/10.1089/end.2000.14.419.
16. Chan DY, Jarrett TW. Techniques in Endourology mini-percutaneous Nephrolithotomy. J Endourol. 2000;14(3):269–73. https://doi.org/10.1089/end.2000.14.269.
17. Sung YM, Choo SW, Jeon SS, Shin SW, Park KB, Do YS. The “mini-perc” technique of percutaneous Nephrolithotomy with a 14-Fr Peel-away sheath: 3-year results in 72 patients. Korean J Radiol. 2006;7(1):50. https://doi.org/10.3348/kjr.2006.7.1.50.
18. Giusti G, Piccinelli A, Taverna G, et al. Miniperc? No, thank you! Eur Urol. 2007;51(3):810–5. https://doi.org/10.1016/j.eururo.2006.07.047.
19. Lahme S, Bichler KH, Strohmaier WL, Götz T. Minimally invasive PCNL in patients with renal pelvic and calyceal stones. Eur Urol. 2001;40(6):619–24. https://doi.org/10.1159/000049847.
20. Nagele U, Horstmann M, Sievert K-D, et al. A newly designed Amplatz sheath decreases Intrapelvic irrigation pressure during mini-percutaneous Nephrolitholapaxy: an *in-vitro* pressure-measurement and microscopic study. J Endourol. 2007;21(9):1113–6. https://doi.org/10.1089/end.2006.0230.
21. Li L-Y, Gao X, Yang M, et al. Does a smaller tract in percutaneous nephrolithotomy contribute to less invasiveness? A prospective comparative study. Urology. 2010;75(1):56–61. https://doi.org/10.1016/j.urology.2009.06.006.
22. Hu G, Guo Z, Liu H, et al. A novel minimally invasive percutaneous nephrolithotomy technique: safety and efficacy report. Scand J Urol. 2015;49(2):174–80. https://doi.org/10.3109/21681805.2014.961545.
23. Druskin SC, Ziemba JB. Minimally invasive (“mini”) percutaneous Nephrolithotomy: classification, indications, and outcomes. Curr Urol Rep. 2016;17(4):30. https://doi.org/10.1007/s11934-016-0591-5.
24. Jackman SV, Hedican SP, Peters CA, Docimo SG. Percutaneous nephrolithotomy in infants and preschool age children: experience with a new technique. Urology. 1998;52(4):697–701. https://doi.org/10.1016/S0090-4295(98)00315-X.
25. Chan DY, Jarrett TW. Techniques in Endourology mini-percutaneous Nephrolithotomy. J Endourol. 2000;14(3):269–73. https://doi.org/10.1089/end.2000.14.269.
26. Mi F, et al. Prospective randomized study of various techniques of percutaneous Nephrolithotomy. Urology. 2001 Sep;58(3):345–50. https://doi.org/10.1016/s0090-4295(01)01225-0.
27. Lipsky MJ, Shapiro EY, Cha DY, Gupta M. Modified-PCNL without modified instruments: a description of technique. J Endourol. 2013;27(6):684–7. https://doi.org/10.1089/end.2012.0604.
28. Desai J, Solanki R. Ultra-mini percutaneous Nephrolithotomy (UMP): one more armamentarium: ultra-mini PCNL. BJU Int. 2013;112:1046–9. https://doi.org/10.1111/bju.12193.
29. Song L, Chen Z, Liu T, et al. The application of a patented system to minimally invasive percutaneous

Nephrolithotomy. J Endourol. 2011;25(8):1281–6. https://doi.org/10.1089/end.2011.0032.
30. Shah K, Agrawal MS, Mishra DK. Superperc: a new technique in minimally-invasive percutaneous nephrolithotomy. Indian J Urol. 2017;33:48–52.
31. Bader MJ, Gratzke C, Seitz M, Sharma R, Stief CG, Desai M. The "all-seeing needle": initial results of an optical puncture system confirming access in percutaneous Nephrolithotomy. Eur Urol. 2011;59(6):1054–9. https://doi.org/10.1016/j.eururo.2011.03.026.
32. Sabnis R, Ganesamoni R, Ganpule A, et al. Current role of microperc in the management of small renal calculi. Indian J Urol. 2013;29(3):214. https://doi.org/10.4103/0970-1591.117282.
33. Zeng G, Zhao Z, Wan S, et al. Minimally invasive percutaneous Nephrolithotomy for simple and complex renal Caliceal stones: a comparative analysis of more than 10,000 cases. J Endourol. 2013;27(10):1203–8. https://doi.org/10.1089/end.2013.0061.
34. Li X, He Z, Wu K, et al. Chinese minimally invasive percutaneous Nephrolithotomy: the Guangzhou experience. J Endourol. 2009;23(10):1693–7. https://doi.org/10.1089/end.2009.1537.
35. Zeng G, Mai Z, Zhao Z, et al. Treatment of upper urinary calculi with Chinese minimally invasive percutaneous nephrolithotomy: a single-center experience with 12,482 consecutive patients over 20 years. Urolithiasis. 2013;41(3):225–9. https://doi.org/10.1007/s00240-013-0561-z.
36. He Z, Li X, Chen L, Zeng G, Yuan J. Minimally invasive percutaneous nephrolithotomy for upper urinary tract calculi in transplanted kidneys. BJU Int. 2007;99(6):1467–71. https://doi.org/10.1111/j.1464-410X.2007.06768.x.
37. Volker Z, Peter L, Sven L. 1930 minimal invasive pcnl (mpcnl)—proven efficiency and safety after more than 650 consecutive patients. J Urol. 2011;185(4S):e772. https://doi.org/10.1016/j.juro.2011.02.2111.
38. Nagele U, Schilling D, Anastasiadis AG, et al. Closing the tract of mini-percutaneous nephrolithotomy with gelatine matrix hemostatic sealant can replace nephrostomy tube placement. Urology. 2006;68(3):489–93. https://doi.org/10.1016/j.urology.2006.03.081.
39. Nagele U, Anastasiadis AG, Schilling DA, Sievert KD, Kuczyk MA, Stenzl A. Introducing a new sealant applicator for easy, safe, and quick closure of a mini-percutaneous Nephrolitholapaxy access tract. J Endourol. 2007;21(4):393–6. https://doi.org/10.1089/end.2006.0244.
40. Low RK. Nephroscopy sheath characteristics and intrarenal pelvic pressure: human kidney model. J Endourol. 1999;13(3):205–8. https://doi.org/10.1089/end.1999.13.205.
41. Hennessey DB, Kinnear NK, Troy A, Angus D, Bolton DM, Webb DR. Mini PCNL for renal calculi: does size matter? BJU Int. 2017;119:39–46. https://doi.org/10.1111/bju.13839.
42. Nagele U, Schilling D, Anastasiadis AG, et al. Minimal-invasive perkutane Nephrolitholapaxie (MIP). Urol. 2008;47(9):1066. https://doi.org/10.1007/s00120-008-1814-2.
43. Nagele U, Schilling D, Sievert K-D, Stenzl A, Kuczyk M. Management of Lower-Pole Stones of 0.8 to 1.5 cm maximal diameter by the minimally invasive percutaneous approach. J Endourol. 2008;22(9):1851–4. https://doi.org/10.1089/end.2008.9791.
44. Bergmann T, Herrmann TRW, Schiller T, Zimmermann U, Burchardt M. Implementation of minimally invasive percutaneous nephrolithotomy (MIP): comparison of the initial learning curve with the later on clinical routine in a tertiary Centre. World J Urol. 2017;35(12):1933–8. https://doi.org/10.1007/s00345-017-2069-6.
45. Mager R, Balzereit C, Reiter M, et al. Introducing a novel *in vitro* model to characterize hydrodynamic effects of percutaneous Nephrolithotomy systems. J Endourol. 2015;29(8):929–32. https://doi.org/10.1089/end.2014.0854.
46. Mager R, Balzereit C, Hüsch T, et al. Clearance of stone fragments and stone dust by continuous flow hydrodynamics in percutaneous renal surgery: an *in vitro* study. J Endourol. 2016;30(4):441–6. https://doi.org/10.1089/end.2015.0572.
47. Omar M, Noble M, Sivalingam S, et al. Systemic inflammatory response syndrome after percutaneous Nephrolithotomy: a randomized single-blind clinical trial evaluating the impact of irrigation pressure. J Urol. 2016;196(1):109–14. https://doi.org/10.1016/j.juro.2016.01.104.
48. Hong YM, Loughlin KR. The use of Hemostatic agents and sealants in urology. J Urol. 2006;176(6):2367–74. https://doi.org/10.1016/j.juro.2006.07.128.
49. Lee DI, Uribe C, Eichel L, et al. Sealing percutaneous Nephrolithotomy tracts with Gelatin matrix Hemostatic sealant: initial clinical use. J Urol. 2004;171(2):575–8. https://doi.org/10.1097/01.ju.0000103501.98597.b7.
50. Shah HN, Hegde S, Shah JN, Mohile PD, Yuvaraja TB, Bansal MB. A prospective, randomized trial evaluating the safety and efficacy of fibrin sealant in tubeless percutaneous Nephrolithotomy. J Urol. 2006;176(6):2488–93. https://doi.org/10.1016/j.juro.2006.07.148.
51. Canales B, Pugh J. New instrumentation in percutaneous nephrolithotomy. Indian J Urol. 2010;26(3):389. https://doi.org/10.4103/0970-1591.70579.

# Fragmentation Devices: Lithotripters, Lasers and Other Advances

6

Sudheer Kumar Devana and Aditya P. Sharma

## 6.1 Introduction

In mini percutaneous nephrolithotomy (mini-PCNL), after gaining safe access into the pelvicalyceal system (PCS), renal stones are ablated by intracorporeal lithotripsy (ICL). ICL during miniPCNL can be done effectively using fragmentation devices like lithotripters and lasers [1]. Paralleling the advancement in miniaturization of nephroscopes during the past few decades, a significant development in the fragmentation devices has also taken place. ICL involves either smash and extract or smash and go techniques. Smash and extract technique involves breaking larger stones into smaller stone fragments and then extracting them out of the PCS. During miniPCNL these stone fragments can be retrieved via the smaller sized percutaneous tract passively with the vacuum cleaner effect, actively with saline flushing of stone fragments using the ureteric catheter or by applying active suction to innovative mini nephroscope sheaths like shah sheath or clear petra systems (Well Lead Medical Co., Ltd., China) [2]. Stone fragments can also be retrieved using stone grasping forceps and baskets. Smash and go technique involves ablating the larger stone into fine stone dust without the need for using forceps or baskets. The stone dust automatically gets cleared due to saline irrigation or active suction or if left will be cleared up spontaneously in the postoperative period. During miniPCNL as the size of the percutaneous tract is smaller, majority of the endourologists prefer to dust the major bulk of the stone using various fragmentation devices (lithotripters and lasers) and then clear the smaller residual stone fragments left at the end for achieving complete stone clearance.

S. K. Devana (✉) · A. P. Sharma
Department of Urology, Post Graduate Institute of Medical Education and Research, Chandigarh, India

## 6.2 Lithotripters

Various intracorporeal lithotripters were invented for ablating the renal stones since the inception of PCNL. These lithotripters differ based on the type of energy source like electro hydraulic, pneumatic and ultrasonic lithotripsy [3, 4]. Recently newer generation lithotripters have been developed, which use combination of ballistic and ultrasonic energies for better and faster fragmentation of renal stones.

### 6.2.1 Electro Hydraulic Lithotripters (EHL)

These were the first intracorporeal lithotripters introduced in 1955 for treating bladder stones that were subsequently extended to breaking ureteric and renal stones as well. They work by the genera-



M. S. Agrawal et al. (eds.), *Minimally Invasive Percutaneous Nephrolithotomy*,
https://doi.org/10.1007/978-981-16-6001-6_6

tion of spark between two electrodes leading to the formation of a cavitation bubble. Collapse of this bubble generates a shock wave that helps in fragmentation of the stones. Significant retropulsion of the stone and tissue perforation are the drawbacks of this modality [5]. Because of this, use of EHL is hardly ever practiced in modern-day practice for treating renal stones.

### 6.2.2 Mechanical or Ballistic Lithotripters

These lithotripters work similarly to a jackhammer where the projectile inside the hand piece is accelerated either using electromagnetic energy or pneumatic energy (compressed air). Pneumatic lithotripters are the most commonly used mechanical lithotripter device for breaking renal stones. Using compressed air, ballistic energy is generated which gets transferred onto a metallic probe which further breaks the stone like a hammer and chisel effect. It breaks all types of stones irrespective of their composition but stone fragments generated are larger which have to be manually retrieved. The probe vibrates longitudinally either in single or multiple pulses [6]. The Swiss Lithoclast®(Electro medical systems, EMS) was first introduced in 1991 which was further improvised in 2005, Swiss Lithoclast® 2(Electro Medical Systems, EMS) with better fragmentation and lesser pushback effect. The lithoclast probes come in various sizes and lengths for use in standard PCNL, miniPCNL, and semirigid ureteroscopic surgery. Probes specifically designed for use in miniPCNL are smaller in size ranging from 0.8 mm to 2 mm. Recently, flexible pneumatic probes of size 0.89 mm and length 600–940 mm were also introduced for use in retrograde intrarenal surgery (RIRS). During PCNL both the frequency and the air pressure can be adjusted according to the hardness of the stone for optimal fragmentation. The major disadvantage of pneumatic lithotripters is a significant amount of retropulsion and also bleeding due to friction between the stone and the pelvicalyceal mucosa while breaking the stones.

### 6.2.3 Ultrasonic Lithotripters

These lithotripters convert electrical energy into mechanical energy with the help of piezo ceramic elements. A very high frequency of 20,000 Hz will be transmitted to the probe which helps in breaking the stone into smaller fragments and also generation of fine dust. This high-frequency oscillations can lead to generation of heat, which might risk damaging the scopes. Hence continuous cooling of the generator is achieved by continuous saline irrigation and also suctioning. Simultaneous suctioning helps in the clearance of stone fragments and stone dust at a faster speed leading to decreased operation times. Isolated ultrasonic lithotripters are not commonly used in day-to-day practice. Lithotripters with both pneumatic and ultrasonic energy facilities have been shown to be having superior efficiency than used alone in stone fragmentation [7]. Examples of such lithotripters include Swiss Lithoclast® Master/Ultra (EMS, Switzerland), Swiss Lithoclast® Select TM(EMS), and Calcuson Lithotripter® (Karl Storz). Swiss Lithoclast® Master, as shown in Fig. 6.1, has a facility for both pneumatic and ultrasonic lithotripters. Special handpieces such as Vario for ultrasonic lithotripsy and PN3 handpiece for pneumatic lithotripsy are used. For combined use of pneumatic and ultrasonic energy compatible solid pneumatic probes are available which pass inside

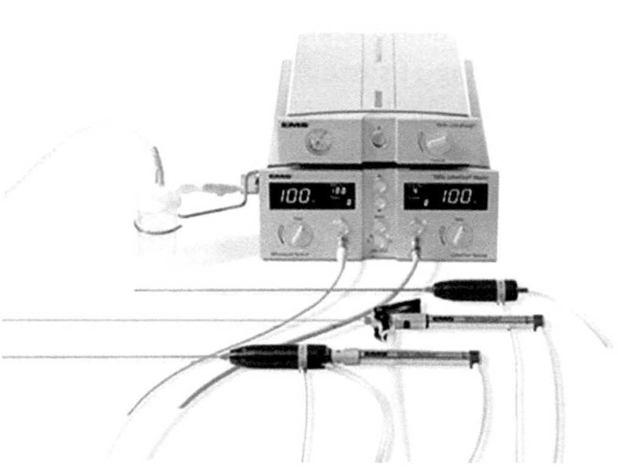

**Fig. 6.1** Swiss Lithoclast® Master (EMS) having combined pneumatic and ultrasonic lithotripter facility. Also depicted in the figure are three handpieces from above downward (Vario handpiece, PN3 handpiece and combined)

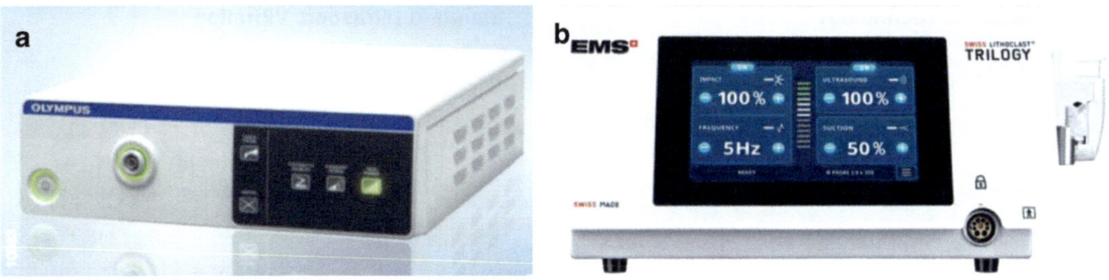


**Fig. 6.2** Showing newer generation dual-energy lithotripters (**a**) Shock Pulse Stone Eliminator™ (Olympus, Japan); (**b**) Swiss Lithoclast®Triology (EMS, Switzerland)

the hollow ultrasonic probes. The ultrasound probes are of larger diameter (3.3–3.8 mm), have added facility of suctioning and are generally used in standard PCNL. They cannot be passed through a 12 Fr mini nephroscope with a working channel of 6Fr. However, recently ultrasound probes of size less than 2 mm have been introduced for use in miniPCNL. Xiong et al. have designed a Micro Ultrasonic probe (HuifuKangCo.Ltd., China) of size 2 mm, which combines the high efficiency of ultrasonic lithotripsy while retaining the ability to pass through mini nephroscopes as well [8]. CyberWand™ (Gyrus ACMI, Southborough, MA, USA) is another fixed dual-probe lithotripter where the inner ultrasonic probe vibrates at 21000 Hz with suction and the outer probe (size 3.3 and 3.8 mm) vibrates at 1000 Hz. However, this cannot be passed through mini nephroscope due to larger size of the probe. Retropulsion is significantly less with ultrasonic lithotripters but they are not effective in hard stones.

### 6.2.4 New Generation Dual Lithotripters

Lithotripters like Swiss Lithoclast® Master or CyberWand™ have double probes (inner and outer probes) for providing both pneumatic and ultrasonic energies for fragmenting and suctioning of stone fragments. Newer generation dual-energy lithotripters with single probes were developed with better fragmentation/dusting and faster stone clearance rates. These include Shock Pulse Stone Eliminator™ (Olympus, Japan) and Swiss Lithoclast®Triology (EMS) (Fig. 6.2). They have single lumen probes with larger inner lumen compared to dual-probe lithotripters leading to better suctioning of even larger stone fragments without the need for active removal of stone fragments. Both these lithotripters have plug and play facility and have handpiece to which single lumen probes of various sizes are attached for use in standard or miniPCNL and ureteroscopic surgery (URS). Effective and variable suction facility with these lithotripters greatly reduces the operating times.

Shock Pulse Stone Eliminator™ simultaneously delivers constant ultrasonic energy with intermittent high-frequency bursts (as high as 300 Hz) of ballistic or mechanical energy for fragmenting as well as aspirating renal stones (Fig. 6.3) [9]. Standard and high power modes buttons are provided on the handpiece for use, according to the hardness of the stone. Single and reusable probes are available with this equipment. For use in miniPCNL, a single or reusable 1.83 mm probe of length 418 mm is available.

Swiss Lithoclast®Triology delivers electromagnetically generated impact and ultrasonic energy along with suction capability. Unlike Shock Pulse, in Lithoclast®Triology there is an option to use either ultrasonic or mechanical or both energies. Pistol grip handpiece and integrated active cooling mechanism for handpiece are also available (Fig. 6.4). Stone catcher with integrated suction facility minimizes the risk of clogging of single lumen probes and also helps in collecting stone dust or fragments for stone analysis. For use in miniPCNL, probe sizes 1.1, 1.5, and 1.9 mm are available. However, the probes

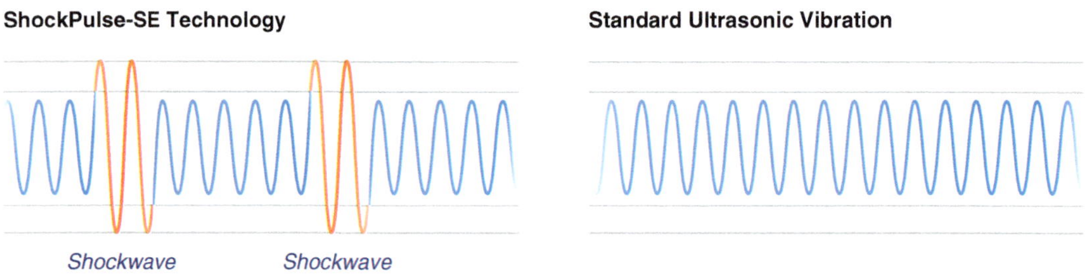


**Fig. 6.3** Mechanism of generation of constant ultrasonic energy with intermittent high-frequency ballistic pulses in Shock Pulse Stone Eliminator™ (Olympus, Japan) when compared to standard ultrasonic vibration

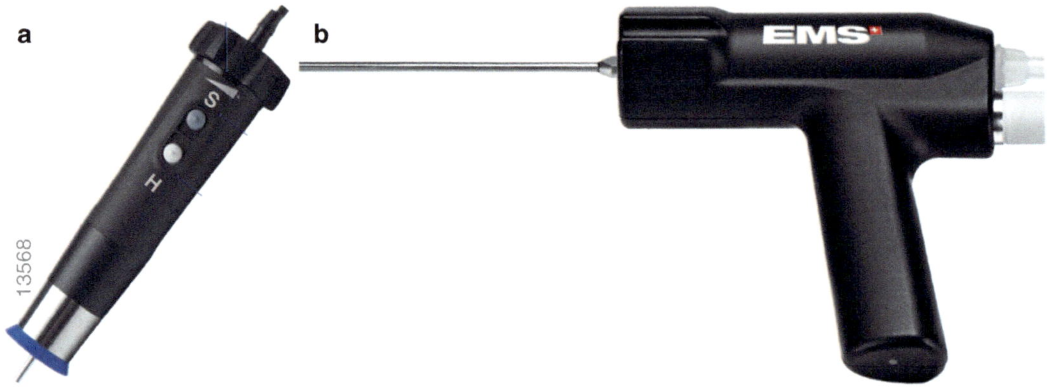


**Fig. 6.4** (**a**) Handpiece used in Shock Pulse Stone Eliminator™ (Olympus, Japan) with surgeon controls; (**b**) Pistol grip handpiece used in Swiss Lithoclast®Triology (EMS, Switzerland) without any surgeon control buttons on it

used in Lithoclast®Triology are disposable for single use, thus adding to increased cost of treatment. Lithoclast®Triology has been shown to be faster than Shock pulse in in vitro studies due to 16 times more ultrasonic probe tip displacement (0.041 mm Vs 0.0025 mm), greater tip displacement during impact or function (0.25 mm Vs 0.01 mm) and larger probe tip diameter [10, 11] (Table 6.1).

### 6.2.5 Cordless Lithotripters

For ease of use and portability, handheld lithotripters were also developed. The Stone Breaker™ (Laryngeal mask airway company Switzerland; distributed by COOK Medical, Bloomington, IN) is a cordless handheld lithotripter that generates ballistic energy using a compressed carbon dioxide cartridge. Lithobreaker®(EMS) is an electrokinetic handheld lithotripter that works using four AAA batteries. Probe sizes of 1 mm and 2 mm are available for use in PCNL as well as URS. These lithotripters have shown to be as effective as conventional lithotripters [12].

## 6.3 Lasers

Laser energy devices are the most versatile lithotripters available. Developed over a period of 6 decades, a lot of research has gone into optimization of type of laser and laser settings for both soft tissue ablation and for stone fragmentation [13]. Lasers providing pulsed mode are best suited for lithotripsy as compared to continuous mode lasers, which are better suited for soft tissue ablation [14].

Holmium: YAG laser is the most commonly used laser for lithotripsy and is the current gold standard for laser intracorporeal lithotripsy (ICL) [15]. Modes commonly used in miniPCNL are dusting and fragmentation. In case of fragmentation as mentioned earlier the vacuum cleaner

**Table 6.1** Various Lithotripters of use during miniPCNL

| S. No. | Lithotripter | Probe type | Available probe sizes |
|---|---|---|---|
| 1. | Swiss Lithoclast® 2 (EMS) | Pneumatic probe | 0.8 mm × 410 mm<br>1.3 mm × 410 mm<br>2.0 mm × 425 mm |
| 2. | Swiss Lithoclast® Master(EMS) | Ultrasound probe<br>Combination of pneumatic with ultrasound probe in miniPCNL | 1.5 mm × 573 mm<br>1.9 mm × 360 mm<br>Not available |
| 3. | Swiss Lithoclast®Triology (EMS) | Combined pneumatic and ultrasound single-use probes | 1.5 mm × 440 mm (5Fr)<br>1.9 mm × 341 mm (6Fr) |
| 4. | Shock Pulse Stone Eliminator™ (Olympus) | Combined pneumatic and ultrasound single and reusable probes | 1.83 mm × 440 mm(5.5Fr) |

EMS, Electro Medical Systems; PCNL, Percutaneous nephrolithotomy

effect in addition to the use of forceps/baskets for active removal of fragments is used [16]. Moses effect which improves the transmission of laser energy through water is the latest advancement in Ho:YAG laser [17, 18]. The Thulium Fiber laser is another emerging diode-based laser that provides new options to treat stone disease [19].

The laser provides a range of techniques of lithotripsy that include dusting, fragmentation, popcorning and pop-dusting [13, 17]. The modulation of pulse energy, pulse frequency and pulse width provide this wide range of modes of lithotripsy while using laser technology. These aspects of laser lithotripsy in the perspective of miniPCNL are discussed in the following section.

### 6.3.1 Settings of Laser and Lasing Techniques

The Ho: YAG laser provides a wide range of settings for power output. Based upon the permutation and combination in frequency, energy and pulse width the laser can be used to dust the stone, to fragment it into small pieces or to create a popcorn effect [20]. Fragmentation and dusting are two most commonly used lithotripsy techniques in miniPCNL.

Dusting is carried out at low energy, high-frequency settings (0.2–0.5 J × 20–80 Hz) [21]. Dusting although a little time consuming creates powder of sub-centimetric size of the stone, which does not require active removal. On the other hand, fragmentation entails the use of higher energy, low frequency and shorter pulse width so as to create fragments, which require active removal (08–1.2 J × 6–10 Hz). Pinning the stone against the wall of the calyx helps in fragmentation of stone safely. The removal of fragments is most commonly done using Bernoulli's principle or the Vacuum Cleaner effect [16]. The stone fragments themselves migrate along the sheath with the eddy current formation. The use of a small fibered laser also helps in continued irrigation to create this effect. The other methods of fragment retrieval include the use of suction, forceps and baskets for stone retrieval. The exit strategies may also be determined by the modality or the technique used for lithotripsy in addition to the stone size and achievement of complete stone clearance.

Devices such as lithAssist (Cook Medical, Bloomington, IN) and laser suction handpiece devices are handheld devices tailor-made to suck fragments created by laser [22]. LithAssist has a 11.6 Fr dual lumen stainless steel cannula for suction with a 5 Fr coaxial inner lumen to allow passage of Laser fiber. In contrast to this device, the laser suction handpiece device has a 12 Fr lumen for suction and a separate working channel for laser fiber [23]. These devices have helped in extending the use of laser lithotripsy to bigger stones including staghorn stones.

### 6.3.2 Laser Fiber

Laser fiber is a particularly important determinant of the laser lithotripsy technique. In contrast to flexible ureteroscopy, a larger diameter fiber is preferred for miniPCNL (300 or 550/600 microns). Large diameter fibers help in using higher energies and cause lesser retropulsion as compared to smaller fibers [24]. On the other hand, small fiber allows for irrigation fluid to egress easily through the sheath, thus improving the vision, efficiency and operating times. The smallest caliber laser fibers (100 microns) are available with Thulium Fiber laser as compared to Ho-YAG where the smallest fiber diameter available is 200 microns only [25]. This is much advantageous with miniaturized version of PCNL.

Ball tip laser fibers have been proposed to provide easy insertion in scopes and also prevent damage to flexible scopes. However, the ball tip degrades due to burn back effect within a few seconds of surgery. Thus, this effect is useful in the setting of single-use fibers. The single-use fibers have been claimed to decrease the overall cost of procedure [26]. There has been much ado about whether the fiber's outer cladding should be stripped or not. The advantages and disadvantages of both are highlighted in Table 6.2. Optimal use of laser fiber is extremely important to obtain the optimal outcome at the same time preventing damage to scopes and operation room (OR) staff as discussed later.

### 6.3.3 Newer Advances in Lasers

#### 6.3.3.1 Moses Effect and Moses Technology

Moses effect is a phenomenon of deformation of the surface of a diamagnetic liquid by application of a magnetic field [27]. As mentioned in the Old testament, Moses crossed the red sea and divided the water holding his staff as the Israelites crossed the sea [28]. Similarly, the Holmium laser, which is absorbed by water due to its properties, creates a vapor tunnel parting the "Sea" of water and blood. Moses technology capitalizes on this principle by using 2 consecutive pulses (Figs. 6.5 and 6.6a) [29]. The first pulse imparts the energy to create a vapor bubble while the second wave travels through this bubble to cause maximal effect over the stone. There are both in vitro and in vivo studies comparing Moses technology to Standard Ho:YAG pulse mode for URS as well as its efficacy for miniPCNL [30, 31]. It has shown to decrease retropulsion and consequently a reduction in procedure duration in preclinical studies [18]. However, cost and single manufacturer remains a drawback for its wider adoption.

#### 6.3.3.2 Thulium Fiber Laser

Thulium Fiber laser (TFL) has been called so as the energy is generated in a chemically doped small fiber and has a wavelength of 1940 nm (Fig. 6.6b) [32]. The wavelength provides a high absorption peak in water and is hence proposed to have better fragmentation properties with almost 1.5 to 4 times faster ablation of stone [33]. Further, it can be easily coupled with smaller fibers with diameter as low as 100 microns. This helps in easy maneuverability and better irrigation while doing lithotripsy.

### 6.3.4 Laser Vs. Other Modalities for miniPCNL—Head to Head Comparison

Tangal et al. and Ganesamoni et al. have compared Laser versus ballistic lithotripsy [34, 35]. The fragmentation time, stone-free rates and complications were comparable between both the groups. However, Ganesamoni et al. found higher stone migration, higher use of forceps for stone retrieval and difficult fragment retrieval when using ballistics [35]. Tangal et al. in addition had a combined group in which the operative time was found to be significantly shorter than either of the groups [34]. They stated that it is better to fragment large size stones using ballistic to around a size of 1 cm each and then use laser for either dusting or fragmentation to smaller pieces, which can be retrieved easily. In a comparative study by Akbulut et al. on laser vs ultrasonic lithotripter, they found that there was higher stone-free rate in laser group as compared to ultrasonic group although it did not reach statistical significance. They further found laser to be much cost effective as compared to ultrasonic lithotripter [36].

**Table 6.2** Summary of the advances or technical aspects of laser lithotripsy[a]

| Laser Parameter | Technical aspect | Benefit | Verdict |
|---|---|---|---|
| Laser settings and Technique | Fragmentation | Faster ablation of primary stone<br>Fragments removed using vacuum cleaner effect | Excellent technique |
| | Dusting | Sub centimetric powdered fragments<br>• No need for active removal | Ablation itself takes more time, compensated by other time gains<br>• Ultra-high-frequency lithotripters further<br>Shorten surgical time |
| | Pop Corning & Pop Dusting | Ideal for multiple smaller stone<br>Fragments in an enclosed space such as calyx<br>Avoids endless chase of fragments | Helpful technique, complementing other Lithotripsy methods |
| Laser lithotripter | Long pulse length (pulse duration or pulse width) | • Less fiber tip degradation<br>• Less stone retropulsion<br>• Smaller residual fragments<br>• Ideal for "dusting" | Gradual rise in its use |
| | Moses effect (modulated laser pulse) | More ablative (in vitro)<br>• Less retropulsion | No significant difference between lasingand procedural time in vivoSingle manufacturer)<br>• Cost is an issue |
| | Thulium fiber laser | More ablative than Ho:YAG<br>• Less retropulsion<br>Coupled with small fiber | Limited availability<br>Lack of randomized trials |
| Laser fibers | Ball tip fiber | Easier insertion in deflected scope | Initial benefit lost after a few seconds with degradation |
| | Tip cleaving tools | All were equivalent | Simple scissors are equally effective |
| | Coated fiber | Greater stone ablation<br>• Easier to pass in the scope<br>• Safer than stripped fiber | More advantageous than stripped fibersin several categories |
| | Stripping of fibers | Debatable higher stone ablation | Significantly less advantages than coated Fibers |

[a] Adapted from Kronenberg P et al. Curr Urol Rep. 2018 (13)

### 6.3.5 Complication and Safety Concerns

The complications of miniPCNL using laser lithotripsy are no different from the use of any other intracorporeal lithotripsy technique. The complications such as bleeding and infection are more related to the surgical procedure itself rather than the use of laser ICL [37]. In fact, in one of the recent studies from our center we found no difference in clinically significant blood loss or infection rate in standard vs miniPCNL [38]. Thus, these common complications and few others such as pelvicalyceal injury, pleural injury, solid organ injury, or bowel injury are more related to access rather than the type of lithotripsy used.

However, unique to Laser lithotripsy is safety concerns for OR staff and surgeons associated with its use in OR. The eyes remain the most vulnerable organ, which can be damaged by laser, especially when it is brought in very close con-

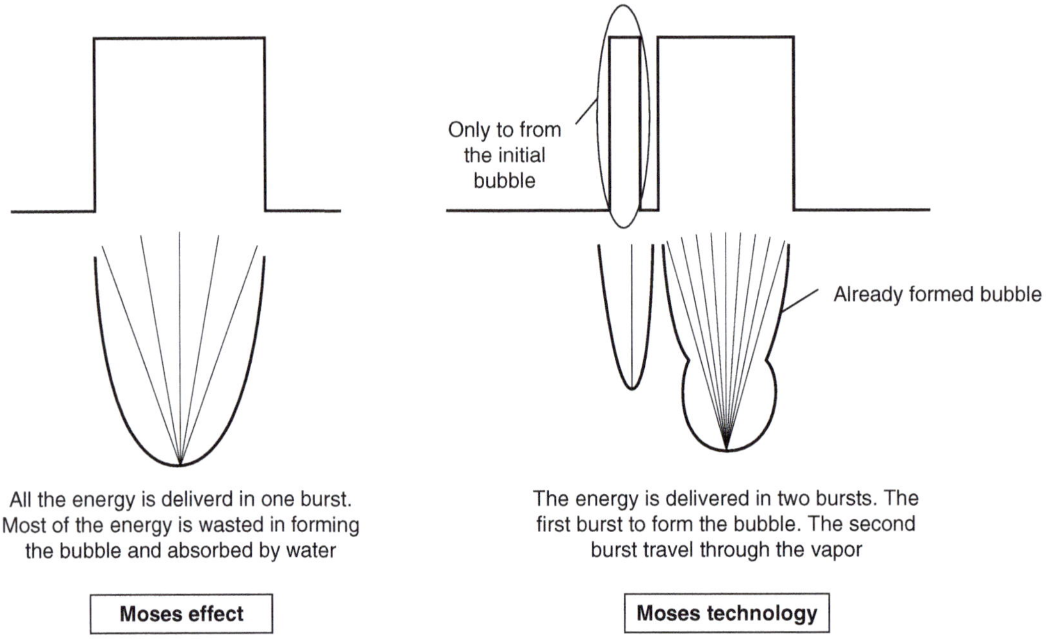


**Fig. 6.5** Moses effect and Moses Technology for Ho:YAG laser (From: Aldoukhi AH, Black KM, Ghani KR. Emerging Laser Techniques for the Management of Stones. Urol Clin North Am. 2019 May;46(2):193–205)

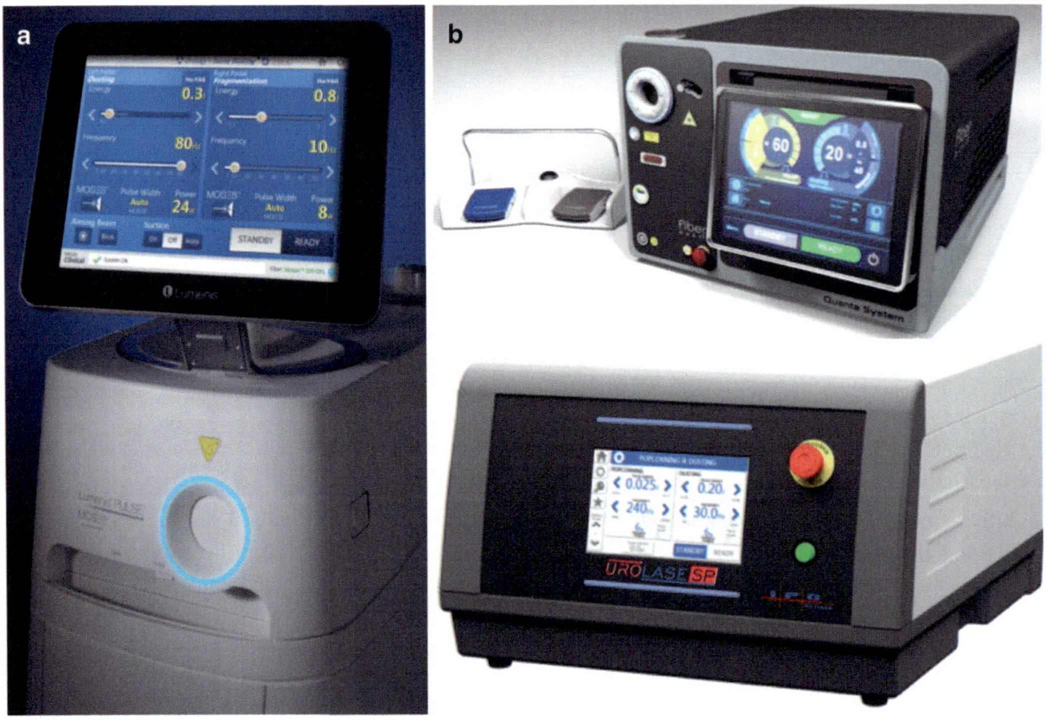


**Fig. 6.6** Laser Generators (**a**) Moses™ Technology from Lumenis™ Pulse (Yokneam, Israel). (**b**) Thulium Fiber Lasers from Quanta™ (Samarate, Italy) and Intercardia Life Sciences™ (Delhi, India)

tact to the eye without any protective covering for the eyes. Simple eyeglasses are equally effective as special Laser protective glasses [39]. The eye injury is a zero event and has never been reported in literature yet.

Another important collateral damage of laser energy is to delicate scopes used in endourology. It is more common for flexible scopes used during URS or RIRS rather than to the rigid scopes used in miniPCNL. Still, the laser fiber should be kept in vision at all times, especially when activating the laser. The fiber should be kept at an adequate distance from the optical end of the scope [40]. Other recommendations include keeping the fiber tip covered and regular cleaving of fiber.

## 6.4 Other Advances

To overcome the high complication rate because of the generated shockwaves with EHL, a newer lithotripter named nanosecond electro pulse lithotripter (NEPL) (Urolith-105 M device) was developed by Lithotech Medical Ltd. (Israel). It produces electric pulses of high voltage being discharged in nanosecond duration, which gets transferred onto the stone. This generates tensile thermomechanical stress in the stone leading to fragmentation of stone. NEPL was found to be better than EHL in an in vitro study by Martov et al. [41]. Martov et al. also have shown in another in vitro study that NEPL was more effective and requires significantly less energy and time for stone disintegration than holmium laser [42]. Flexible probes of various sizes 2.7 to 4.5 Fr are available for use with cystoscope, semirigid ureteroscope, and flexible ureteroscopes [43]. Studies done using this technology in miniPCNL are not available so far in the existing literature.

## 6.5 Conclusions

Miniaturization of fragmentation devices has accompanied the miniaturization of PCNL procedure. Currently Ho:YAG Laser remains the gold standard for stone ablation in miniPCNL. Moses technology and Thulium Fiber laser are showing promising results in terms of faster stone ablation. Newer generation lithotripters with thin probes are tailor-made to decrease retropulation and are being combined with effective suction mechanism for a better clearance rate.

## References

1. Lingeman JE, Beiko D, Cleveland RO, Evan AP, Gettman MT, Kohrmann KU, Liatsikos E, Matlaga BR, McAteer JA, Monga M, Tailly G, Timoney A (2008) Stone technology: shock wave and intracorporeal lithotripsy. In: J Denstedt, S Khoury, editors. Stone disease. 2nd international consultation on stone disease, vol 4, 21st edn. Health Publications Committee, UK, pp. 85–136. ISBN 0–9546956–7-4.
2. Zanetti SP, Lievore E, Fontana M, Turetti M, Gallioli A, Longo F, Albo G, De Lorenzis E, Montanari E. Vacuum-assisted mini-percutaneous nephrolithotomy: a new perspective in fragments clearance and intrarenal pressure control. World J Urol. 202;39(6):1717–23.
3. Scotland KB, Kroczak T, Pace KT, Chew BH. Stone technology: intracorporeal lithotripters. World J Urol. 2017 Sep;35(9):1347–51.
4. Alken P. Intracorporeal lithotripsy. Urolithiasis. 2018 Feb;46(1):19–29.
5. Vorreuther R, Corleis R, Klotz T, Bernards P, Engelmann U. Impact of shock wave pattern and cavitation bubble size on tissue damage during ureteroscopic electro hydraulic lithotripsy. J Urol. 1995;153(3 Pt 1):849–53.
6. Hemal AK, Goel A, Aron M, Seth A, Dogra PN, Gupta NP. Evaluation of fragmentation with single or multiple pulse setting of lithoclast for renal calculi during percutaneous nephro- lithotripsy and its impact on clearance. Urol Int. 2003;70(4):265–8.
7. Auge BK, Lallas CD, Pietrow PK, Zhong P, Preminger GM. In vitro comparison of standard ultrasound and pneumatic lithotrites with a new combination intracorporeal lithotripsy device. Urology. 2002 Jul;60(1):28–32.
8. Xiong L, Huang X, Ye X, Chen L, Ma K, Liu J, Hong Y, Xu Q, Wang X. Micro ultrasonic probe combined with ultrasound-guided Minipercutaneous nephrolithotomy in the treatment of upper ureteral and renal stones: a consecutive cohort study. J Endourol. 2020 Apr;34(4):429–33.
9. Chew BH, Matteliano AA, de Los RT, Lipkin ME, Paterson RF, Lange D. Bench top and initial clinical evaluation of the shock pulse stone eliminator in percutaneous nephrolithotomy. J Endourol. 2017;31:191–7.
10. Carlos EC, Wollin DA, Winship BB, Jiang R, Radvak D, Chew BH, Gustafson MR, Simmons WN, Zhong P,

Preminger GM, Lipkin ME. In vitro comparison of a novel single probe dual-energy lithotripter to current devices. J Endourol. 2018 Jun;32(6):534–40.
11. Sabnis RB, Balaji SS, Sonawane PL, Sharma R, Vijayakumar M, Singh AG, Ganpule AP, Desai MR. EMS Lithoclast trilogy™: an effective single-probe dual-energy lithotripter for mini and standard PCNL. World J Urol. 2020 Apr;38(4):1043–50.
12. Wang AJ, Baldwin GT, Gabriel JC, Cocks FH, Goldsmith ZG, Iqbal MW, Astroza GM, Simmons WN, Zhong P, Preminger GM, Lipkin ME. In-vitro assessment of a new portable ballistic lithotripter with percutaneous and ureteroscopic models. J Endourol. 2012 Nov;26(11):1500–5.
13. Kronenberg P, Somani B. Advances in lasers for the treatment of stones—a systematic review. Curr Urol Rep. 2018;19(6):45.
14. Pal D, Ghosh A, Sen R, Pal A. Continuous-wave and quasi-continuous wave thulium-doped all-fiber laser: implementation on kidney stone fragmentations. Appl Opt 2016 Aug;55(23):6151–6155. https://www.osapublishing.org/ao/abstract.cfm?URI=ao-55-23-6151.
15. Leveillee RJ, Lobik L. Intracorporeal lithotripsy: which modality is best? Curr Opin Urol. 2003 May;13(3):249–53.
16. Mager R, Balzereit C, Gust K, Hüsch T, Herrmann T, Nagele U, et al. The hydrodynamic basis of the vacuum cleaner effect in continuous-flow PCNL instruments: an empiric approach and mathematical model. World J Urol. 2016 May;34(5):717–24.
17. Aldoukhi AH, Black KM, Ghani KR. Emerging laser techniques for the Management of Stones. Urol Clin North Am. 2019;46(2):193–205.
18. Elhilali MM, Badaan S, Ibrahim A, Andonian S. Use of the Moses Technology to improve holmium laser lithotripsy outcomes: a preclinical study. J Endourol. 2017 Jun;31(6):598–604.
19. Traxer O, Keller EX. Thulium fiber laser: the new player for kidney stone treatment? A comparison with holmium:YAG laser. World J Urol. 2020 Aug;38(8):1883–94.
20. Matlaga BR, Chew B, Eisner B, Humphreys M, Knudsen B, Krambeck A, et al. Ureteroscopic laser lithotripsy: a review of dusting vs fragmentation with extraction. J Endourol. 2018 Jan;32(1):1–6.
21. Doizi S, Keller EX, De Coninck V, Traxer O. Dusting technique for lithotripsy: what does it mean? Nat Rev Urol. 2018 Nov;15(11):653–4.
22. Okhunov Z, del Junco M, Yoon R, Labadie K, Lusch A, Ordon M. In vitro evaluation of LithAssist: a novel combined holmium laser and suction device. J Endourol. 2014 Aug;28(8):980–4.
23. Dauw CA, Borofsky MS, York N, Lingeman JE. A usability comparison of laser suction handpieces for percutaneous nephrolithotomy. J Endourol. 2016 Nov;30(11):1165–8.
24. Kang HW, Lee H, Teichman JMH, Oh J, Kim J, Welch AJ. Dependence of calculus retropulsion on pulse duration during ho: YAG laser lithotripsy. Lasers Surg Med. 2006 Sep;38(8):762–72.
25. Fried NM, Irby PB. Advances in laser technology and fibre-optic delivery systems in lithotripsy. Nat Rev Urol. 2018 Sep;15(9):563–73.
26. Shin RH, Lautz JM, Cabrera FJ, Shami CJ, Goldsmith ZG, Kuntz NJ, et al. Evaluation of novel ball-tip holmium laser fiber: impact on ureteroscope performance and fragmentation efficiency. J Endourol. 2016 Feb;30(2):189–94.
27. Bormashenko E. Moses effect: physics and applications. Adv Colloid Interf Sci. 2019 Jul;269:1–6.
28. Book of Exodus. In: The Bible: Old Testament. p. 13:17–14:2.
29. Ibrahim A, Badaan S, Elhilali MM, Andonian S. Moses technology in a stone simulator. Can Urol Assoc J = J l'Association des Urol du Canada. 2018 Apr;12(4):127–30.
30. Mekayten M, Lorber A, Katafigiotis I, Sfoungaristos S, Leotsakos I, Heifetz EM, et al. Will stone density stop being a key factor in endourology? The impact of stone density on laser time using Lumenis laser p120w and standard 20 W laser: a comparative study. J Endourol. 2019 Jul;33(7):585–9.
31. Leotsakos I, Katafigiotis I, Lorber A, Sfoungaristos S, Sabler IM, Yutkin V, et al. Initial experience in combined ultra-mini percutaneous nephrolithotomy with the use of 120-W laser and the anti-retropulsion "Moses effect": the future of percutaneous nephrolithotomy? Lasers Med Sci. 2020 Dec;35(9):1961–6.
32. Blackmon RL, Irby PB, Fried NM. Holmium:YAG (lambda = 2120 nm) versus thulium fiber (lambda = 1908 nm) laser lithotripsy. Lasers Surg Med. 2010 Mar;42(3):232–6.
33. Rapoport LM, Gazimiev MA, Korolev DO, Tsarichenko DG, Svetikova YUA, Enikeev ME, et al. Flexible ureteroscopy for lower pole renal stones: novel super pulse thulium (TM) fiber laser lithotripsy. Urologiia. 2020 Dec;(6):89–92.
34. Tangal S, Sancı A, Baklacı U, Babayiğit M, Karaburun MC, Kubilay E, et al. What is the optimum lithotripsy method for high density stones during mini-PNL? Laser, ballistic or combination of both. Lasers Med Sci. 2020;35(8):1765–8.
35. Ganesamoni R, Sabnis RB, Mishra S, Parekh N, Ganpule A, Vyas JB, et al. Prospective randomized controlled trial comparing laser lithotripsy with pneumatic lithotripsy in miniperc for renal calculi. J Endourol. 2013 Dec;27(12):1444–9.
36. Akbulut F, Kucuktopcu O, Kandemir E, Sonmezay E, Simsek A, Ucpinar B, et al. Comparison of efficacy of laser lithotripter with ultrasonic lithotripter in mini percutaneous nephrolithotomy. Arch Ital di Urol Androl organo Uff [di] Soc Ital di Ecogr Urol e Nefrol. 2016 Jan;87(4):276–9.
37. Althunayan AM, Elkoushy MA, Elhilali MM, Andonian S. Adverse events resulting from lasers used in urology. J Endourol. 2014 Feb;28(2):256–60.
38. Thakur A, Sharma AP, Devana SK, Parmar KM, Mavuduru RS, Bora GS, et al. Does miniaturization

actually decrease bleeding after percutaneous nephrolithotomy? A single-center randomized trial. J Endourol. 2021;35(4):451–56.
39. Villa L, Cloutier J, Compérat E, Kronemberg P, Charlotte F, Berthe L, et al. Do we really need to Wear proper eye protection when using holmium:YAG laser during endourologic procedures? Results from an ex vivo animal model on pig eyes. J Endourol. 2016 Mar;30(3):332–7.
40. Talso M, Emiliani E, Haddad M, Berthe L, Baghdadi M, Montanari E, et al. Laser fiber and flexible Ureterorenoscopy: the safety distance concept. J Endourol. 2016 Dec;30(12):1269–74.
41. Martov A, Gudkov A, Diamant V, Chepovetsky G, Lerner M. Investigation of differences between nanosecond electropulse and electrohydraulic methods of lithotripsy: a comparative in vitro study of efficacy. J Endourol. 2014 Apr;28(4):437–45.
42. Martov A, Diamant V, Borisik A, Andronov A, Chernenko V. Comparative in vitro study of the effectiveness of nanosecond electrical pulse and laser lithotripters. J Endourol. 2013 Oct;27(10):1287–96.
43. Gudkov A, Boshchenko V, Petlin A, Afonin V, Diamant V, Lerner M. Retrograde endoscopic lithotripsy using the innovative nanosecond electropulse method. Springerplus. 2013 Oct 17;2:538.

# Part III

# Anesthesia Considerations and Positioning

# 7 Anesthesia in Mini-PCNL

Handattu M. Krishna and Savan Kumar Nagesh

## 7.1 Introduction

It is intuitive to believe that mini-PCNL would offer many benefits from the perspective of anesthesia. The flexibility with patient positioning and the reduction in surgical invasiveness are the main reasons behind it. It enables us to juggle with different modalities of anesthesia and choose the best one for a particular patient. But, are these perceptions supported by evidence from literature? Do the facts that mini-PCNL with its small incision, reduced surgical invasiveness, and hence the pain, ability to do in prone or supine position translate to better patient outcomes? We seek to explore.

## 7.2 Anesthetic Concerns for Mini-PCNL

The patient-related concerns would remain the same, whether it is PCNL or mini-PCNL. These include the comorbidities of the patient like diabetes mellitus, hypertension, coronary artery disease, impaired renal function, dyselectrolytemia, and age-appropriate considerations (pediatric, geriatric).

H. M. Krishna (✉) · S. K. Nagesh
Department of Anesthesiology, Kasturba Medical College, Manipal, Manipal Academy of Higher Education, Manipal, Karnataka, India

The surgical stress in the intraoperative and postoperative period during mini-PCNL was assumed to be lesser than standard PCNL, due to mini-PCNL being less invasive. It was claimed that the lower surgical stress would then translate to a better perioperative course, even in patients with above-mentioned comorbidities. The evidence to support this claim is contrasting. Li LY et al. demonstrated that both regular and mini-PCNL resulted in comparable surgery-related tissue damage [10]. Traxer O et al. also concluded that postoperative scarring and renal parenchymal loss were similar between mini-PCNL and standard PCNL [19]. Clinically though, it has been shown that patients undergoing mini-PCNL have lower blood loss, lesser need for transfusion, and shorter in-hospital stay [14].

PCNL is most commonly performed in the prone position. Hence, it is accompanied by the concerns associated with prone positioning, like alteration of ventilation and hemodynamics, pressure effects on the soft tissues, threat of dislodgement of tracheal tube, and venous access [4]. Mini-PCNL performed in prone position also faces the same concerns of prone position and requires the same attentive care.

Mini-PCNL can also be performed in modified supine position, avoiding the problems seen with prone positioning. Sakr A et al. reported improved safety of mini-PCNL in supine position compared to standard PCNL [15]. The position


M. S. Agrawal et al. (eds.), *Minimally Invasive Percutaneous Nephrolithotomy*,
https://doi.org/10.1007/978-981-16-6001-6_7

chosen to perform mini-PCNL dictates the concerns and precautions to be taken.

A smaller incision in mini-PCNL means lesser postoperative pain, lower blood loss, and increased incidence of tubeless PCNL. When taken together, these have led to a shorter postoperative hospital stay [18]. As an extension of this idea, an ambulatory or overnight stay tubeless mini-PCNL can be considered in selected patients. Anesthetic concerns for an ambulatory or overnight stay surgery would be appropriate patient selection, use of short-acting anesthetic agents, and good pain control, which is known to improve patient satisfaction, reduce cost, and hospital resource utilization [9].

The time duration for mini-PCNL depends on the stone characteristics and the surgical experience. It is intuitive to guess that the surgical duration for mini-PCNL would be less than that for PCNL and it would result in lesser exposure to anesthetics and reduced cost. But most studies show equal time duration for both or mini-PCNL taking longer time [7, 21].

## 7.3 Available Anesthetic Techniques for Mini-PCNL

Mini-PCNL can be performed under general anesthesia, central neuraxial (spinal/epidural) anesthesia, or local anesthesia (Table 7.1). The advent of ultrasound-guided nerve blocks has also kindled interest in ultrasound-guided truncal blocks for mini-PCNL. The patient's position in which the procedure is planned (supine vs. prone), patient comorbidities that determine the modality of anesthesia best tolerated by the patient, stone characteristics influencing the duration of the procedure, and the extent of tissue handling determine the choice of anesthesia.

**Table 7.1** Anesthetic options for mini-PCNL

| |
|---|
| General anesthesia with tracheal intubation |
| General anesthesia with supraglottic device |
| Spinal/epidural anesthesia |
| Local anesthesia with Monitored Anesthesia Care (MAC) |
| Ultrasound-guided truncal blocks (paravertebral block, erector spinae block) |

General anesthesia is as popular for mini-PCNL as for PCNL. Fentanyl-propofol-atracurium/vecuronium-isoflurane/sevoflurane in air/nitrous oxide–oxygen mixture—paracetamol-based general anesthesia is commonly used. Patients are usually intubated with tracheal tube to have a secure airway, especially for prone position procedures. However, laryngeal mask airway or I gel can be used instead of tracheal tube for procedures in the supine position. The use of these supraglottic devices for prone position surgeries has been reported [11]. Secure airway, better control of hemodynamics, better control over oxygenation and ventilation of the patient, lack of awareness of the procedure and surrounding environment to the patient, no limitation to the surgical duration are some of the advantages of general anesthesia. The disadvantages of general anesthesia are that it is expensive, masks some of the warning symptoms the patient would have reported had he been awake (like pressure over soft tissues), risks of instrumenting the airway, and aspiration.

Mini-PCNL done in supine position can be done under spinal or epidural anesthesia. Hyperbaric bupivacaine with or without additives like fentanyl, buprenorphine, and clonidine is the commonly used drug for spinal anesthesia while bupivacaine, ropivacaine, and levobupivacaine are widely used for epidural anesthesia. Combining central neuraxial block with sedation enhances patient comfort. The advantages of central neuraxial block are it avoids polypharmacy (and hence the side effects of the multiple drugs) as seen in general anesthesia, less expensive, better intraoperative and postoperative analgesia, the ability of the awake patient to report the symptoms which can provide early warning, protection against deep venous thrombosis by improving the rheologic properties of blood, reduced procedural bleeding due to accompanying reduction in blood pressure. The disadvantages of central neuraxial block are hypotension, especially if the block height ascends above $T_6$ segment, bradycardia secondary to blockade of cardio accelerator fibers due to high block, awareness of the surrounding by the patient which could be unpleasant, breakthrough pain, especially with the ungentle handling of the deeper tissues, limited duration (2–3 h) with spinal anesthesia. A sensory level of blockade up to at least $T_4$ segment is required for PCNL. Hemodynamic changes like hypotension and bradycardia are expected to occur with this height of blockade. Spinal anesthesia is not always a safe alternative to general anesthesia. Having an awake patient does not necessarily mean enhanced safety.

There are centers that perform mini-PCNL and PCNL in prone position under spinal anesthesia. But this requires special precautions and experience. Data for the feasibility of regional anesthesia in prone PCNL surgeries are mostly single-center randomized controlled trials (RCT) done in patients undergoing standard PCNL. However, this data can be extrapolated to patients undergoing mini-PCNL as the surgical indication, duration of surgery, and anesthetic techniques are similar. Mehrabi S et al. reviewed 160 patients who underwent standard PCNL surgery in prone position under spinal anesthesia safely. There were no major complications. Six patients complained of postoperative headache, and only eight patients complained of mild pain intraoperatively [12]. An RCT done by Movasseghi G et al. compared 30 patients each under spinal and general anesthesia undergoing PCNL. They found spinal anesthesia to be equally feasible as general anesthesia, with more stable hemodynamics, lesser postoperative pain, and lower blood loss in the spinal anesthesia arm [13]. Cicek T et al. also retrospectively compared patients who underwent PCNL surgery under spinal and general anesthesia and concluded both to be equally safe techniques [2]. Studies comparing epidural and spinal–epidural anesthesia with general anesthesia, as the primary anesthetic technique for standard PCNL, also showed similar efficacy and safety [8, 16, 17]. While overall, the data does suggest lower surgical time, lesser postoperative pain, and more stable hemodynamics with regional anesthesia, we have to keep in mind that these are single-center studies, where there might be requisite setup and training to manage patients undergoing regional anesthesia in the prone position, which may add bias to these studies.

Mini-PCNL can be performed under local anesthesia as well. A cooperative patient, gentle urologist, and a vigilant anesthesiologist to monitor the vital parameters make this technique successful. Lignocaine 1–2% with 1:200000 adrenaline, bupivacaine0.25%, levo-bupivacaine 0.25%, ropivacaine 0.2% are commonly used for local anesthetic infiltration of the puncture site. Deeper infiltration is made as one proceeds. Attention must be paid to the maximum permissible dose of these local anesthetics to prevent local anesthetic toxicity (4 mg/kg for plain lignocaine, 7 mg/kg for lignocaine with adrenaline, and 2–3 mg/kg for bupivacaine, levo-bupivacaine, and ropivacaine). Aravantinos et al. performed 25 mini-PCNL under local anesthesia, all of whom tolerated the procedure well with some mild sedation and intravenous analgesics [1]. Ding et al. also performed mini-PCNL in 40 patients under local anesthesia successfully [3]. Local anesthetic technique is useful in sick patients who would not tolerate general or spinal anesthesia. Still, it should be borne in mind that the pain results not only from the skin incision but also from the surgical dissection in the deeper tissues.

Ultrasound-guided erector spinae block and paravertebral block have been described for mini-PCNL. The paravertebral block involves injecting local anesthetic around spinal nerve roots as they exit from the intervertebral foramen and offer superior analgesic quality compared to local anesthetic infiltration technique without the hemodynamic changes seen with spinal anesthesia. This technique requires multilevel injections to block $T_{10}$–$T_{12}$ segments using 0.25–0.5% ropivacaine or bupivacaine. The disadvantages of this technique include the requirement of multiple injections, ipsilateral lower limb weakness, long duration for the onset of anesthesia (10–20 min), risk of failed block, risk of pneumothorax, and local anesthetic systemic toxicity due to the high dose of local anesthetic used. Yang et al. performed mini-PCNL in 45 patients under paravertebral block and mild sedation. All patients tolerated the procedure well [20].

Erector spinae plane block relies on a high volume of local anesthetic injected below the erector spinae muscle and spread of the local anesthetic along the erector spinae plane, thereby blocking the spinal nerves as they emerge out from the intervertebral foramen. Large volumes (20–40 mL) of local anesthetic are required for adequate spread along the correct plane, and hence it is less reliable than paravertebral block as a sole anesthetic technique. It can also be used as a technique for postoperative analgesia as a part of multimodal analgesia and has been shown to provide a safe and effective analgesic technique [5, 6].

## 7.4 Specific Anesthetic Problems Encountered During Mini-PCNL

The option to do mini-PCNL in supine position avoids all the problems associated with the prone position. Problems with the prone position are discussed in detail in another chapter. A high puncture can result in pneumothorax even with mini-PCNL as well. Nitrous oxide is avoided if there is a suspicion of pneumothorax, and postoperative chest X-ray is required to rule out pneumothorax. If significant, it might require the insertion of an intercostals drain tube. For prolonged procedures, significant fluid absorption, blood loss (and its estimation), hypothermia, need to convert spinal anesthesia to general anesthesia could be problematic.

## 7.5 Conclusion

Does your anesthesiologist like mini-PCNL? Yes, if there is a flexibility to do it in the supine or prone position, to choose the right modality of anesthesia which suits the best for the patient, if the duration of the procedure is shorter, if the accompanying surgical stress response is lower, if the postoperative pain is lower, if the postoperative recovery is faster resulting in earlier discharge from the hospital. Above all, if it is safe and results in better patient satisfaction, an anesthesiologist, undoubtedly would welcome mini-PCNL wholeheartedly.

## References

1. Aravantinos E, Kalogeras N, Stamatiou G, Chantzi E, Moutzouris G, Zygoulakis N, Melekos M. 'Single puncture'mini-percutaneous nephrolithotomy under assisted local anesthesia. Curr Urol. 2010;4(4):177–81.
2. Cicek T, Gonulalan U, Dogan R, Kosan M, Istanbulluoglu O, Gonen M, Ozturk B, Ozkardes H. Spinal anesthesia is an efficient and safe anesthetic method for percutaneous nephrolithotomy. Urology. 2014;83(1):50–5.
3. Ding Q, Wang W, Shao W, Chen X. Local anesthesia effect of minimally invasive percutaneous nephrolithotomy on systemic inflammatory response and renal function damage. Int J Clin Exp Med. 2017;10(2):3747–51.
4. Edgcombe H, Carter K, Yarrow S. Anaesthesia in the prone position. Br J Anaesth. 2008;100(2):165–83.
5. Gultekin MH, Erdogan A, Akyol F. Evaluation of the efficacy of the erector spinae plane block for postoperative pain in patients undergoing percutaneous nephrolithotomy: a randomized controlled trial. J Endourol. 2020;34(3):267–72.
6. Ibrahim M, Elnabtity AM. Analgesic efficacy of erector spinae plane block in percutaneous nephrolithotomy: a randomized controlled trial. Anaesthesist. 2019;68(11):755–61.
7. Jones P, Elmussareh M, Aboumarzouk OM, Mucksavage P, Somani BK. Role of minimally invasive (micro and ultra-mini) PCNL for adult urinary stone disease in the modern era: evidence from a systematic review. Curr Urol Rep. 2018;19(4):27.
8. Karacalar S, Bilen CY, Sarihasan B, Sarikaya S. Spinal-epidural anesthesia versus general anesthesia in the management of percutaneous nephrolithotripsy. J Endourol. 2009;23(10):1591–7.
9. Kulkarni S, Harsoor SS, Chandrasekar M, Bhaskar SB, Bapat J, Ramdas EK, Valecha UK, Pradhan AS, Swami AC. Consensus statement on anaesthesia for day care surgeries. Indian J Anaesth. 2017;61(2):110–24.
10. Li LY, Gao X, Yang M, Li JF, Zhang HB, Xu WF, Lin Z. Does a smaller tract in percutaneous nephrolithotomy contribute to less invasiveness? A prospective comparative study. Urology. 2010;75(1):56–61.
11. Lopez AM, Valero R. Use of supraglottic airway devices in patients positioned other than supine. Trends Anesthesia Crit Care. 2012;2(2):65–70.
12. Mehrabi S, Shirazi KK. Results and complications of spinal anesthesia in percutaneous nephrolithotomy. Urol J. 2010;7(1):22–5.
13. Movasseghi G, Hassani V, Mohaghegh MR, Safaeian R, Safari S, Zamani MM, Nabizadeh R. Comparison between spinal and general anesthesia in percutaneous nephrolithotomy. Anesth Pain Med. 2013;4(1):e13871.
14. Proietti S, Giusti G, Desai M, Ganpule AP. A critical review of miniaturized percutaneous nephrolithotomy: is smaller better? Eur Urol Focus. 2017;3(1):56–61.

15. Sakr A, Salem E, Kamel M, Desoky E, Ragab A, Omran M, Fawzi A, Shahin A. Minimally invasive percutaneous nephrolithotomy vs standard PCNL for management of renal stones in the flank-free modified supine position: single-center experience. Urolithiasis. 2017;45(6):585–9.
16. Singh V, Sinha RJ, Sankhwar SN, Malik A. A prospective randomized study comparing percutaneous nephrolithotomy under combined spinal-epidural anesthesia with percutaneous nephrolithotomy under general anesthesia. Urol Int. 2011;87(3):293–8.
17. Tangpaitoon T, Nisoog C, Lojanapiwat B. Efficacy and safety of percutaneous nephrolithotomy (PCNL): a prospective and randomized study comparing regional epidural anesthesia with general anesthesia. Int Braz J Urol. 2012;38(4):504–11.
18. Thapa BB, Niranjan V. Mini PCNL over standard PCNL: what makes it better? Surg J (N Y). 2020;6(1):e19–23.
19. Traxer O, Smith TG 3rd, Pearle MS, Corwin TS, Saboorian H, Cadeddu JA. Renal parenchymal injury after standard and mini percutaneous nephrostolithotomy. J Urol. 2001;165(5):1693–5.
20. Yang H, Yu X, Hu J, Peng E, Li C, Cui L, Zhao C, Wang S, Wei C, Mei W, Wang S, Ye Z. Usage of multilevel paravertebral block as the main anesthesia for mini-invasive PCNL: retrospective review of 45 cases with large stones. Urol Int. 2017;99(3):326–30.
21. Zhu W, Liu Y, Liu L, Lei M, Yuan J, Wan SP, Zeng G. Minimally invasive versus standard percutaneous nephrolithotomy: a meta-analysis. Urolithiasis. 2015;43(6):563–70.

# 8 Positioning for MIP (Prone and Supine)

Abhishek Singh

## 8.1 Introduction

Percutaneous nephrolithotomy (PCNL) is the treatment of choice for stones larger than 1.5–2.0 cm [1]. The procedure has evolved manifold since its inception in 1976 [2]. There has been modification and progress in each and every step of the procedure, the instrumentation has also greatly developed [3]. If you consider access techniques, they have changed, so have the instruments, miniaturization has become the order of the day. Energy sources have become more efficient and quicker [3].

Patient positioning has also come a long way, the initial position described by Fernstorm was in prone position and it is still the most popular position for PCNL surgery [2, 4]. Modifications in patient positioning started as early as the late 80s when Valdivia et al. described PCNL in supine position [5]. Since then many variations in patient positioning have been described. All the positions have merits and demerits. Between supine and the prone position there is no clear winner, as all the operative parameters are comparable in both the positions [6]. The positioning time may potentially make the supine position more time efficient, but this does not translate into better perioperative outcomes like stone free rate and complications [6].

In the following text we shall try to understand various patient positions that have been described for mini PCNL. The patient positioning for standard PCNL and mini PCNL remains the same. The details of each of the positioning technique, their advantages and disadvantages will be described.

## 8.2 Classification of Positioning in Mini PCNL

- 8.2.1 Classical Prone position.
- 8.2.2 Modification of Prone position.
  - 8.2.2.1 Reverse lithotomy.
  - 8.2.2.2 Prone split leg position.
  - 8.2.2.3 Prone flex position.
- 8.2.3 Complete supine position.
- 8.2.4 Modifications of supine position.
  - 8.2.4.1 Double S position.
  - 8.2.4.2 Valdivia position.
  - 8.2.4.3 Galdakao-Modified Valdivia position.
  - 8.2.4.4 Bart's position for PCNL.
  - 8.2.4.5 Modified Bart's flank free position.
  - 8.2.4.6 Supine oblique position.
  - 8.2.4.7 Semi supine position.
- 8.2.5 Lateral position for PCNL.
- 8.2.6 Sitting position for PCNL.

A. Singh (✉)
Department of Urology, Muljibhai Patel Urological Hospital (MPUH), Nadiad, Gujarat, India



M. S. Agrawal et al. (eds.), *Minimally Invasive Percutaneous Nephrolithotomy*,
https://doi.org/10.1007/978-981-16-6001-6_8

### 8.2.1 Prone Position

PCNL was first described in prone position by Fernstorm et al. [2]. After this for many decades it was done in prone position only [4].

In the prone position the patient lies on his belly. The legs are adducted, the arms are hyper abducted and placed by the side of the head, slightly flexed at the level of elbow. The head is placed on a pillow and turned to one side. A bolster is placed below the lower chest and at the level of pelvis/hips so that the abdomen falls forward and abdominal compression does not give rise to cardio-respiratory embarrassment [7, 8]. All the pressure points are well padded and secured. These points include the knee, dorsum of feet, the elbows, forehead, shoulder, and eyes.

**Positioning Technique**

1. The patient is anesthetized on a trolley/stretcher and after intubation the patient is turned prone on to the operating table.
2. Patient is anesthetized on the operating table, then shifted on to the stretcher and then again turned back on to the operating table.
3. Patient is anesthetized on the operating table and then turned prone on the same table (Fig. 8.1a and b). This technique is labor intensive and requires experienced manpower. A minimum of three adults may be required to turn a relatively heavy adult (80 kg) (Fig. 8.1a and b).

As the patient is being turned prone, the circulating staff nurse places two bolsters below the lower chest and hip (Figs. 8.1a, b, 8.2 and 8.3). Commercially available gel filled mattress can also be used, they support the lower chest and the pelvis, so that abdominal compression does not occur. This also allows the abdominal viscera to fall forward, whereas the kidney which is fixed to the retroperitoneum remains behind (Fig. 8.4a and b).

Montreal mattress is an example of a PCNL positioning mattress [9] (Fig. 8.5). It is a rectangular mattress with a central hollow, this hollow accommodates the abdomen and prevents abdominal compression [9]. At the cranial end there is a groove which accommodates the head of the patient; this also ensures that the neck is under slight flexion. The head can also be protected by a prone helmet. The caudal end has a slope for the thighs to rest upon.

**Advantages of Prone Positioning**

This position provides the widest surface area to work with for percutaneous access [10–12]. Posterior calyceal entry in this position is very easy. Multiple calyceal entry becomes easy as there is a large working space. Larger space for movement of nephroscope allows access of upper pole with a lower calyceal puncture and vice versa [10–12]. The irrigation fluid does not drain out keeping the PCS (pelvicalyceal system) relatively filled, making movement of the nephroscope and the accessories possible in PCS. In complex system with multiple branched calyx, prone position is beneficial as it provides better mobility of the scope with reasonable distension of the pelvicalyceal system [11, 12].

In the prone position, upper polar puncture is easier as the upper pole is located close to the posterior wall than the lower pole, though it is more medial than the lower pole.

In the prone position both fluoroscopic and ultrasound guided access are possible and equally effective. This is not true with all the positions in PCNL. In some of the variation of supine position, where the flank and chest are torqued, the kidney overlies the spine and the fluoroscopy guided access becomes impossible.

In prone position bilateral simultaneous PCNL is possible and has been demonstrated by Desai et al. [13].

**Disadvantage of Prone Position**

1. Retrograde access is not possible in the conventional prone position.
2. For ureteric catheterization the patient has to be first placed in the lithotomy position and then shifted to prone position.
3. Due to the change in position that is required the overall operative time increases [6, 11, 12, 14].

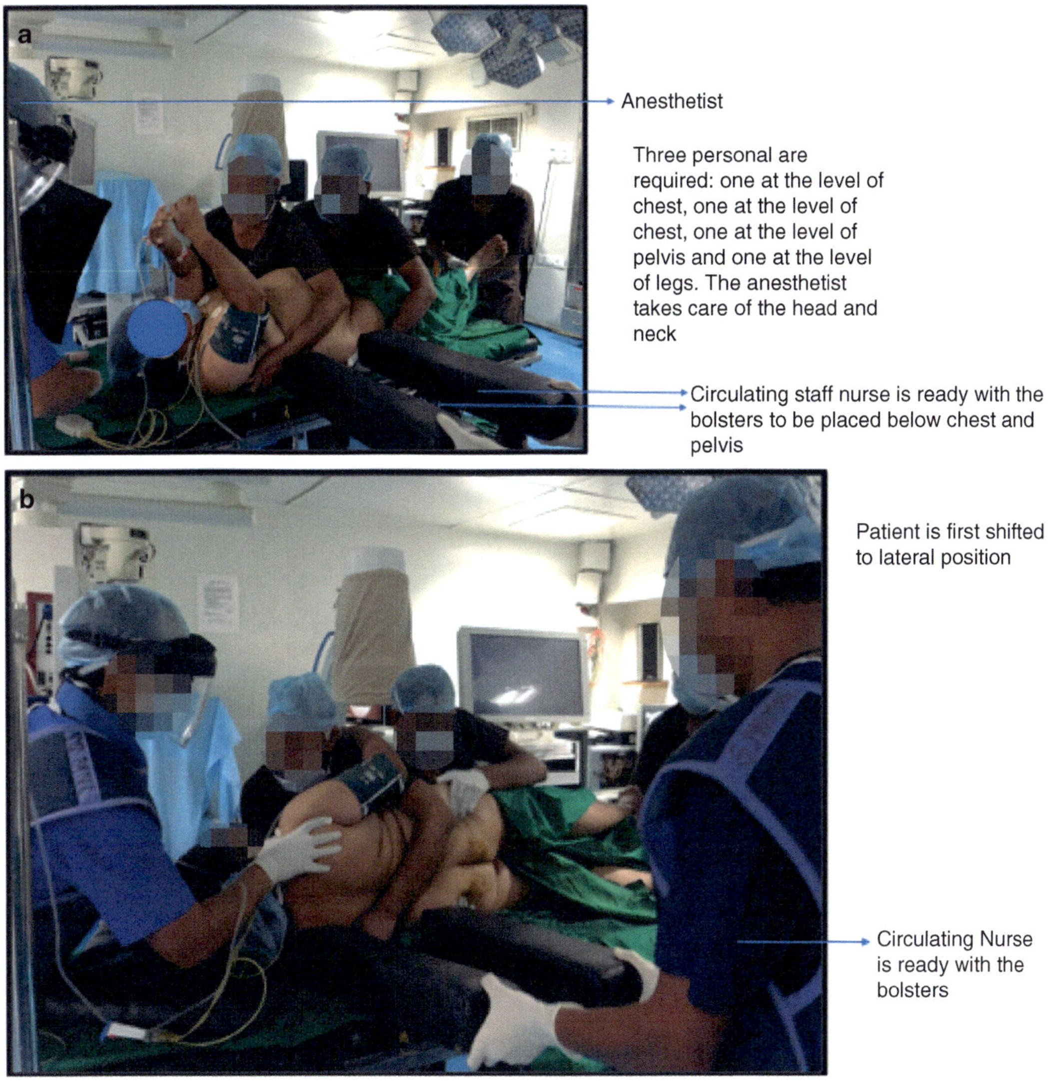


**Fig. 8.1** Figure showing technique of turning the patient prone (**a** and **b**)

**Fig. 8.2** Prone position for PCNL patient cranio-caudal view

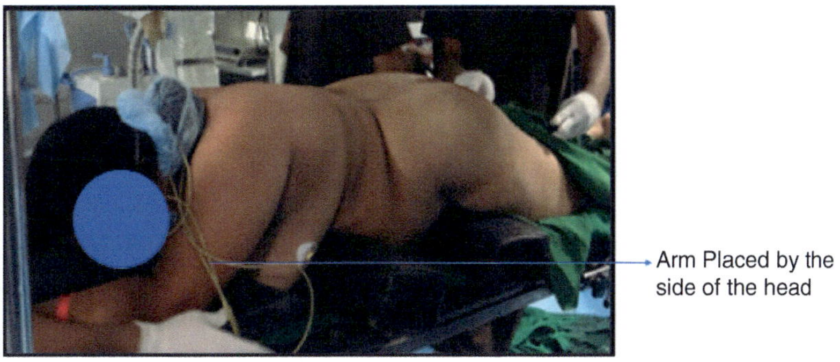

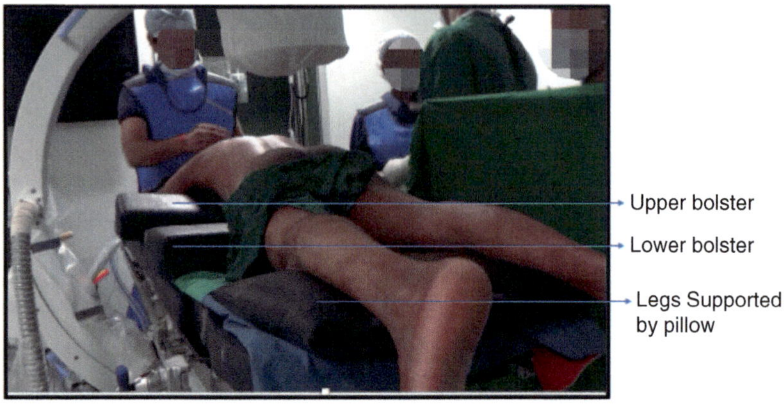


**Fig. 8.3** Prone position for PCNL caudo-cranial view

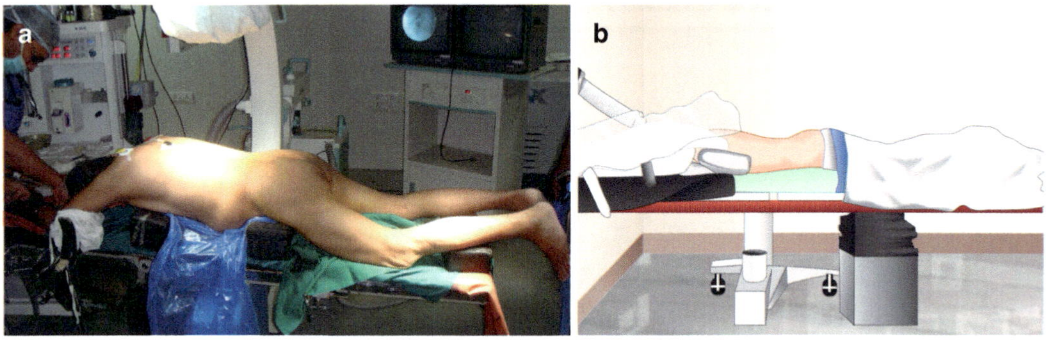


**Fig. 8.4** Prone position for PCNL lateral view (**a** and **b**)

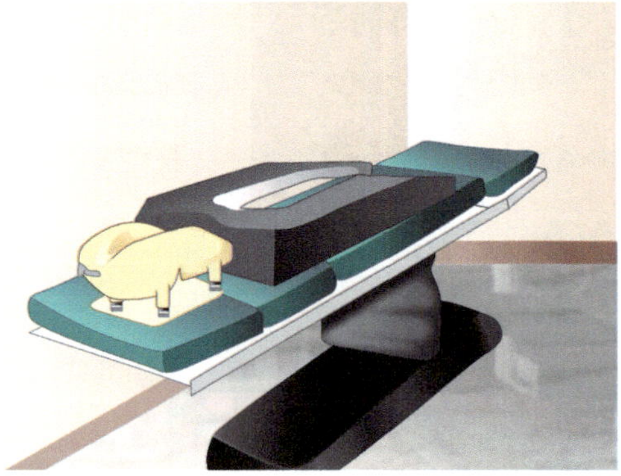

**Fig. 8.5** Montreal mattress with helmet

4. Turning the patient prone or rolling him over may cause injury to cervical spine.
5. The prone position can lead to corneal abrasions, increased pressure on the eye leading to increased intraocular pressure, consequently neuropathic and vascular effects on eye. Optic atrophy and vision loss have also been reported.
6. Injury to brachial plexus can occur if the axilla is not padded and the arms are not positioned diligently.
7. It is relatively difficult to maintain the airway access in prone position. Abdominal compression may lead to cardio-respiratory embarrassment. There is a possibility that the airway pressures may rise, and the ventilation may decrease. The cardiac index may decrease in prone position.

### 8.2.2 Modification of Prone Positions

#### 8.2.2.1 Reverse Lithotomy

Reverse lithotomy is also known as Sky divers' position [15]. Patient is given a general anesthesia and placed in prone position. Patients thighs and knees are placed in molded cradle made of plastic. The caudal end of the table is taken down to the lowest feasible position and the

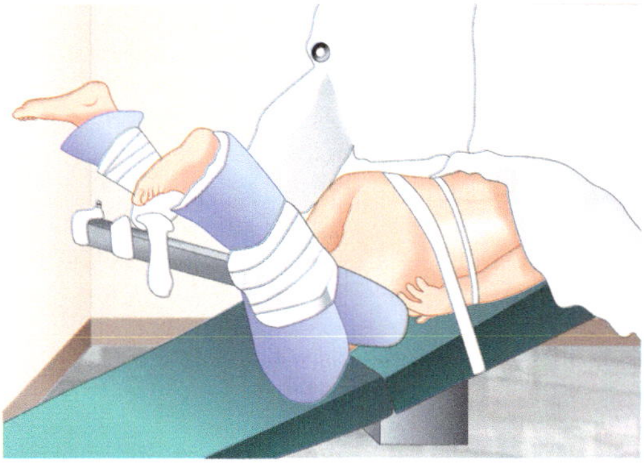

**Fig. 8.6** Reverse lithotomy

limbs are abducted at hip and flexed at knee (Fig. 8.6). Both the legs on the cradle are adequately padded [15].

**Advantage**
This position allows simultaneous access to the urethra. Single position can be used for the entire procedure.

**Disadvantage**
It is a cumbersome procedure. The positioning process is labor intensive and there are risks of pressure injuries. The ureteroscopic surgeon may require some time to get oriented to the anatomy.

#### 8.2.2.2 Prone Split Leg Position

This position was initially described by Grasso et al. [16], the patient is anesthetized on a stretcher and then turned prone as he is shifted on the operating table. The genitalia are exposed and placed at the caudal edge of the table. Both the legs are padded and placed on the adapters which enable abduction/splitting legs up to 45° in the same plane as the level of the table (Fig. 8.7a–d) [16].

This position allows a retrograde access to the kidney along with large flank exposure, enabling puncture and dilatation to be achieved in a more conventional way.

**Advantages**
A single positioning for entire procedure is adequate. This position allows the retrograde access to the PCS. As the flank is well exposed, the puncture and dilation can proceed with ease. Large working area makes nephroscopic manipulation easier.

**Disadvantages**
Splitting of legs may not be possible in patients with hip issues.

#### 8.2.2.3 Prone Flex Position

In this position, the patient is placed in prone position and at the level of the flank the table is flexed to 30° [17] (Fig. 8.8). This position increases the distance between the 12th rib and the iliac crest by 2.9 cm on an average and the distance between 11th rib and the iliac crest increased by a mean of 3.0 cm.

Authors described a caudal displacement of upper calyx by 1.5 cm and this led to a decrease in the supracostal punctures and the punctures above the 11th rib could be decreased by 45.5% [17].

The imaging studies showed that the liver and spleen rotated laterally in this position, so if the surgeon used a bull's eye technique the chance of injury would theoretically decrease [17].

**Advantages**
The working space for PCNL increases and better manipulation of instruments can be achieved. There is a decreased chance of visceral organ and pleural injury.

**Disadvantage**
Anesthetic challenges increase as the IVC (inferior vena cava) gets compressed in addition to the abdomen. In morbidly obese patients the airway pressures increase with this position. On occasions to achieve a lower airway pressure, one may have to decrease the flexion.

### 8.2.3 Completely Supine Position

Completely supine PCNL has been described by Falahatkar et al. [18]. The patient is placed supine on the ipsilateral edge of the operating table, with the flank exposed (Fig. 8.9). The legs are kept straight and adducted [18, 19]. Ipsilateral arm is

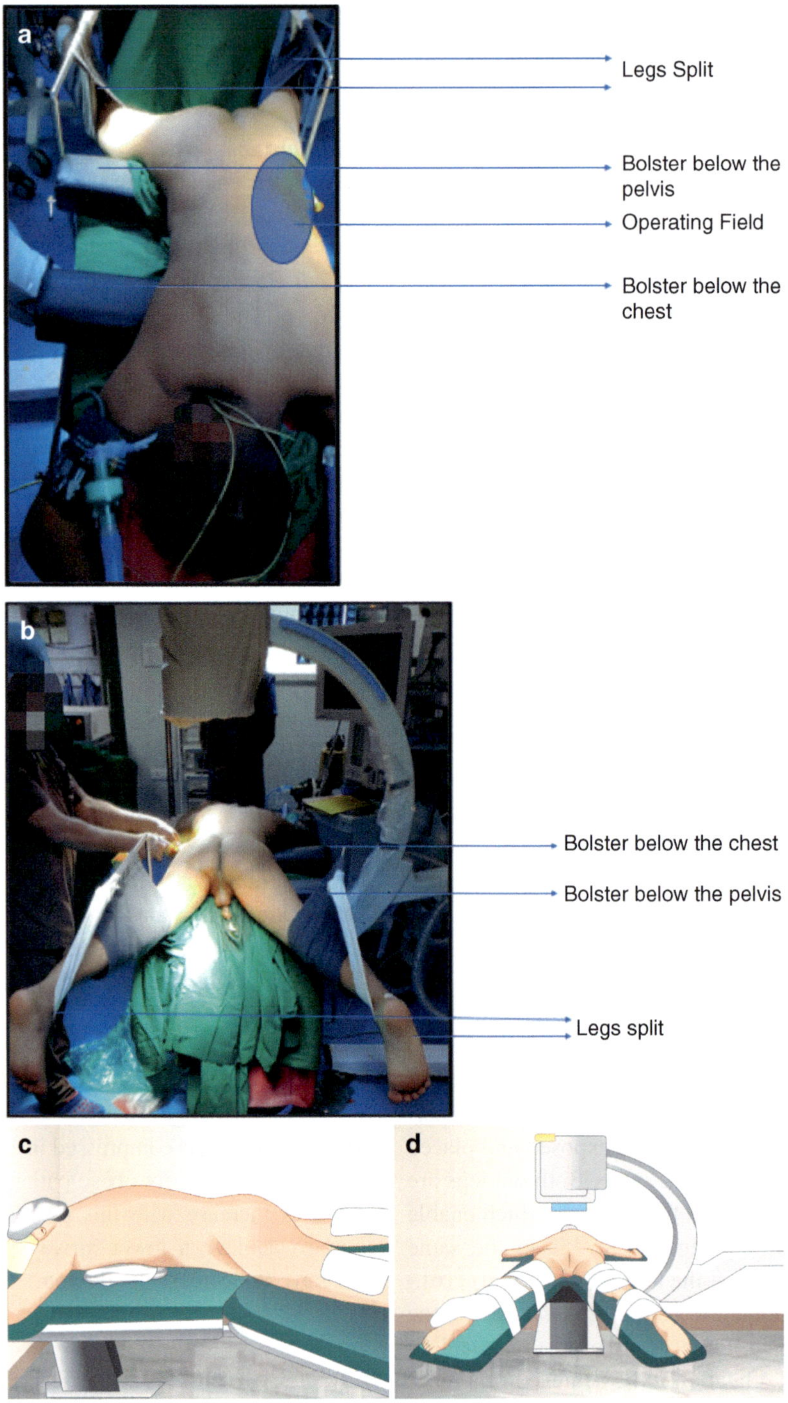


**Fig. 8.7** Split leg prone position (**a**–**d**)

folded over the chest and contralateral hand is placed on an arm rest.

**Advantage**

Advantage in this position is that the spine does not overlap with kidney and fluoroscopic visualization can be achieved.

**Disadvantage**

Simultaneous retrograde access is not possible and the working space in the flank region is also limited.

### 8.2.4 Modifications of Supine Position

#### 8.2.4.1 Double S Position

The patient is placed on the operating table with buttocks at the lower edge. Patient should be placed away from the metallic part as it may be radiopaque [20, 21]. The legs of the patient are split, and the hips are abducted, but not flexed. The split leg position allows retrograde access [20, 21]. The ipsilateral arm is folded over the thorax and fixed to the opposite arm by a bandage tied to the wrist of the ipsilateral arm [20]. The contralateral arm is abducted and placed on an arm rest. The ipsilateral side thorax is rotated by 30°.

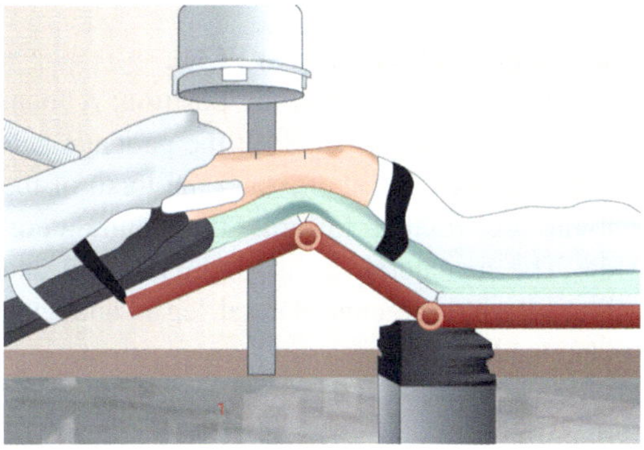

**Fig. 8.8** Prone flex

All the rotations can be measured by using the Protractor™ app on smart phone [20] (Exa Mobile S.A Poland).

**Advantages of Double S Position**

1. This position of course allows a simultaneous retrograde access. Lesser number of operating room personnel need, to shift a lighter load [20, 21].
2. The distance between ribs and iliac crest increases in this position increasing the flank exposure giving a better working space to the surgeon for puncture, dilatation, etc.
3. The support is placed under the shoulder in this technique as compared to the Valdivia position where it is placed under the lumbar region. The lumbar support may lead to a cranial migration of the kidney making an upper pole access difficult, this is less likely to happen in a double S position [20, 21].
4. The thoracic rotation is only 30°, this does not interfere with the fluoroscopic visualization of the kidney, as the vertebral column is still away from the kidney at this angle.

**Fig. 8.9** Completely supine position

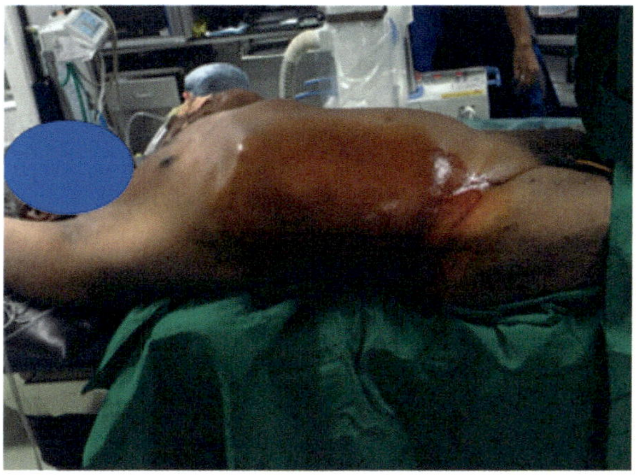

5. The knees are not flexed in this position, so the pressure injuries to structures around the knee will not occur.

**Disadvantage**

The distance between the two legs is less in this position, so the effective working space for the retrograde access surgeon may be less.

#### 8.2.4.2 Valdivia Position

Patient is placed supine and a three-liter collapsible saline bag is placed below the flank [5, 22]. The legs are adducted and fully stretched, and the patient lies supine (Fig. 8.10). Any thoracic or flank rotation should be avoided. The ipsilateral hand is folded over the thorax and the contralateral hand is extended for iv access and placed on armrest [5, 22].

The ureteric catheterization requires a flexible cystoscope and is done in supine position.

**Advantages**

Single and simple positioning for the entire procedure is required. There is a decreased need for manpower.

**Disadvantages**

Simultaneous retrograde access is not possible. Decreased working space and hyper mobile kidney may be very difficult to handle in this position.

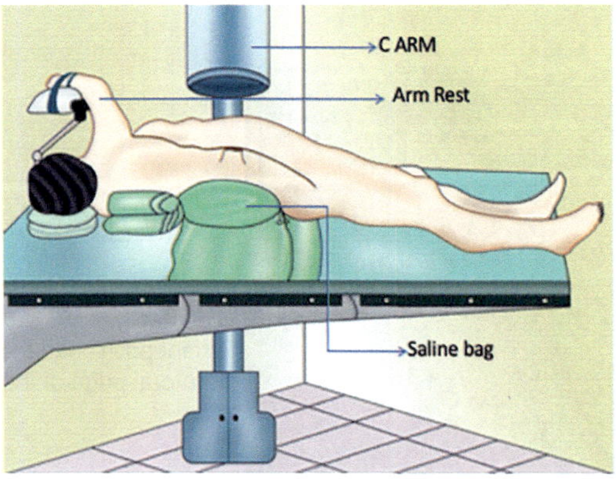


**Fig. 8.10** Valdivia position

#### 8.2.4.3 Galdakao-Modified Valdivia Position

The patient is positioned supine with a 3-L saline bag filled with air placed below the ipsilateral flank (Fig. 8.11). The amount of air can be varied to achieve desired elevation. Ipsilateral leg is extended, and contralateral leg is slightly flexed and abducted [23]. Both the legs are in essence separated from each other and placed on padded stirrups. The ipsilateral hand is folded over the thorax and the contralateral hand is extended and placed over an arm rest for IV access.

**Advantage**

Single position can accomplish the complete procedure. It is less labor intensive and simultaneous retrograde access possible [23].

**Disadvantage**

Decreased working space. Hyper mobile kidney may be very difficult to handle.

#### 8.2.4.4 Bart's Position for PCNL

Patient is placed in lithotomy position; A foam wedge is used to raise and tilt the patient's pelvis to 45° [24]. The thorax and the torso of the patient are rotated towards the contralateral side. The ipsilateral leg is slightly flexed and adducted, and the contralateral leg is abducted and extended [24].

**Advantages**

This positioning provides an excellent exposure of the flank. Simultaneous percutaneous and retrograde access can be achieved. Single positioning can be used to complete the surgery. It is less labor intensive. Operating surgeon has a larger number of access points to choose from and also choose a steeper angle to puncture.

**Disadvantage**

Significant rotation occurs in this positioning which can give rise to pain post operatively. The kidney overlies the spine in fluoroscopic imaging, so on occasions an ultrasound guided access may be the only way to gain access (Fig. 8.12). Increased obliquity may disorient the operating

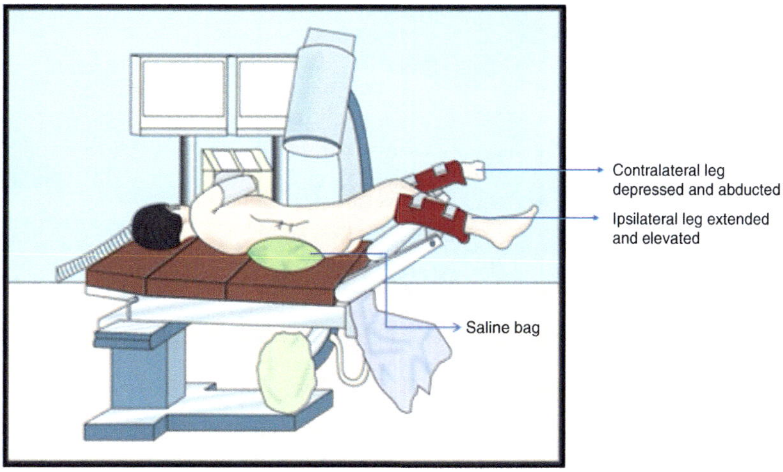


**Fig. 8.11** Galdakao-modified Valdivia position

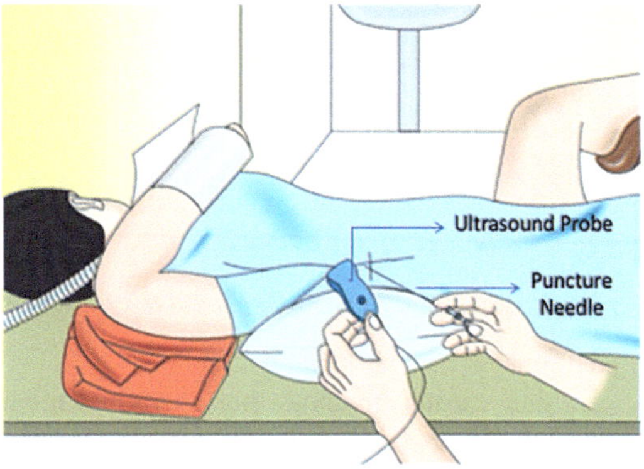


**Fig. 8.12** USG guided puncture in Bart's position

surgeon. Patients with musculoskeletal abnormalities cannot be subjected to so much torsion.

#### 8.2.4.5 Bart's Flank Free Modified Supine Position

This position was developed to overcome the shortcomings of Bart's positioning. In this position patient is placed in lithotomy position, a saline bag is placed under ipsilateral rib cage and gel pad below ipsilateral hip, this helps achieve a 15° flank tilt [25] (Fig. 8.13a–c). As no support is placed below the flank, a greater working space is achieved in the flank region. The legs are placed on stirrups with the ipsilateral leg extended and contralateral leg is abducted and in an elevated position. The ipsilateral hand is folded on to the chest and the contralateral hand is placed on a hand rest for IV access.

Using this modified positioning, Bach et al. treated 37 patients in their first series and clearance rate of 86.5% could be achieved [25].

**Advantages**

The absence of cushion below the flank and cushion below the rib cage and hip increases the working space between the costal margin and the iliac crest. This provides larger space for puncture, dilatation, and manipulation of the nephroscope. The position by virtue of the saline bag below the rib cage stabilizes the kidney and decreases mobility. This leads to the puncture and dilatation becoming easier. This position makes a posterior calyceal puncture possible even in supine position.

**Disadvantages**

The tract is more horizontal in this position as compared to Valdivia position and the original Bart's position, which may make space for nephroscope limited.

#### 8.2.4.6 Supine Oblique Position

In this position the patient is kept oblique at 45° to the operating table [26]. No cushions are used but instead two rolls each of 25 cm length is placed below the scapula and hip [26]. Patient leans on to the table at an angle of 45° and his body is secured with two tapes one at the level of thorax and other at the level of trochanter.

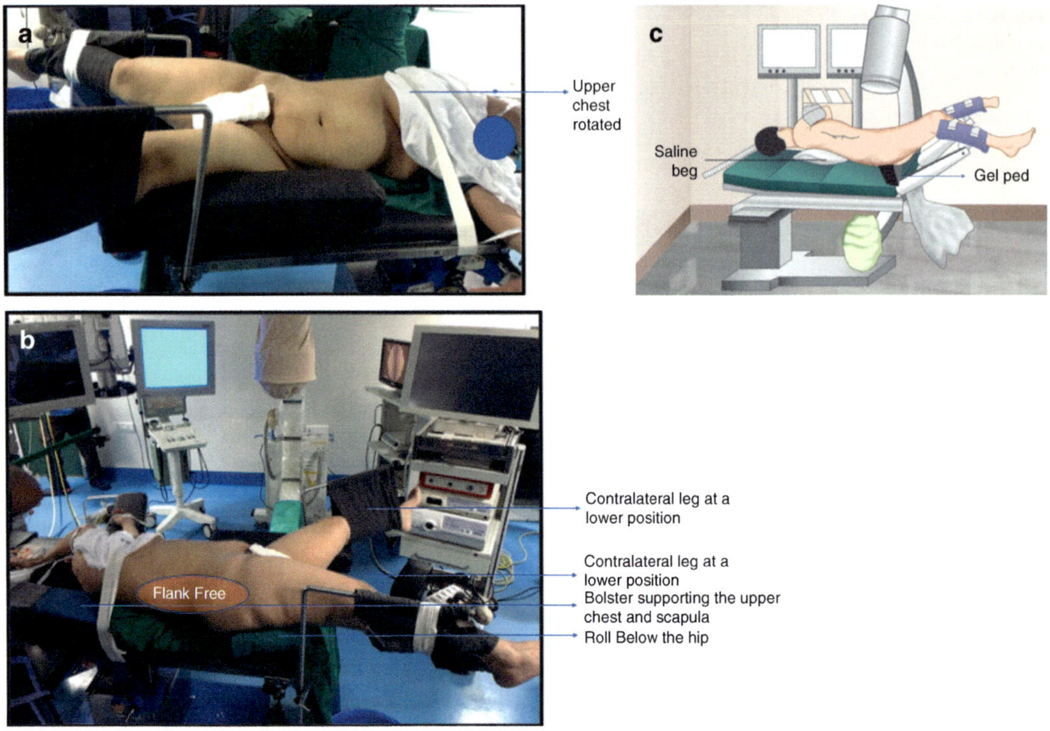


**Fig. 8.13** Flank free position (**a**–**c**)

Ultrasound is used for initial puncture and initial puncture is behind the posterior axillary line. It is a good procedure to use in emergency situation [26].

**Advantage**
Flank exposure is good.

**Disadvantage**
Spine will overlie the kidney. Simultaneous retrograde access is not possible.

#### 8.2.4.7 Semi Supine Position

Xu et al. described three methods to keep patient semi supine or at 45° [27].

Method 1: a wooden plank with a 40 cm × 20 cm area cutout to expose the flank was used to position the patient. This plank was mounted on a wooden base. The angle of the plank could be altered to achieve any degree of inclination and to achieve a semi supine position it was kept at 45° [27].

In the second method the operating team designed a special table, the table could be adjusted to an inclination of 45° and the area corresponding to the flank was cutout.

The third method described was a standard flank position of 60° inclination and the patient was strapped to the table at the level of chest and thighs. The kidney bridge was raised, and the patients was tilted 15° to achieve a net inclination of 45°. The back and hips were supported by metal baffles [27].

A success rate of 92.2% for single calculus and 72.9% for staghorn calculus has been described using this position [27]. It was possible to achieve a superior calyceal puncture in 12.1% patients using this positioning [27].

**Advantages**
The flank exposure is good. Monitoring of the patient under anesthesia is more convenient. The hands of the operating surgeon do not come in the field of fluoroscopy. Low pressure in the PCS can be maintained while doing nephroscopy.

**Disadvantage**
Positioning has to be done after ureteric catheter placement. Kidney may overlie the spine, making visualization difficult.

### 8.2.5 Lateral Position

This position was first described by Kerbl et al. [28]. The patient is positioned in lateral decubitus with the ipsilateral side facing upwards and on the ipsilateral edge of the table (Fig. 8.14). The kidney bridge is raised, and the table is flexed at the level of flank; this increases the exposure of the flank. The patient is strapped to the table at the level of chest and flank. The C arm is placed in a "u" configuration. Using this position Gan et al. described a retrospective review of 347 patients [29]. The upper calyceal puncture in this series was 77.4% and the stone clearance rate was 82.7% [29].

This positioning is very useful in patients with morbid obesity and kyphoscoliosis as neither can these patients lie supine nor can they be turned prone [30].

**Advantages**
This position can give advantages of both supine and prone. The raised kidney bridge and table break give excellent flank exposure.

**Disadvantage**
Flexible cystoscopy is needed to put in a ureteric catheter. If rigid cystoscope is used, it needs to be done in lithotomy position. Simultaneous retrograde access is not possible.

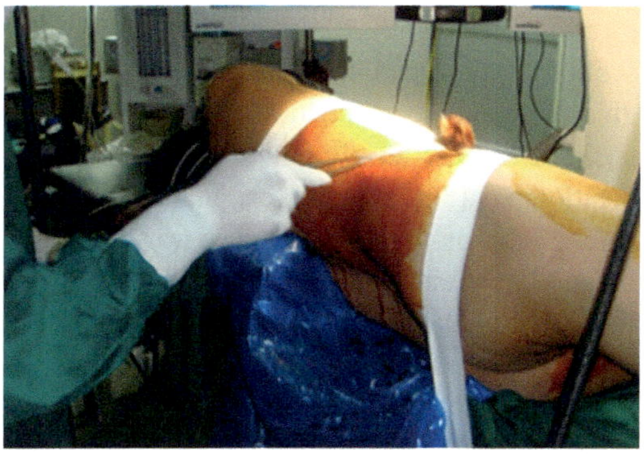

**Fig. 8.14** Lateral position

### 8.2.6 Sitting Position

Sitting position is an extremely unergonomic position for PCNL, surgeons use it only when pushed to the wall.

**Indications**
Severe COPD where the patient cannot lie down in supine or flank position. Musculoskeletal abnormality like osteogenesis imperfecta. Where the patient cannot lie down in supine, prone or flank position [31].

**Patient Positioning**
A chair is placed at the end of the operating table with the head rest facing the headend of the table [31]. The patient is seated on the chair with the chest facing the back rest. Both the hands of the patient rest on the operating table and the patient is leaning on the operating table. This forward leaning increases the intercostal space and makes the puncture easier. The puncture is done under ultrasound guidance. The ureteric catheterization is done with flexible cystoscopy.

**Disadvantage**
The procedure has to be accomplished in local anesthesia, general anesthesia and airway control is not possible in this position. Retrograde access is of course not possible.

**So, how do you decide which position is suitable for an index patient?**
After understanding the technicalities of the patient positioning, it is critical to understand that patient positioning in PCNL is a shared decision that the surgical team, the anesthetist, and the nursing team should make. There is nothing like a best position, rather horses for courses approach and what fits the bill is more important.

So, the ideal position for mini PCNL in a given case could be tradeoff between a position that is best to gain access and what the patient can actually tolerate (Table 8.1). All the positions can

**Table 8.1** Comparison of various features of each of the positions in mini PCNL

| | Features of each position | | | | | |
|---|---|---|---|---|---|---|
| Positions | Ease of positioning | Retrograde access possible | Puncture guidance | Ease of puncturing | Tract dilatation | Multiple punctures |
| Classic prone | Labor intensive | No | Fluoroscopic and USG | Routine | Routine, shorter tracts easy dilatation | Possible as large operative working space |
| Reverse lithotomy | Labor intensive | Yes | Fluoroscopic and USG | Routine | Routine, shorter tracts easy dilatation | Possible as large operative working space |
| Prone split leg | Labor intensive | Yes | Fluoroscopic and USG | Routine | Routine, shorter tracts easy dilatation | Possible as large operative working space |
| Prone flex | Labor intensive | No | Fluoroscopic and USG | Routine | Routine, shorter tracts easy dilatation | Possible as large operative working space |
| Classic supine | Simple | No | Fluoroscopic and USG | Routine | Longer tract, but otherwise routine | Difficult as limited space |
| Double S | Simple | Yes | Fluoroscopic and USG | Rotation makes puncture challenging | Kidney mobile, hence difficult | Possible as flank well exposed |
| Valdivia | Simple | No | Fluoroscopic and USG | Rotation makes puncture challenging | Kidney mobile, hence difficult | Difficult as limited space |
| Galdakao-modified Valdivia | Simple | Yes | Fluoroscopic and USG | | Kidney mobile, hence difficult | Difficult as limited space |
| Bart' s position | Simple | Yes | USG may be easier | Rotation makes puncture challenging | Kidney mobile, hence difficult | Possible as flank well exposed |
| Flank free position | Simple | Yes | Fluoroscopic and USG | Routine | Kidney less mobile than other supine positions | Possible as flank well exposed |

cause certain physiological changes that may affect the patient's outcome. Like if we consider prone position, it causes decrease in cardiac index as IVC is compressed and venous return compromised. The splinting and cranial displacement of diaphragm can cause increase in airway pressures and decrease the pulmonary compliance [32]. But in the absence of abdominal compression, the prone position may have benefit as the functional residual capacity increases [33, 34]. In spite of the discussion going around the prone positioning, it is still the most popular position for PCNL [35]. But patients with kyphoscoliosis, obese patients, and patients with marginal lung and heart function do not tolerate this position and are absolute indications for supine positioning [36]. In the originally described supine position the working space was limited, so the modifications of supine position are effective in increasing the space and allowing a retrograde access, these modifications make supine more a more effective position.

**How do you compare Supine to prone positioning in terms of perioperative variables?**

There are about six meta-analysis comparing the supine to prone positioning in PCNL [6, 37–41]. The earlier meta-analysis concluded that the operating time was lesser in supine PCNL with no difference in the perioperative variables like stone clearance and complications [37, 38].

In the analysis by Zang et al. and Yaun et al., the operative time was still less in supine group, but the stone clearance was inferior [38, 39]. The meta-analysis by Falhatkar et al. concluded that though stone clearance is comparable, but the incidence of fever and blood transfusion is less in supine position.

These studies do not specify the type of supine position used, so it is difficult to compare apples and oranges, also the cases have not been stratified according to BMI and comorbidities making any recommendation difficult.

**Learning Points**

1. Patient positioning is a combined decision of surgeon, anesthetist, and nursing team.
2. Familiarity of a surgeon with a procedure in a particular position may determine the outcome.
3. A surgeon should be well versed with technical details of all the positions in PCNL, as he may need any of the positions sometimes or the other.
4. No guidelines have opined on a best positioning for PCNL.
5. The patient positioning at present should be tailored to the patients' profile, i.e. stone burden, location, anatomy and his comorbidities.

## References


1. Sabler IM, Katafigiotis I, Gofrit ON, Duvdevani M. Present indications and techniques of percutaneous nephrolithotomy: what the future holds? Asian J Urol. 2018 Oct 1;5(4):287–94.
2. Fernstrom I, Johansson B. Percutaneous pyelolithotomy. A new extraction technique. Scand J Urol Nephrol. 1976;10:257–9.
3. Ghani KR, Andonian S, Bultitude M, et al. Percutaneous nephrolithotomy: update, trends, and future directions. Eur Urol. 2016;70:382–96.
4. Alken P, Hutschenreiter G, Günther R, Marberger M. Percutaneous stone manipulation. J Urol. 2017 Feb;197(2S):S154–7.
5. Valdivia Uría JG, Lachares Santamaría E, Villarroya Rodríguez S, et al. [Percutaneous nephrolithectomy: simplified technic (preliminary report)]. Arch Esp Urol. 1987;40:177–180.
6. Li J, Gao L, Li Q, Zhang Y, Jiang Q. Supine versus prone position for percutaneous nephrolithotripsy: a meta-analysis of randomized controlled trials. Int J Surg. 2019 Jun 1;66:62–71.
7. Turner CD, Anderson J, Gerber GS. Improved patient positioning for percutaneous nephroscopic procedures using a surgical saddle. J Urol. 2000;163:199–200.
8. Papatsoris A, Masood J, El-Husseiny T, et al. Improving patient positioning to reduce complications in prone percutaneous nephrolithotomy. J Endourol. 2009;23:831–2.
9. Addla SK, Rajpal S, Sutcliffe N, Adeyoju A. A simple aid to improve patient positioning during percutaneous nephrolithotomy. Ann R Coll Surg Engl. 2008 Jul;90(5):433–4.
10. Karaolides T, Moraitis K, Bach C, et al. Positions for percutaneous nephrolithotomy: thirty-five years of evolution. Arab J Urol. 2012;10:307–16.
11. Mak DK-C, Smith Y, Buchholz N, El-Husseiny T. What is better in percutaneous nephrolithotomy—prone or supine? A systematic review. Arab J Urol. 2016;14:101–7.
12. Patel RM, Okhunov Z, Clayman RV, Landman J. Prone versus supine percutaneous nephrolithotomy: what is your position? Curr Urol Rep. 2017;18:26.
13. Desai M, Grover R, Manohar T, Ganpule A. Simultaneous bilateral percutaneous nephrolithotomy: a single-center experience. J Endourol. 2007;21:508–14.
14. Mourmouris P, Berdempes M, Markopoulos T, Lazarou L, Tzelves L, Skolarikos A. Patient positioning during percutaneous nephrolithotomy: what is the current best practice? Res Rep Urol. 2018;10:189.
15. Lehman T, Bagley DH. Reverse lithotomy: modified prone position for simultaneous nephroscopic and ureteroscopic procedures in women. Urology. 1988;32:529–31.
16. Grasso M, Nord R, Bagley DH. Prone split leg and flank roll positioning: simultaneous antegrade and retrograde access to the upper urinary tract. J Endourol. 1993 Aug;7(4):307–10.
17. Ray AA, Chung DG, Honey RJ. Percutaneous nephrolithotomy in the prone and prone-flexed positions: anatomic considerations. J Endourol. 2009 Oct 1;23(10):1607–14.
18. Falahatkar S, Asli MM, Emadi SA, Enshaei A, Pourhadi H, Allahkhah A. Complete supine percutaneous nephrolithotomy (csPCNL) in patients with and without a history of stone surgery: safety

and effectiveness of csPCNL. Urol Res. 2011 Aug 1;39(4):295–301.
19. Falahatkar S, Allahkhah A. UroToday Int J Apr;5(2):art 12.
20. Giusti G, De Lisa A. Supine percutaneous nephrolithotripsy in double-S position. Adv Urol. 2018 Mar 11;2018:7193843.
21. Giusti G, De Lisa A. PCNL in the prone position VS PCNL in the modified supine double-S position: is there a better position? A prospective randomized trial. Urolithiasis. 2020 Feb;48(1):63–9.
22. Uría JV, Gerhold JV, López JL, Rodriguez SV, Navarro CA, Fabián MR, Bazalo JR, Elipe MS. Technique and complications of percutaneous nephroscopy: experience with 557 patients in the supine position. J Urol. 1998 Dec 1;160(6):1975–8.
23. Ibarluzea G, Scoffone CM, Cracco CM, Poggio M, Porpiglia F, Terrone C, Astobieta A, Camargo I, Gamarra M, Tempia A, Valdivia Uria JG. Supine Valdivia and modified lithotomy position for simultaneous anterograde and retrograde endourological access. BJU Int. 2007 Jul;100(1):233–6.
24. Papatsoris AG, Zaman F, Panah A, Masood J, El-Husseiny T, Buchholz N. Simultaneous anterograde and retrograde endourologic access: "the Barts technique". J Endourol. 2008 Dec 1;22(12):2665–6.
25. Bach C, Goyal A, Kumar P, Kachrilas S, Papatsoris AG, Buchholz N, Masood J. The Barts 'flank-free' modified supine position for percutaneous nephrolithotomy. Urol Int. 2012;89(3):365–8.
26. Arrabal-Polo MA, Arrabal-Martin M, Saz T, Paiz P. Emergency percutaneous nephrostomy in supine-oblique position without cushion. Urol Res. 2011 Dec 1;39(6):521–2.
27. Xu KW, Huang J, Guo ZH, Lin TX, Zhang CX, Liu H, Chun J, Yao YS, Han JL, Huang H. Percutaneous nephrolithotomy in semisupine position: a modified approach for renal calculus. Urol Res. 2011 Dec;39(6):467–75.
28. Kerbl K, Clayman RV, Chandhoke PS, Urban DA, De Leo BC, Carbone JM. Percutaneous stone removal with the patient in a flank position. J Urol. 1994 Mar;151(3):686–8.
29. Gan JJ, Gan JJ, Gan JJ, Lee KT. Lateral percutaneous nephrolithotomy: a safe and effective surgical approach. Indian J Urol. 2018 Jan;34(1):45.
30. Gofrit ON, Shapiro A, Donchin Y, et al. Lateral decubitus position for percutaneous nephrolithotripsy in the morbidly obese or kyphotic patient. J Endourol. 2002;16:383–6.
31. Zhai J, Wang H, Xu X, Liu Z, Man L. PCNL in COPD patient in the sit position under local infiltration anesthesia case report. BMC Urol. 2020 Dec;20(1):1–4.
32. Palmon SC, Kirsch JR, Depper JA, Toung TJ. The effect of the prone position on pulmonary mechanics is frame-dependent. Anesth Analg. 1998;87:1175–80.
33. Zhao Z, Fan J, Liu Y, de la Rosette J, Zeng G. Percutaneous nephrolithotomy: position, position, position! Urolithiasis. 2018 Feb 1;46(1):79–86.
34. Lumb AB, Nunn JF. Respiratory function and ribcage contribution to ventilation in body positions commonly used during anesthesia. Anesth Analg. 1991;73:422–6.
35. de la Rosette JJMCH, Tsakiris P, Ferrandino MN, et al. Beyond prone position in percutaneous nephrolithotomy: a comprehensive review. Eur Urol. 2008;54:1262–9.
36. Pelosi P, Croci M, Calappi E, et al. The prone positioning during general anesthesia minimally affects respiratory mechanics while improving functional residual capacity and increasing oxygen tension. Anesth Analg. 1995;80:955–60.
37. Falahatkar S, Mokhtari G, Teimoori M. An update on supine versus prone percutaneous nephrolithotomy: a meta-analysis. Urol J. 2016;13:2814–22.
38. Zhang X, Xia L, Xu T, et al. Is the supine position superior to the prone position for percutaneous nephrolithotomy (PCNL)? Urolithiasis. 2014;42:87–93.
39. Wu P, Wang L, Wang K. Supine versus prone position in percutaneous nephrolithotomy for kidney calculi: a meta-analysis. Int Urol Nephrol. 2011;43:67–77.
40. Yuan D, Liu Y, Rao H, et al. Supine versus prone position in percutaneous nephrolithotomy for kidney calculi: a meta-analysis. J Endourol. 2016;30:754–63.
41. Liu L, Zheng S, Xu Y, Wei Q. Systematic review and meta-analysis of percutaneous nephrolithotomy for patients in the supine versus prone position. J Endourol. 2010;24:1941–6.

# Part IV

# Renal Access for Mini-PCNL

# 9 Fluoroscopic-Guided Access

Shashi Kiran Pal

## 9.1 Introduction

Percutaneous nephrolithotomy is an established technique since more than 40 years for management of upper tract urolithiasis worldwide. It has stood the test of time and established its undoubted superiority in management of complex and larger renal calculi. A better, more appropriate, and explanatory name for this technique should be *Percutaneous Nephrostolithotripsy*, since the procedure involves creating a hole (os, track) through renal parenchyma to gain access into the collecting system. Establishing an accurate renal access is the first and most crucial step for a successful outcome, be it a standard or a Mini PCNL, initial steps remain the same. Renal access is conventionally obtained under fluoroscopic guidance, right from the first reported description of PCNL technique by Fernstrom I and Johansson B. in 1976 on three cases [1]. This crucial step of accurate renal access under fluoroscopic guidance is the most challenging aspect of PCNL, because it encompasses an accurate imagination and visualization of three-dimensional anatomy on a two-dimensional fluoroscopic screen. This involves a thorough understanding of details of renal anatomy and scope and limitations of fluoroscopic technology. This chapter is aimed to provide a step by step understanding of this complex situation through available published literature and personal experience of author in carrying out this technique on more than 10,000 cases over last 33 years.

## 9.2 Relevant Anatomical Considerations

### 9.2.1 Location

Embryologically, kidneys develop from mesonephros and hence are always located in retroperitoneal space. Even if kidneys have been found in ectopic locations, viz. in pelvis or in thorax, they are always retroperitoneal or retromediastinal, respectively. Only, muscles and fat in different layers are found in relation with the kidneys posteriorly (Fig. 9.1). It appears, as if kidneys are so well positioned and made for percutaneous approach from behind, only. Posterior lumbotomy approach described and practiced in the 1970s and thereafter, for removal of stones from upper tract may be considered first step forward in this direction, which identified this anatomical fact and took proper advantage of this favourable location of the kidneys.

As per surface anatomy, all those calyces, which fall within the outlined space in Fig. 9.2, under fluoroscopic visualization, can safely be approached from posterior aspect, to gain access into pelvicalyceal system.

S. K. Pal (✉)
Indraprastha Apollo Hospital, New Delhi, India



M. S. Agrawal et al. (eds.), *Minimally Invasive Percutaneous Nephrolithotomy*,
https://doi.org/10.1007/978-981-16-6001-6_9

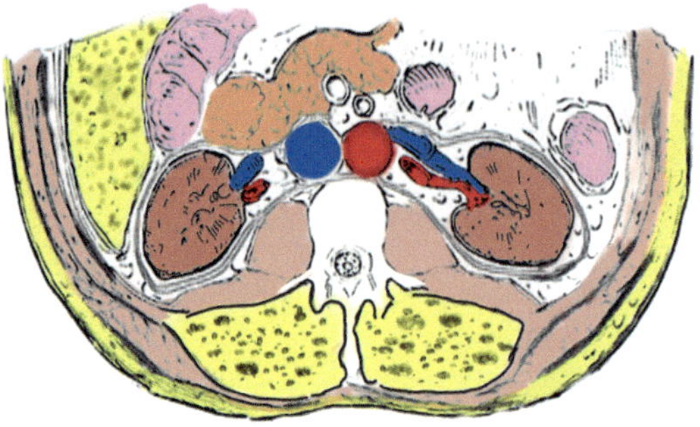

Fig. 9.1 Posterior relations of kidneys

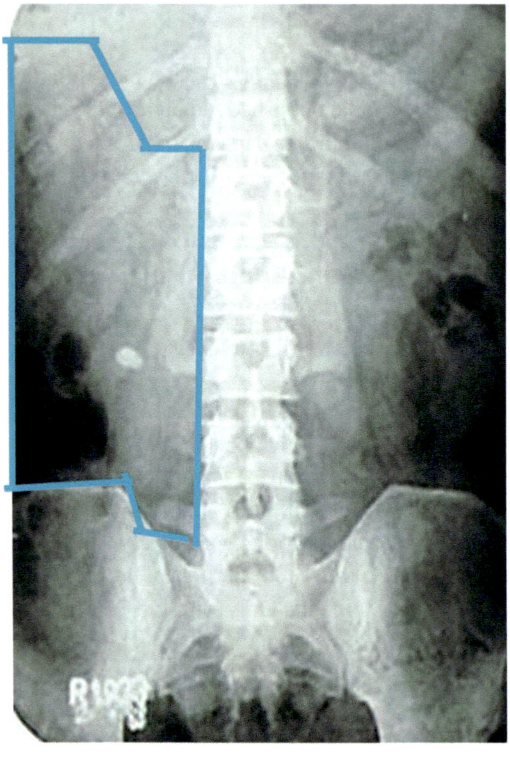

Fig. 9.2 Calyces visualized within outlined space can safely be accessed from behind

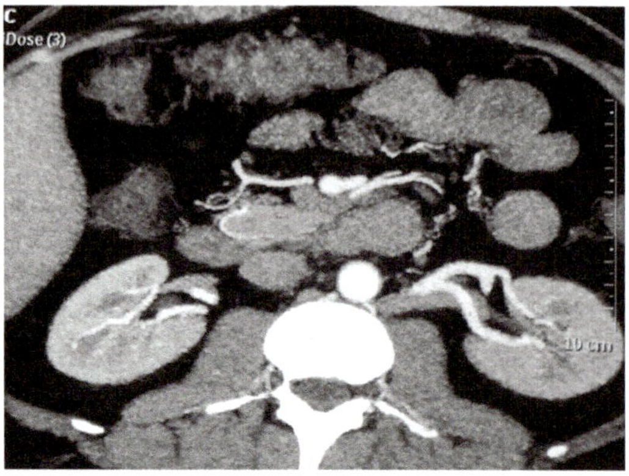


Fig. 9.3 Main renal artery divides into anterior and posterior divisions

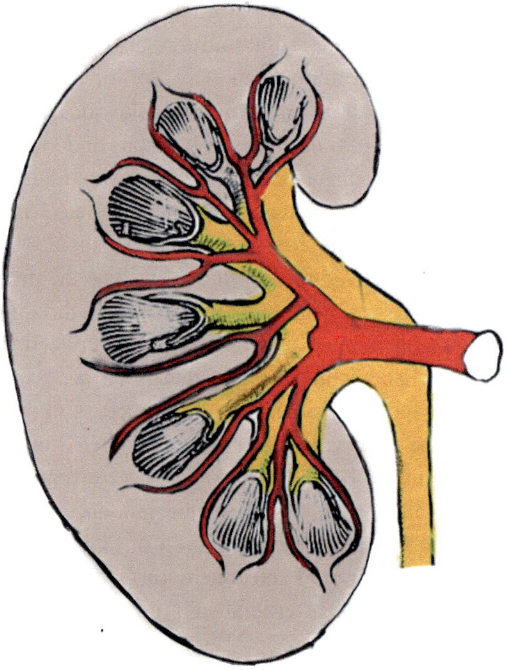

Fig. 9.4 Anterior segmental arteries fan out on the anterior aspect of pelvis and proceed as interlobar arteries surrounding the infundibuli

### 9.2.2 Vascular Anatomy

Kidneys are highly vascular organs. Almost 20% of cardiac output straight goes into the kidneys. As is evident in Fig. 9.3, most often, main renal artery divides into two main branches Anterior and Posterior division. Anterior division, which is usually larger in size, further subdivides into 3 to 5 Anterior segmental arteries, which fan out on the anterior aspect of renal pelvis and further divide and proceed as interlobar arteries adjacent to infundibuli and supply anterior aspect of renal parenchyma and both the poles of the kidney (Fig. 9.4) [2].

In more than 57% of cases Posterior segmental artery courses at neck of the infundibulum of superior calyx, where infundibulum joins the renal pelvis and supplies posterior portion of renal parenchyma (Fig. 9.5) [3]. Due to this ana-

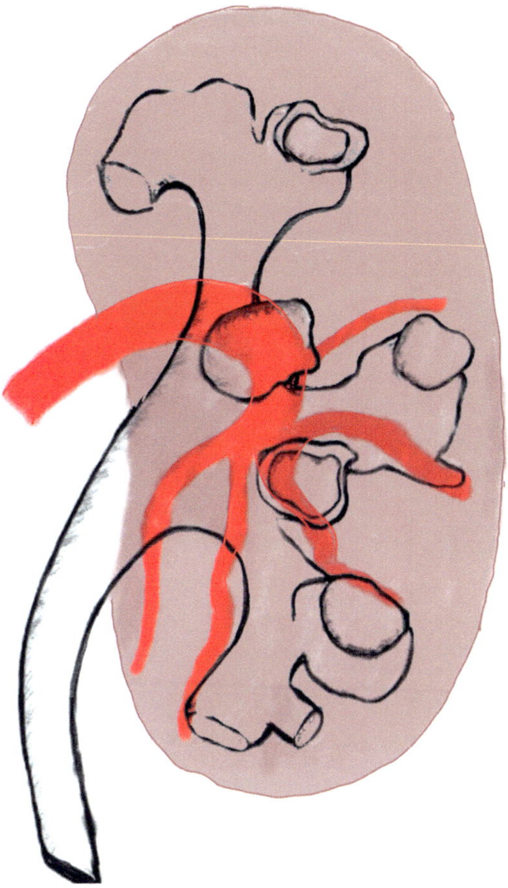

**Fig. 9.5** Close relationship of posterior segmental artery with the infundibular neck of superior calyx

tomical fact, suggested by Sampaio et al., during percutaneous access to the superior calyx, with patient in prone position, special care must be taken, not to come anywhere close to the infundibulum of superior calyx and all punctures must be made, higher up, through the fornices of superior calyx only.

Interlobar arteries gradually get oriented horizontally and curve to form arcuate arteries at corticomedullary junction. Further, finer interlobular arteries branch off from arcuate arteries at right angle and get oriented vertically as shown in Figs. 9.6 and 9.7.

An imaginary Brodel's white line, situated 1 cm posterior to the convex border of the kidney delineates a relatively avascular plane between supplies from anterior and posterior divisions (Fig. 9.8). This is the plane, through which anatrophic nephrolithotomy has been recommended and all efforts must be made to gain percutaneous renal access through this plane only, so as to avoid bleeding complications.

## 9.3 Planning for Fluoroscopic Guided Access

A very meticulous planning must be done for every percutaneous access, in the quite surroundings of the clinic, one day before, rather than just before the surgery in operation theatre. All available images of computed tomography, old and recent X-rays or IVU must be viewed together and a three-dimensional imagination must be constructed in the mind. Although most accurate three-dimensional anatomical details get visualized pre operatively through computed tomography, but practically in operation theatre, we have to depend upon two-dimensional fluoroscopic and/or ultrasonic guidance only. During IVU or CT Urography, it is strongly recommended to get at least few images in prone position, because this is how we are going to visualize the patient on table during prone PCNL.

Once all the films are displayed on the view box together, following points must be carefully looked for, in great details for a perfect planning of percutaneous access:

1. Location of Calculi within Pelvi Calyceal System?
2. Are Calculi Fixed or Changing Position within PCS?
3. Pattern of Colonic Gas Shadows?
4. Which is the Ideal Calyx to Puncture?
5. Any Alternative Calyx?
6. How to Manage Possible Migration of Stone Fragments?

### 9.3.1 Location of Calculi within Pelvi Calyceal System?

Although planning must be aimed for complete clearance of renal calculi, obstructing stones must get tackled on priority basis. Since rigid

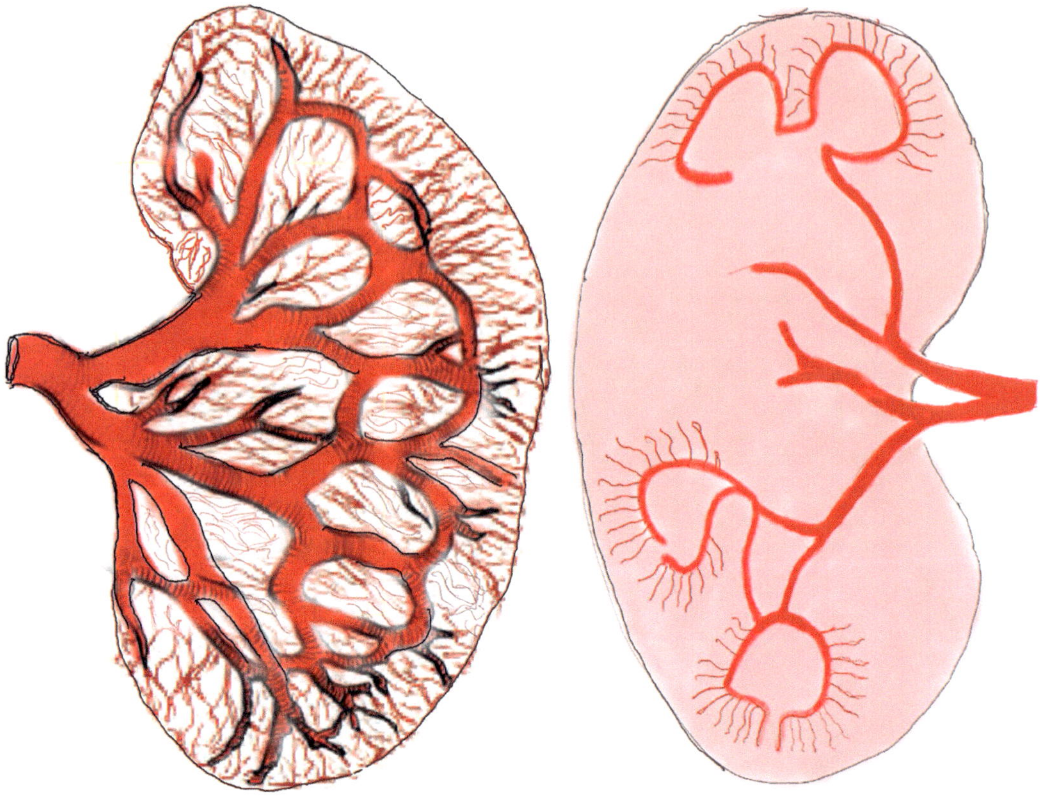

**Figs. 9.6** and **9.7** Interlobar arteries gradually curve to form arcuate arteries at corticomedullary junction. Further, finer interlobular arteries branch off from arcuate arteries at right angle and get oriented vertically

nephroscopes are straight instruments, a planning must be made to create access through those calyces, which are in straight alignment with maximum bulk of the stones. If some stone bulk is extending into those calyces, which are at an angle of more than 70 degrees to the planned primary track, a secondary track may be required during the course of the procedure, and must be planned in advance. Another important factor while planning access up to the stone is width of the infundibulum. All efforts must be made, not to overdilate or injure infundibuli during making of a track or to and fro movements while removing calculi. Preferably a track should be made through that calyx which has a wider infundibulum (Fig. 9.9). Narrow infundibuli will necessitate use of smaller nephroscope and may restrict free movement of rigid nephroscope within pelvicalyceal system. Separate tracks for calculi in different calyces may be required in such cases (Fig. 9.10). Very complex calculi need a meticulous planning. Apart from straight individualized tracks through selected calyces, a Y track may be required in these cases to approach stones in neighbouring calyces (Fig. 9.11).

Staghorn stones, occupying most of the calyces are best approached through access through superior calyx (Figs. 9.12 and 9.13). It is stated that entering pelvicalyceal system (PCS) through superior calyx is similar to entering into the room through the roof. It allows you to inspect and deal with all the objects in the room. At the same time, you can easily access all the stones in anterior as well as posterior calyces of the inferior and middle group along with straight access to PUJ and upper ureter also, through this singular approach.

Entering PCS through PUJ as in RIRS is like entering the room through the door, and through

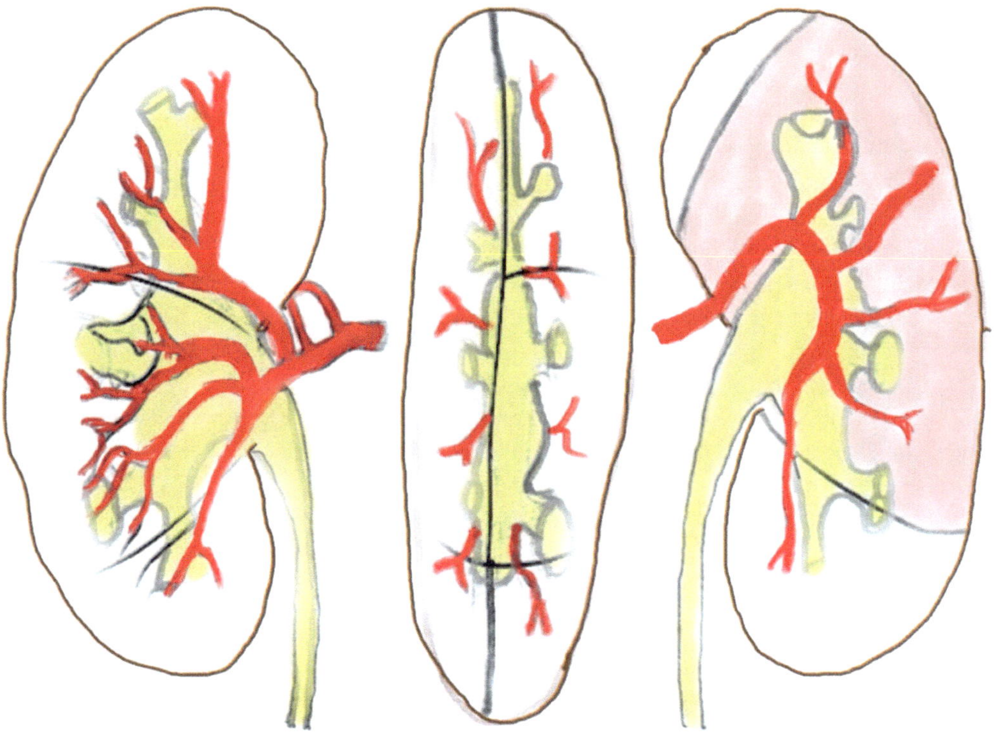

**Fig. 9.8** Renal parenchyma is supplied by Anterior and posterior divisions of renal artery. Brodel's avascular white line is 1 cm. posterior to the convex border of the kidney. Portion of renal parenchyma supplied by posterior division of renal artery is shown as shaded area

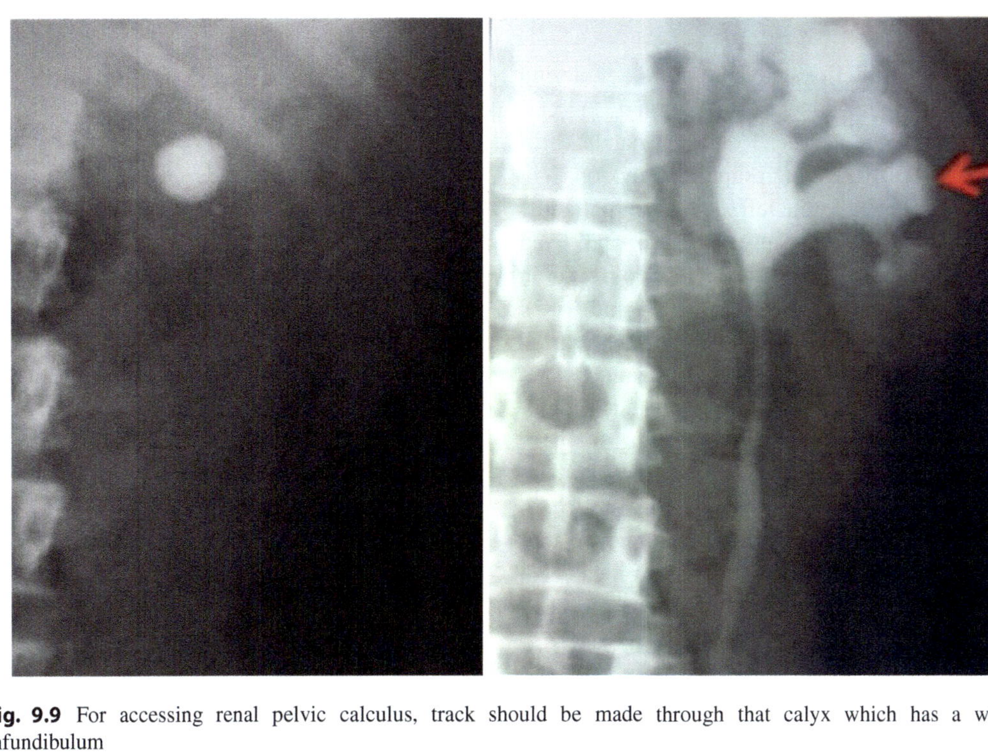

**Fig. 9.9** For accessing renal pelvic calculus, track should be made through that calyx which has a wider infundibulum

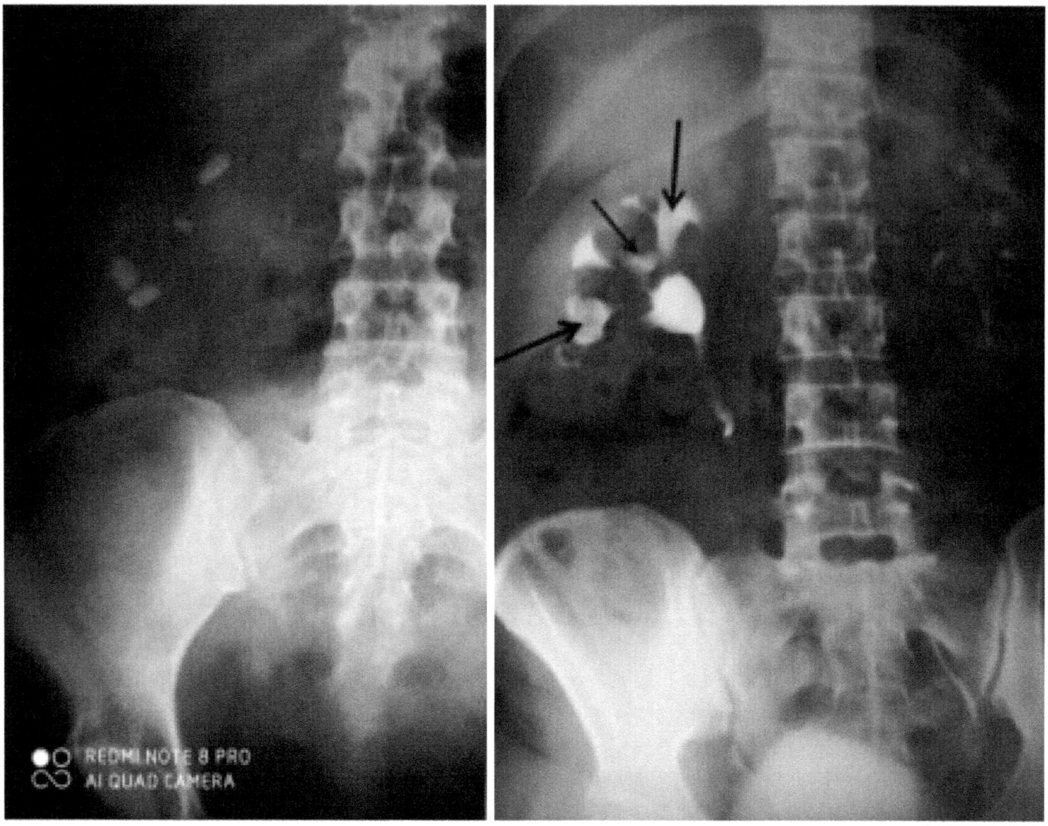

**Fig. 9.10** Narrow infundibuli may restrict free movement of rigid nephroscope within PCS. Separate tracks for calculi in different calyces may be required in such cases

middle and inferior calyces is like entering through windows with a limited access. Anatomically, it is easier for a right-handed urosurgeon to access through superior calyx on right side as compared to the left side, when patient is in prone position because the arm and hand movements of the surgeon are smooth and in alignment with the body (Figs. 9.14 and 9.15). This avoids excessive bending and physical strain on the operating surgeon. As per Tae Kon Hwang, Right-sided kidneys are also situated slightly lower down as compared to the left and their movement with respiration is also more, which avoids pleural complications in supracostal punctures on the right side [2]. This fact must be kept in mind, while planning and superior calyceal access should be preferred for all complex and staghorn stones on the right side by a right-handed urosurgeon and vice versa.

### 9.3.2 Are Calculi Fixed or Changing Position within PCS?

All efforts must be made to collect and display all previous and recent images together to assess relative or absolute movement of any stone within pelvicalyceal system. It is always easier to pick up and remove mobile stones from within the PCS. Those stones which are noticed at different locations within PCS in different images are free and mobile stones in dilated system and can easily be mobilized and pushed with saline jet to move to more appropriate locations for extraction. Since, presence of obstructing stone in renal pelvis or PUJ causes back pressure changes and dilatation of infundibuli and calyces (Fig. 9.16), most of the times it becomes easier to push a calyceal stone with the help of a saline jet, through a selective

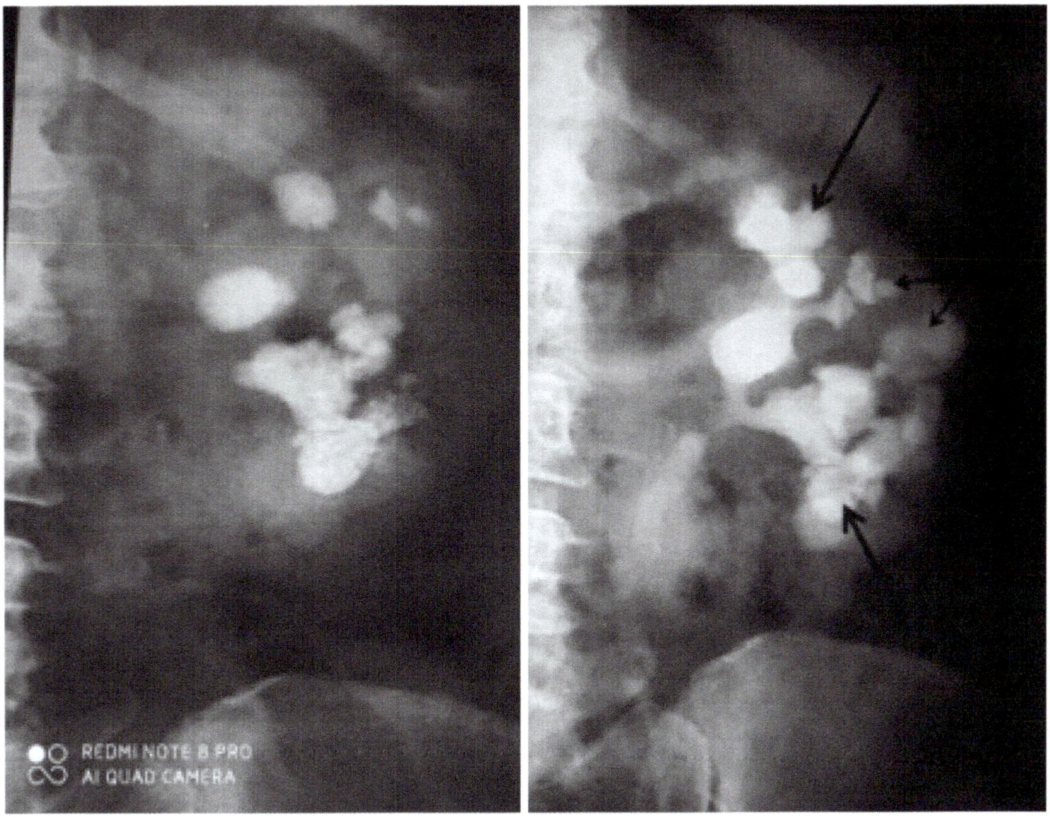


**Fig. 9.11** Very complex calculi need a meticulous planning. Apart from straight individualized tracks through selected calyces, a Y track may be required

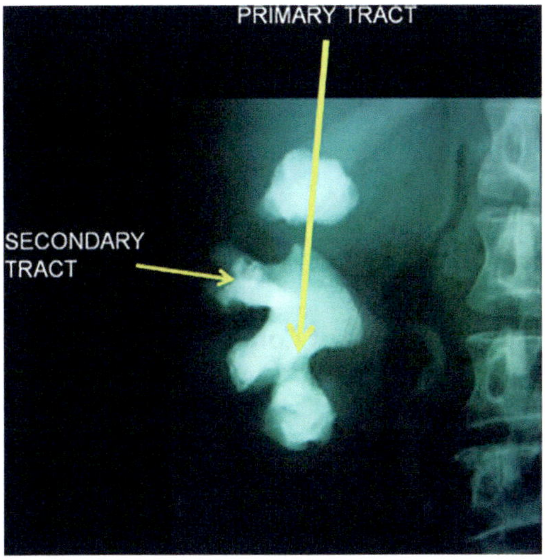


**Fig. 9.12** Superior calyceal access is ideal for managing staghorn stones

calyceal puncture of stone harbouring calyx, with initial puncture needle, from wide infundibulum into the renal pelvis from where the calyceal stone can easily be picked up and removed through original primary tract (Figs. 9.17, 9.18 and 9.19).

Author has been using and demonstrating this saline push technique since more than 25 years, very successfully. This technique greatly helps in reducing the number of additional tracts and ancillary procedures, viz. flexible nephroscopy and laser lithotripsy of calyceal calculi. Since whole stone is pushed in front of Amplatz sheath and is picked up and removed as shown in Figs. 9.20, 9.21 and 9.22, no dust or residual fragments are left behind in the inaccessible calyces as probable nest for early recurrence. Operating time and subsequent bleeding also get reduced by using this

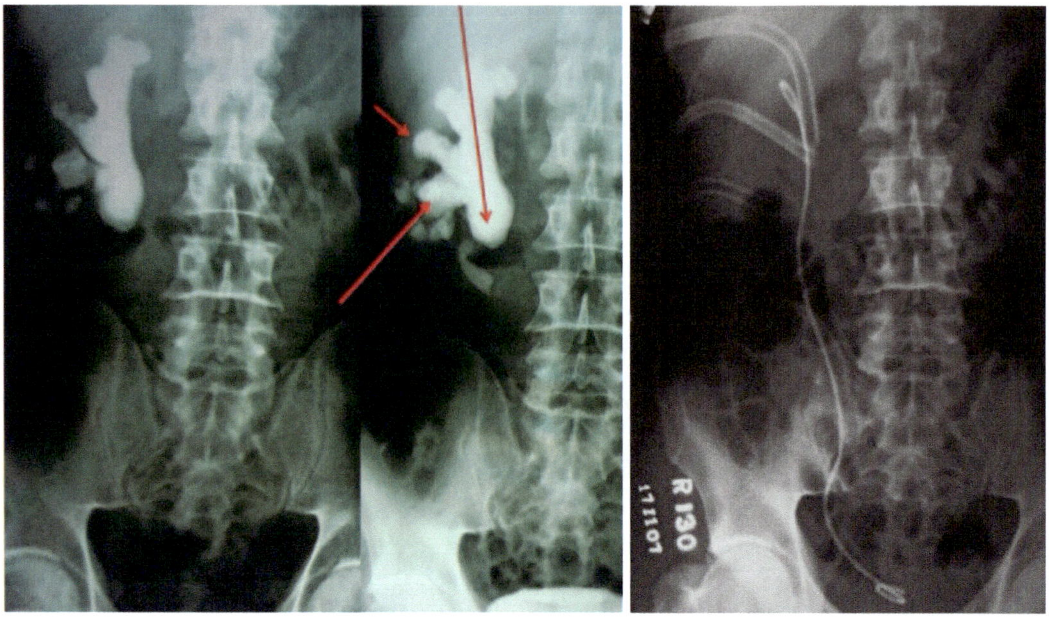

**Fig. 9.13** Primary track should be able to access most of the bulk of the stone. Secondary smaller tracks may be planned to remove the remaining calculi

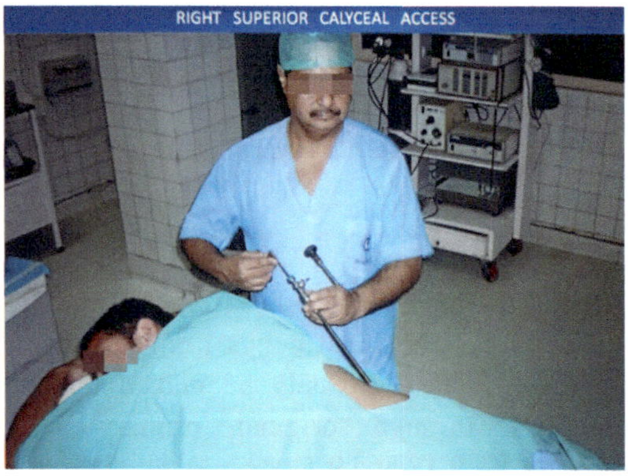


**Fig. 9.14** Comfortable posture of right-handed urosurgeon for right superior calyceal access in prone PCNL

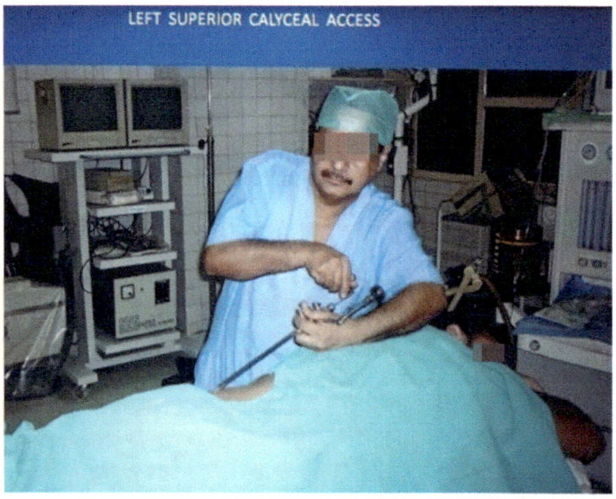


**Fig. 9.15** Left superior calyceal access involves bending and physical strain for right-handed urosurgeon

technique. Only prerequisite for efficient and successful use of this technique is to learn accurate initial puncture technique to be able to place needle tip in the desired calyx, at the lateral aspect of each calyceal stone, chosen for this purpose, as shown in Figs. 9.23, 9.24 and 9.25. During planning of the procedure, with display of all images together, such mobile and pushable calculi can be identified and kept in mind.

### 9.3.3 Pattern of Colonic Gas Shadows

Colon lies in close proximity to the middle portions and lower poles of both the kidneys (Fig. 9.26). When patient lies in supine position, in 1.9% individuals, colon is seen lying either at posterior or postero-lateral relation to the lower pole of the kidneys (Fig. 9.27), where it becomes

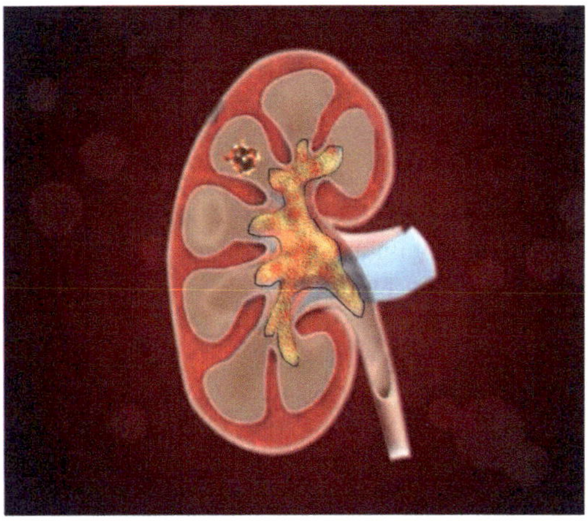

**Fig. 9.16** Presence of staghorn leads to dilatation of calyces and infundibuli

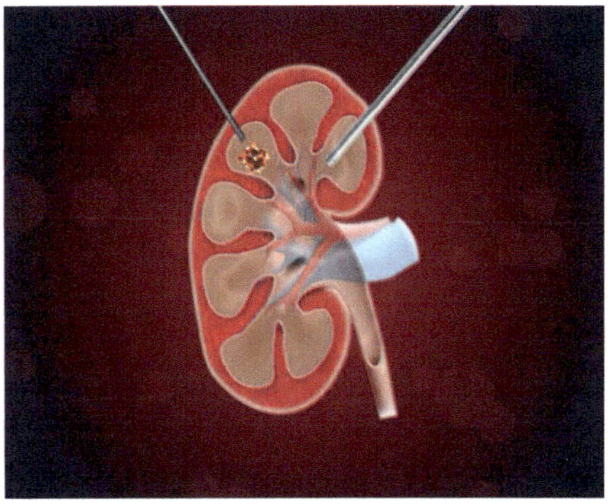

**Fig. 9.17** After extraction of staghorn stone, calyceal puncture is made on lateral aspect of stone

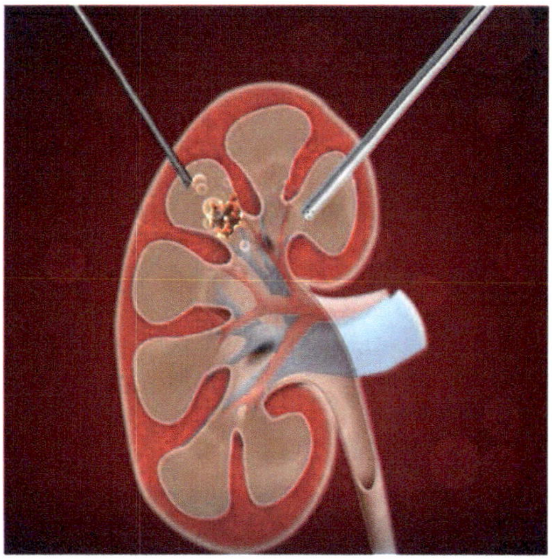

**Fig. 9.18** Forceful injection of saline through puncture needle pushes the calyceal stone into the renal pelvis

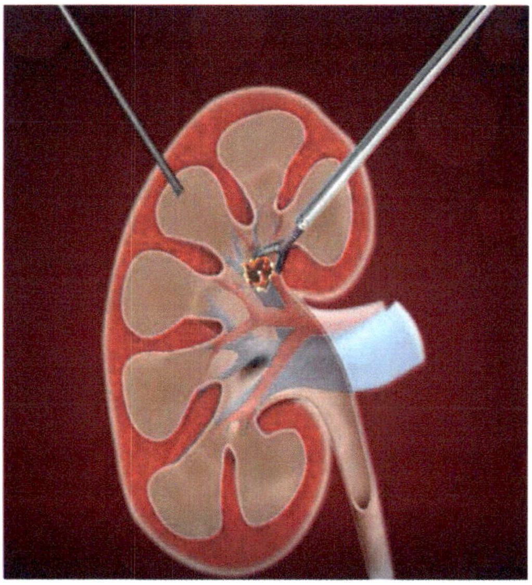

**Fig. 9.19** Pushed and relocated calyceal stone can easily be removed through original tract

vulnerable for getting injured during percutaneous access. When the same patient lies in prone position, colon gets pushed to these locations in 4.7% individuals (Hopper K D et al) [4]. Incidence of partial, or through and through colonic injuries (Fig. 9.28) during percutaneous renal access is very low because colon is a mobile organ and usually moves away or gets pushed away during initial puncture or making a track.

When all available radiological images are displayed together on view box, it becomes imperative to study the location and pattern of colon in relation to the lower pole of the ipsilateral kidney in all the images. Special attention must be paid to assess the movement or fixity of the colon (Fig. 9.29). If colon remains fixed to the lower pole of the ipsilateral kidney in all the images (Fig. 9.30), there are more chances of colonic injury during PCNL, and an alternative plan of gaining access through superior or middle calyx has to be made and very special attention must be paid to keep an eye on the movement of the colonic gas shadows while advancing needle for making an initial puncture or making a track in such a case. Use of ultrasound is highly recommended in such situations.

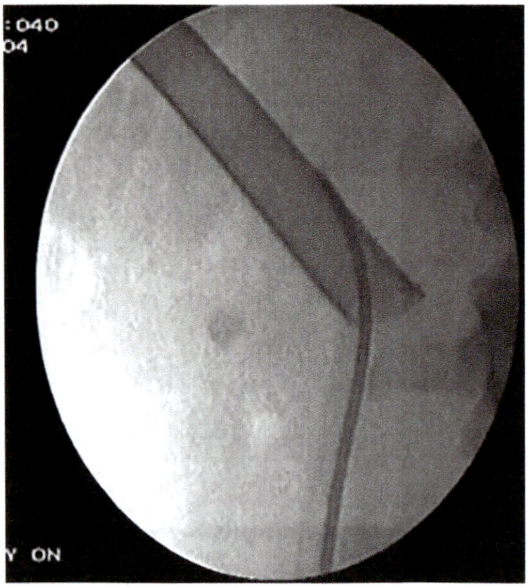

**Fig. 9.20** Inaccessible calyceal calculus far away from Amplatz sheath

Chances of colonic injuries are more in following situations, and special care must be taken to study the radiological images of these patients with predisposing factors:

1. Previously operated patients.
2. Congenital renal anomalies.
3. Very thin or morbidly obese patients.
4. Patients with history of panniculitis or perinephric abscess.
5. Patients with Diabetes.
6. Extremes of ages.
7. Patients with Incisional hernia.

### 9.3.4 Which Is the Ideal Calyx to Puncture?

**1. If calculi are located in renal pelvis, at PUJ or in upper ureter and there are no associated calyceal calculi-**

In such a situation, a most peripheral calyx (lateral) should be chosen which has thin renal

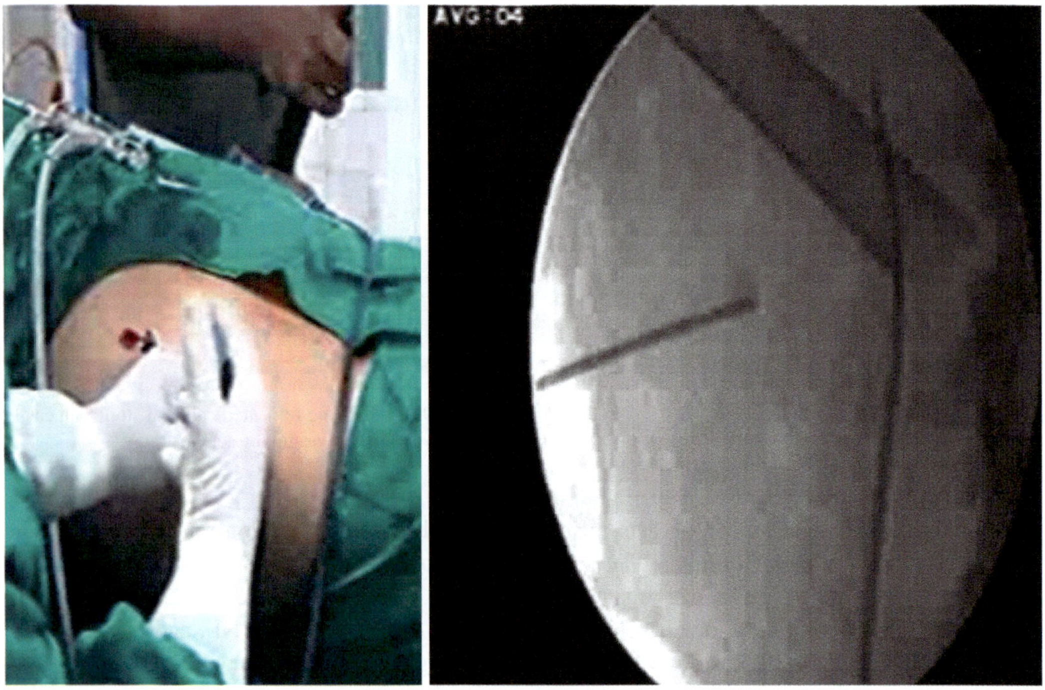


**Fig. 9.21** Selective accurate stone guided puncture is made on lateral aspect of calyceal stone and forceful injection of saline is made to push and relocate the stone

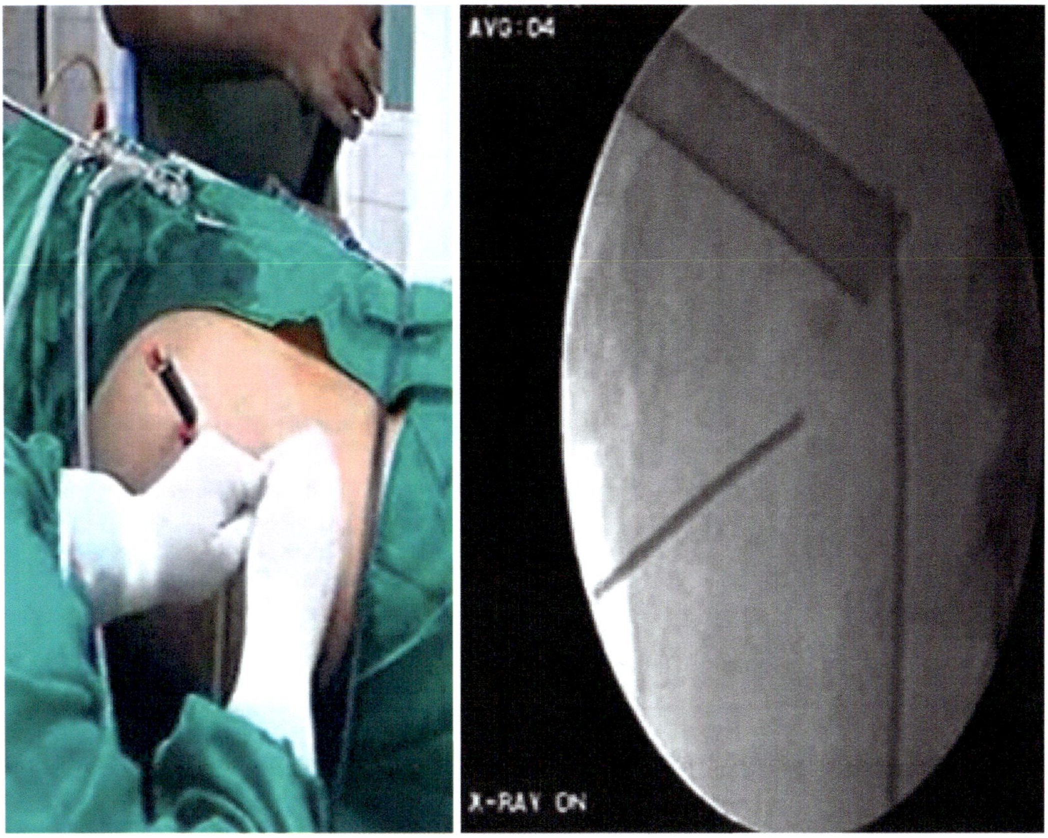


**Fig. 9.22** Relocated calyceal stone nearer to Amplatz sheath is then picked up and removed

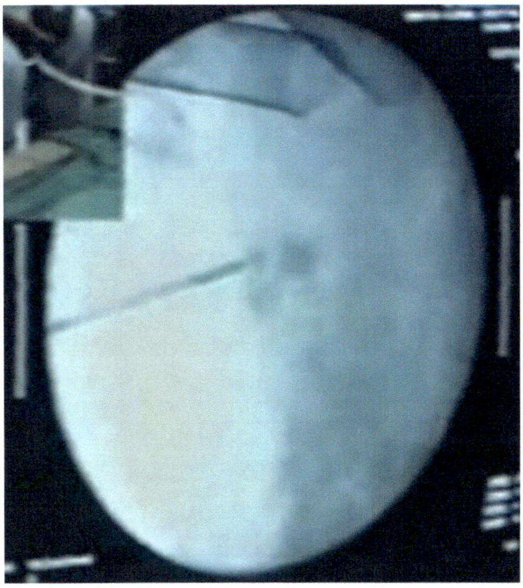

**Fig. 9.23** Few calyceal calculi were inaccessible through two superior calyceal tracts

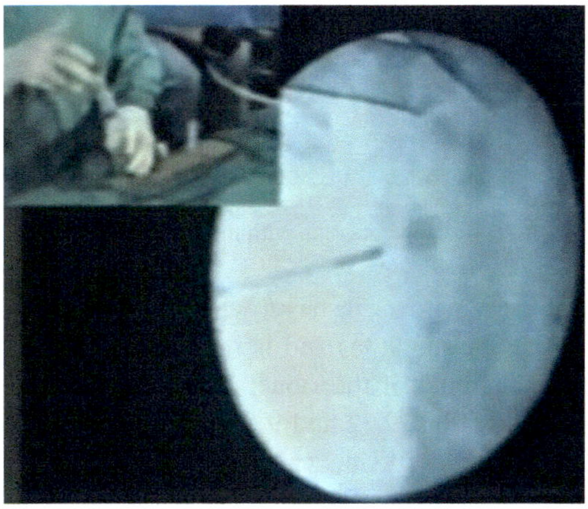

**Fig. 9.24** Selective stone guided punctures were made and all calyceal calculi were pushed with saline jet

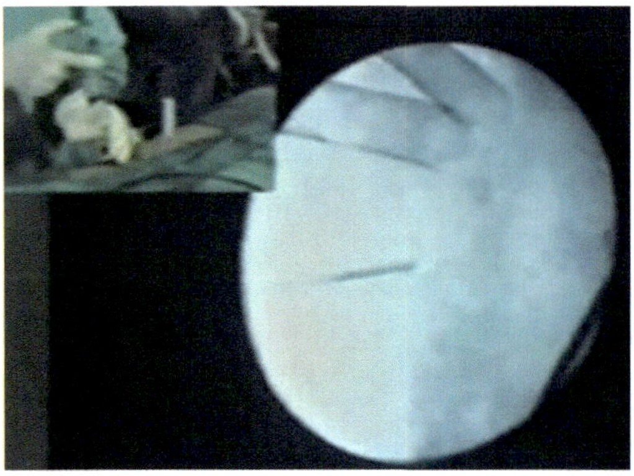

**Fig. 9.25** All calyceal calculi could be flushed and pushed towards the Amplatz sheaths and picked up and removed within no time

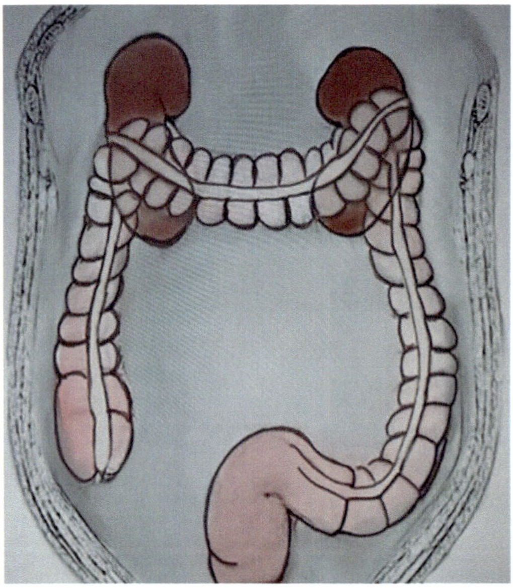

**Fig. 9.26** Relation of colon with the kidneys

parenchyma over it, has a wider infundibulum (Figs. 9.9 and 9.31) and is in direct alignment with the bulk of the stone. In Hodson type of kidneys (Figs. 9.32 and 9.61), which are more common on left side, calyx fulfilling these criteria is mostly an anterior calyx of the lower calyceal group. In contrast to the common teaching of selecting air identified posterior calyx to be the most preferred calyx in all the situations, irrespective of location of the stone, there should not be any hesitation in puncturing the anterior calyx, if it is a lateral calyx and has a wide infundibulum. This leads to the

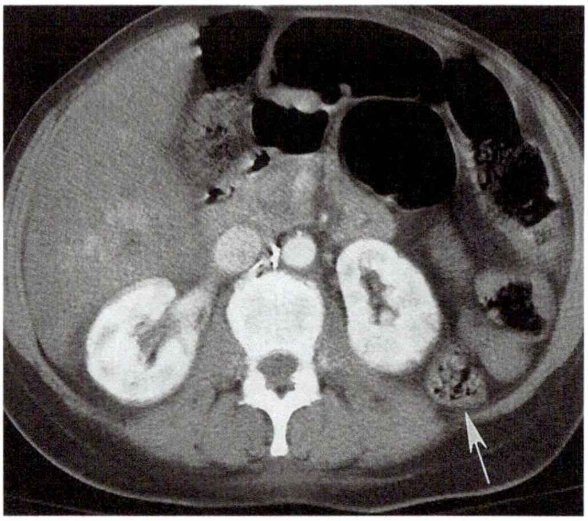

**Fig. 9.27** CT image showing a retrorenal colon, prone to get injured during percutaneous renal access

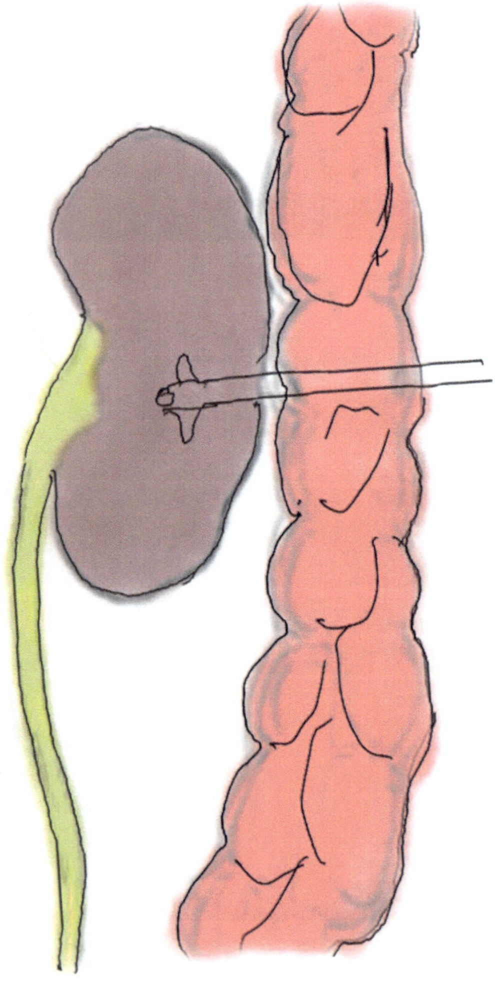

**Fig. 9.28** Transcolonic access to the kidney

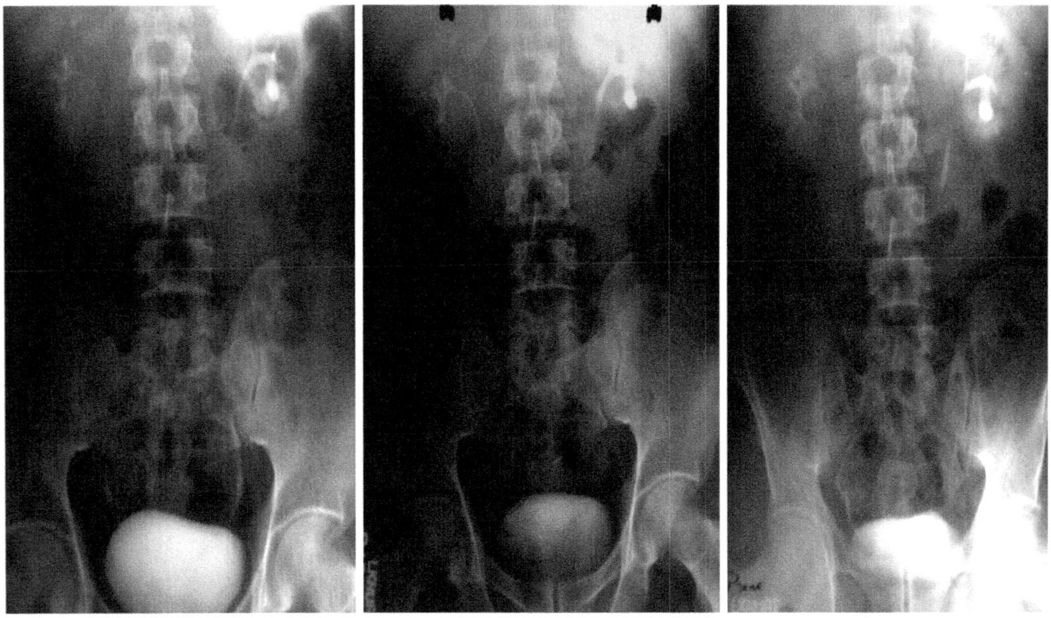

**Fig. 9.29** Colonic gas shadows are seen changing their position in relation to the lower pole of the left kidney in different films taken within a span of 90 min

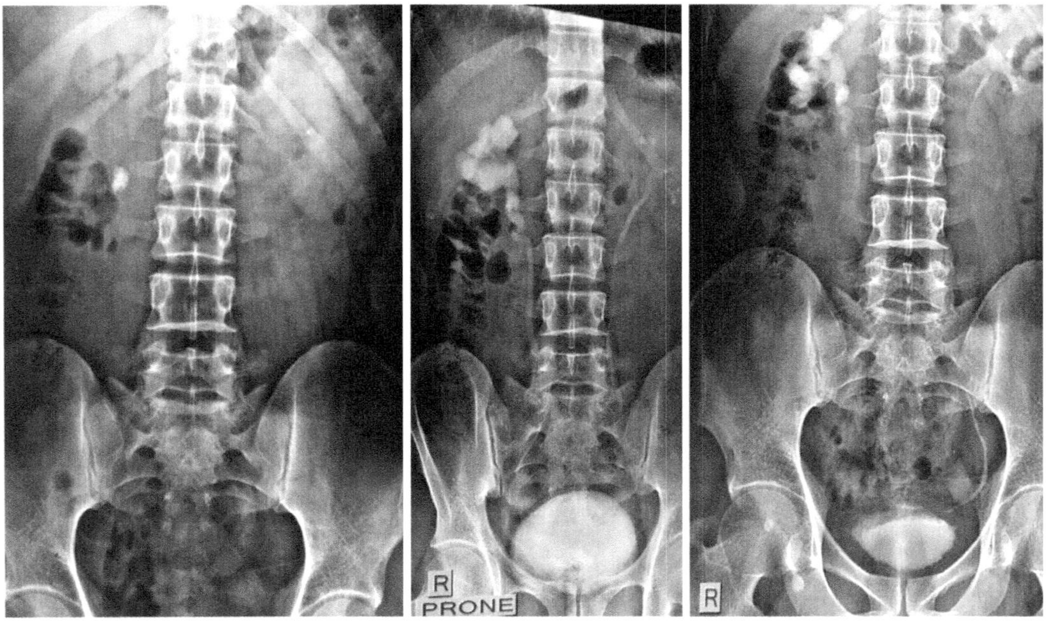


**Fig. 9.30** Colonic gas shadows remain fixed to the lower pole of this previously operated upon right kidney in all the films, making colon vulnerable to injury during PCNL

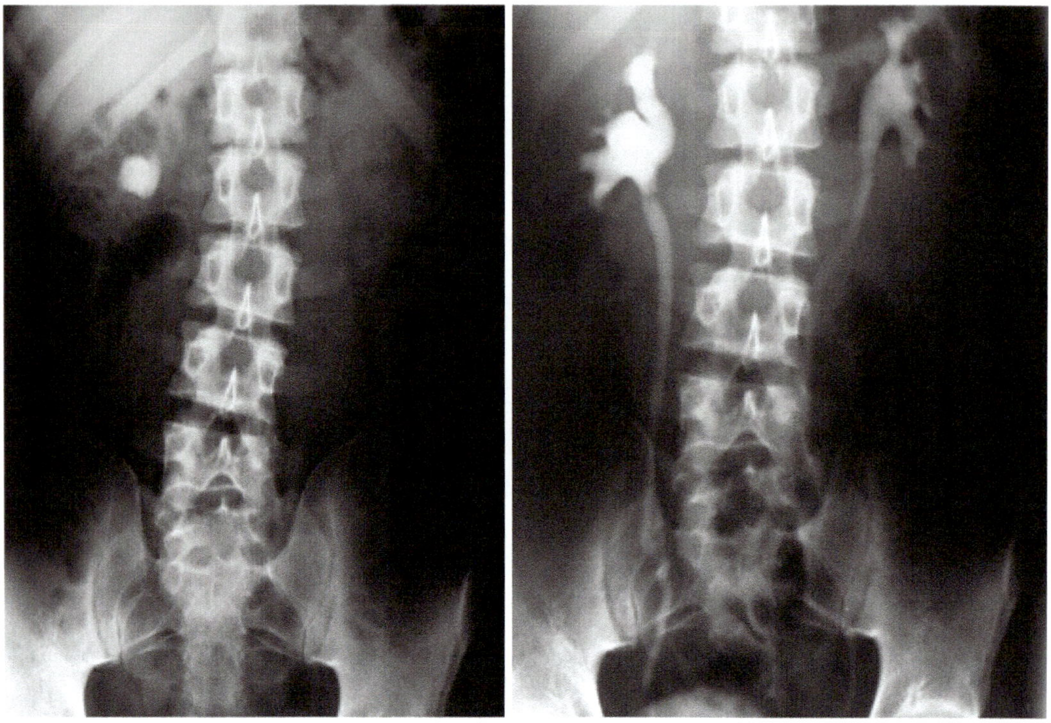

**Fig. 9.31** For renal pelvic calculi, access should be made through most peripheral calyx, which has thin overlying parenchyma and wide infundibulum

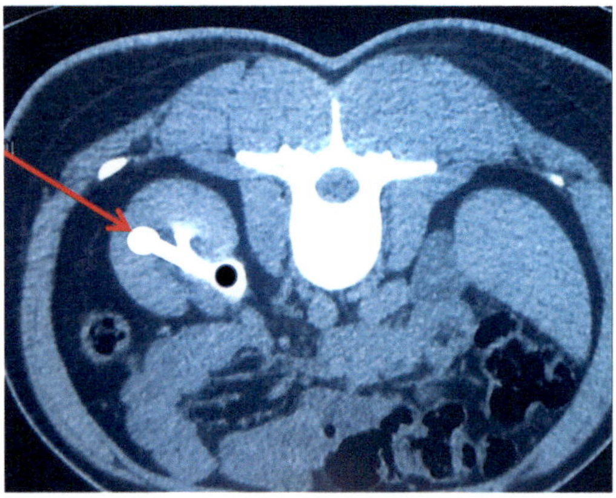

**Fig. 9.32** In Hodson type of kidneys anterior calyces extend laterally

reduction in blood loss if a calyx with thin overlying parenchyma is punctured.

**2. If there is an additional calyceal calculus along with the pelvic calculus**

In such situation stone bearing calyx (Anterior or posterior) must be chosen for making initial puncture (Fig. 9.33) After making a puncture, it needs to be confirmed that stone bearing calyx only has been punctured and none else, by any of the following manoeuvres, before making a tract, so that whole stone bulk gets removed through a single track:

- By confirming the close and constant proximity of needle tip to the calyceal stone in any two planes of the C arm.
- Movement and feeling of the stone by moving the needle.
- Slight movement and displacement of stone/stones by injecting saline through initial puncture needle.
- Movement of stone/stones by the touch of guide wire.

Once successful puncture of stone bearing calyx gets confirmed, guide wire can be placed and PCN track should be established. In such situation, it is better to manage the pelvic calculi first and once that has been done up to satisfaction, the Amplatz sheath should be slowly withdrawn till the entry point in renal calyx to visualize and tackle calyceal calculus later. This policy has been found to be useful on two counts.

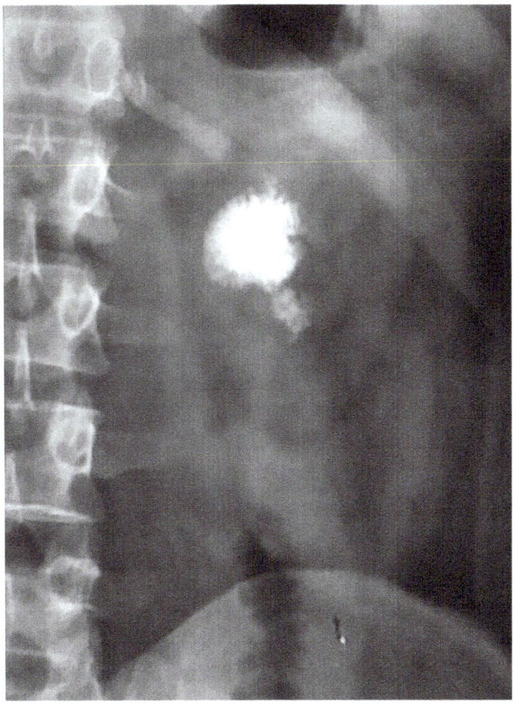

**Fig. 9.33** Planning must be done to puncture stone bearing calyx in such a situation (It may be an anterior or a posterior calyx) and accurate puncture must be confirmed before making a tract by injecting saline and watching movement of the calyceal stone

By keeping the Amplatz sheath well within the PCS for some duration, while managing the pelvic calculus, a good and reasonable haemostasis gets achieved by the tamponade effect of Amplatz sheath and there is reduced blood loss while tackling the calyceal calculus later.

During fragmentation and removal of pelvic calculus, some fragments move away with the irrigation fluid and get settled just below and behind the Amplatz sheath. Later on, when Amplatz sheath is slowly withdrawn till the entry point in PCS, these fragments also become obvious and get managed along with calyceal calculus.

**3. If stones are located within both the anterior and posterior calyces at lower pole with or without calculi in renal pelvis or upper ureter**

It is better to plan access into pelvicalyceal system through superior calyx in such cases (Fig. 9.34). This gives direct, straight, and easy access to these locations simultaneously (Fig. 9.35). In moderately or severely hydronephrotic kidneys, similar access can be obtained through middle calyx also.

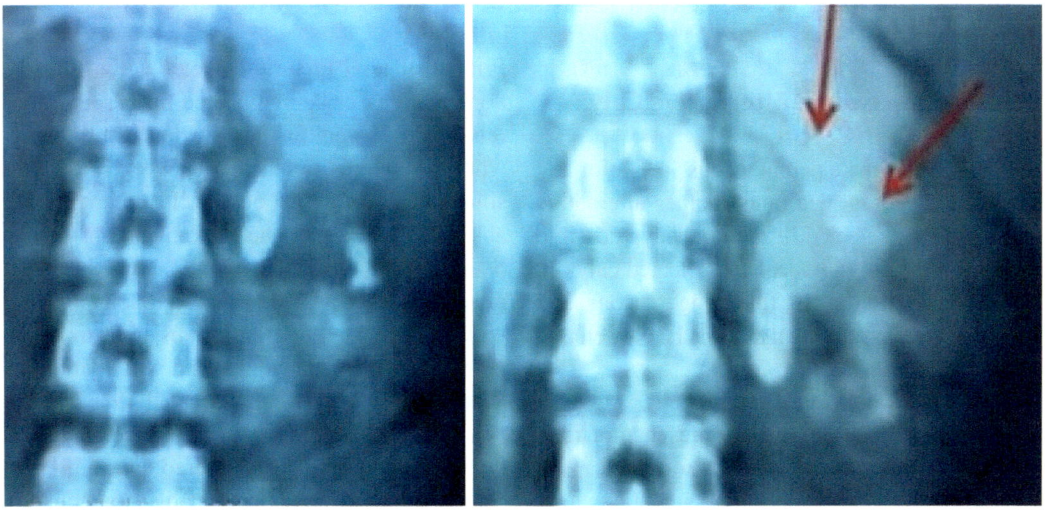

**Fig. 9.34** All calculi in anterior or posterior lower pole calyces, at PUJ and upper ureter are best accessed through superior or middle calyceal puncture

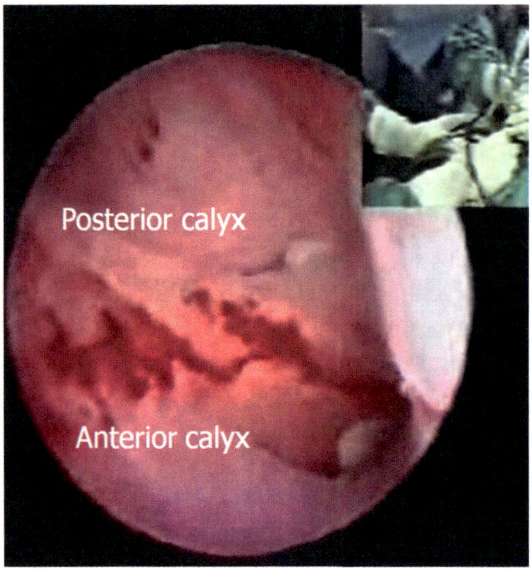


**Fig. 9.35** Superior calyceal track provides easy, direct, and simultaneous access to both the anterior and posterior lower pole calyceal calculi

**4. Staghorn Stones**
It is better to approach staghorn stones through superior calyx. Entering the pelvicalyceal system through superior calyx offers a wider access and helps in reducing the number of ancillary tracts. In those situations, where kidney is located higher up and making a track through superior calyx is likely to cause pleural or pulmonary complications, other options of choosing middle or inferior calyces may be considered.

### 9.3.5 Choice of an Alternative Calyx

During planning of a percutaneous access for any particular case, an ideal and another alternative calyx must be selected. It is not always possible to gain access through ideal and selected calyx in all of the cases due to following reasons and therefore an alternative calyx must be chosen and kept in mind:

1. Anatomical restrictions like presence of ribs, Kyphoscoliosis, contour of buttocks, etc.
2. If the ideal calyx does not get adequately opacified during RGP due to poor entry of contrast caused by blockage of calyx by stone, blood clot, pus flakes, fungal balls, or stone matrix or it is cut off from PCS due to infundibular stenosis.
3. Contrast extravasation during RGP or during repeated attempts of puncture hides or overshadows the desired chosen calyx.
4. If significant bleeding is encountered on puncturing selected calyx, necessitating abandoning of this track.

### 9.3.6 Stone Migration

Mechanical impact of pneumatic lithoclast and fast irrigation during mini PCNL may cause migration of stone and/or stone fragments to other locations within pelvicalyceal system. This fact must be kept in mind during selection of most appropriate calyx for percutaneous access. Chosen route should also provide adequate and straight access to the possible locations of the migratory stone fragments. This problem of possible migration of stone/stone fragments is seen more often in mini PCNL, when fast irrigation is applied for spontaneous extraction of calculi/fragments by whirlpool effect and pelvicalyceal system is moderately or severely hydronephrotic.

## 9.4 Ureteric Catheterization

Prior ipsilateral ureteric catheterization must be done in all cases being planned for percutaneous renal access, even if it is being done for relook or when a previous track is already existing. This simple procedure, first of all helps in confirming absence of any significant anatomical obstructive pathology in the ureter, which might have got missed in other available investigations, prior to making a track. A percutaneous track is never going to heal spontaneously and will continue to leak, if any obstructive ureteric pathology continues to offer distal obstruction. In case, any difficulty or resistance is encountered during ureteric catheterization, an ureteroscopic examination must be done to identify and manage the situation. It is strongly recommended by author, to directly visualize, identify, and manage the situation by ureteroscopic examination and not to inject contrast agent at this time as far as possible. If contrast is injected at this time, it will fill up or outline certain calyces of ipsilateral kidney and the details of stone will get masked, which may create problem in accurate assessment of the bulk and lie of stone/stones, within the kidney and hence in proper planning of the most suitable and appropriate track for removal of the stone. Routinely, contrast should be injected under constant visualization, only after the patient has been positioned and initial puncture needle is indicating the stone bulk.

Some amount of uncertainty always exists in percutaneous renal surgery, in spite of the greatest experience of the operator and hence this surgery must be carried out with all due precautions being observed. This surgical exercise can never be taken for granted. Presence of ureteric catheter well beyond PUJ into the renal pelvis fortifies operators position with significant control over the situation in many ways, even if something goes wrong in the course of this surgery. Uses and advantages of in situ ureteric catheter during and after percutaneous renal surgery are as follows:

1. Opacification of pelvicalyceal system by injecting contrast/air or both.
2. Distension of pelvicalyceal system for better ultrasonic visualization and/or for placement of guide wire in a compact or stone filled system.
3. Confirmation of accurate puncture by obtaining free flow of injected saline.
4. Prevention of migration of stone fragments down into the ureter because of its mechanical presence, when the flow of irrigation is augmented by pressure pump during mini PCNL for obtaining stone clearance by whirlpool effect.
5. Flushing back of those stone fragments into PCS, which accidentally migrate down into the ureter.
6. Easy identification of PUJ in cases with oedema and/or intense congestion of renal pelvis, or when there is malrotation or a very large, dilated renal pelvis.
7. It helps in placement of double J stent.
8. It provides drainage in routine and sometimes in difficult situations, when an accidental tear or partial avulsion at PUJ has taken place.

## 9.5 Use of Bolsters

There is no general agreement or guidelines as regards to use or position of bolsters. At most of the centres, it is planned according to mutual understanding and agreement between anaesthetist and urologist. Basic purpose to place bolsters from anaesthetists point of view is to ensure free movements of abdominal wall and lower chest to ensure proper oxygen saturation in prone position during surgery. Although few operators from Germany demonstrate placement of inflatable bolsters just in the middle of epigastric region, upper abdomen and lower chest, which theoretically should create problem in free movement of abdominal wall. In India, either no bolsters are used or these are positioned in horizontal or vertical orientation. Horizontal placement of bolsters implies, positioning of one bolster across the lower chest and another across iliac crests, so that whole abdomen is totally free and without any compression (Fig. 9.36). In author's opinion, horizontal placement of bolsters allows excessive forward movements of kidney during initial puncture and subsequent dilatation and creation of track.

Author's preference has always been to place bolsters in vertical orientation (Fig. 9.37), paral-

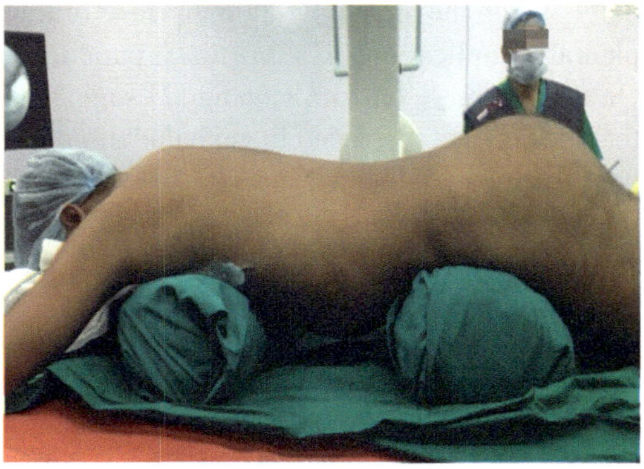

**Fig. 9.36** Horizontal placement of bolsters

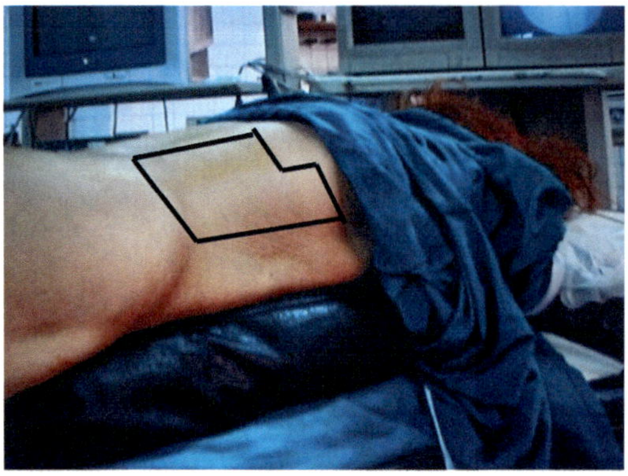

**Fig. 9.37** Vertical placement of bolsters

lel to the body, supporting both flanks, extending from lower chest to the iliac crest on either side. Such placement is supposed to give stability and fixity to the kidney and offers counter pressure to the push by advancing needle and dilators while making a tract. At the same time, this allows free movement of the central portion of abdomen to help maintain the optimum oxygen saturation in prone position.

Most probably the ultimate average length of the track will also be shorter, when bolsters are placed in vertical orientation (Fig. 9.37). Prospective study by Sagalovich D et al. [5] demonstrated increase in kidney to diaphragm, kidney to 12th rib, and kidney to vertebral body distances by placing bolsters in horizontal position but there was no statistically significant difference in the length of the track whether bolsters were placed horizontally or vertically. They concluded that horizontal placement of bolsters allowed kidneys to be displaced caudally, which movement would help in avoiding pleural complications in supracostal punctures. On the contrary, Tae kon Hwang [2] suggested that kidneys get displaced in cephalad direction on placement of bolster under the chest and upper abdomen. In fact, several multicentre studies are needed to address this issue and till then it remains a personal choice of the operator or a mutual agreement between anaesthetist and the urologist.

## 9.6 Placement of Equipments in OR

PCNL procedure has a highly unpredictable course. A case appearing very simple and straightforward may turn into a nightmare. Therefore, urosurgeon who is going to start a PCNL surgery must make himself very comfortable and physically at ease on all counts. Lighting in the operating room should be dim, so as to visualize images on the X-ray image intensifier and Endo monitor better, without straining the eyes. OR temperature should be optimum and all monitors should be right in front of the surgeon, so that he can fix his gaze even for a long time if needed, without straining on his neck.

There are four likely positions for urosurgeon to stand while performing PCNL surgery, two on each side. Supracostal approach is used to access superior calyx and infracostal approach is used to access middle or lower calyces. In both the approaches, both monitors should be placed together right across side to side, just straight in front of and facing the surgeon on appropriate side of the C arm as shown in Figs. 9.38 and 9.39. Energy source for fragmentation of stone should be positioned next to or just behind the trolly for instruments.

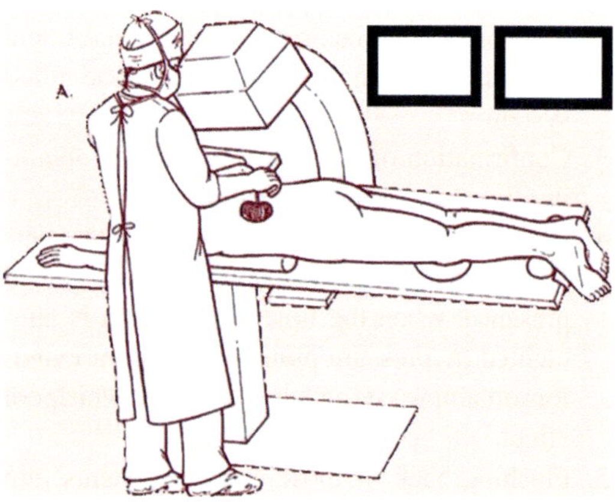


**Fig. 9.38** Placement of both C arm monitor and endoscopic image monitor straight in front of urosurgeon for left superior calyceal access

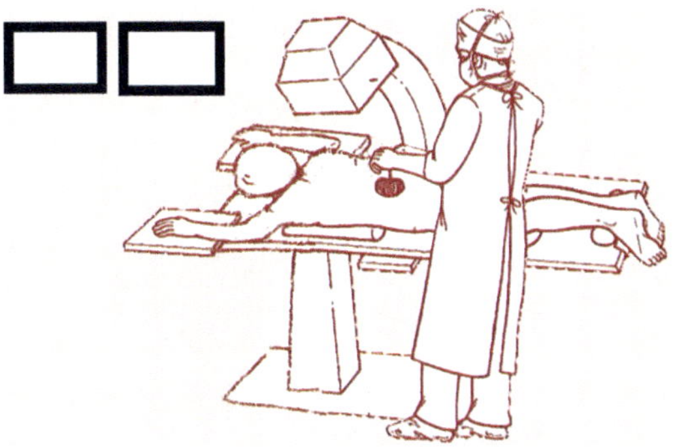

**Fig. 9.39** Placement of both C arm monitor and endoscopic image monitor straight in front of urosurgeon for left inferior calyceal access

## 9.7 How to Place C Arm and Proceed

### 9.7.1 For PCNL in Prone Position

C Arm image intensifier should be wheeled in from the opposite side, right in the middle of the table after the patient has been positioned in prone position following ureteric catheterization (Fig. 9.40). A general assessment of position of stone, ureteric catheter, and pattern of colonic gas shadows in vicinity of ipsilateral kidney is made with C arm in zero degrees position. If ureteric catheter is not draining the drops of urine or if it appears to have got placed much higher up in the superior calyx or has coiled up in dilated PCS, it needs to be slightly withdrawn and straightened under radiological control. About 5 to 10 ml of saline should be injected through ureteric catheter at this time and slow return dripping of saline through ureteric catheter should be noted. It confirms patency and proper placement of ureteric catheter into the space of pelvicalyceal system. If the ureteric catheter has got blocked due to matrix or some blood clot during the time elapsed for positioning of the patient and equipment around the table, injection of saline will encounter resistance. Ureteric catheter must be opened by forceful injection of saline or passage of guide wire or stellate through it or else changed in such a situation. If absence of return dripping of injected saline is noted, following possibilities should be entertained:

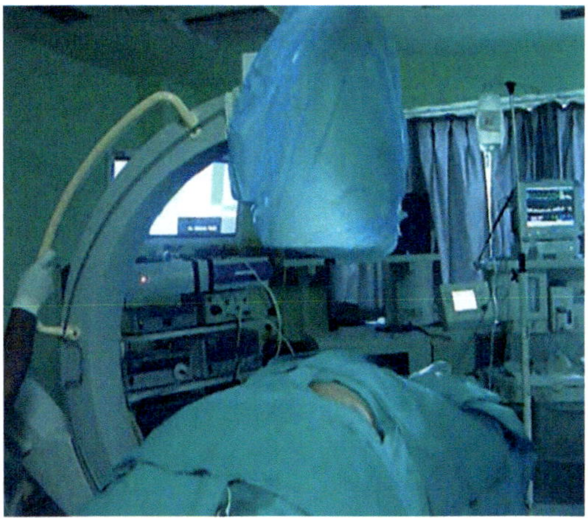

**Fig. 9.40** C arm is wheeled in from opposite side and positioned in zero degree position

- Downward slipping of ureteric catheter into the ureter.
- Tip of ureteric catheter might have created and entered in a submucosal tunnel or perforated and gone out of PCS. This can happen if the ureteric catheter is overenthusiastically pushed too much into a calyx or if stone is densely impacted and there is no sufficient space between the impacted stone and mucosa. Injecting contrast in these situations will result into extravasation and loss of anatomical details.
- Tip of ureteric catheter is in close apposition to the oedematous mucosa in PCS and hence free return of injected saline is compromised.
- Presence of blood clots, thick pus, matrix within PCS.

Once free return dripping from ureteric catheter has been established, cleaning and draping should be done and image intensifier is covered with sterile cover. Now the C arm should be tilted 30 degrees, with image intensifier coming closer to the head of the surgeon and X-ray tube moving far away from the surgeon's body to make an initial puncture as shown in Fig. 9.41. This helps in reducing the radiation exposure to the operating surgeon, assistant, and the scrub nurse.

Positioning of C arm with such 30 degrees tilt also allows the target calyces to be visualized head-on and in most accurate anatomical ways,

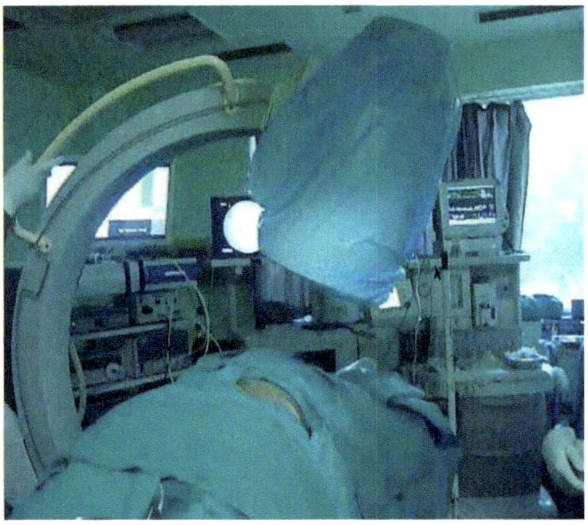

**Fig. 9.41** C arm is tilted 30 degrees to visualize kidney in most appropriate anatomical orientation

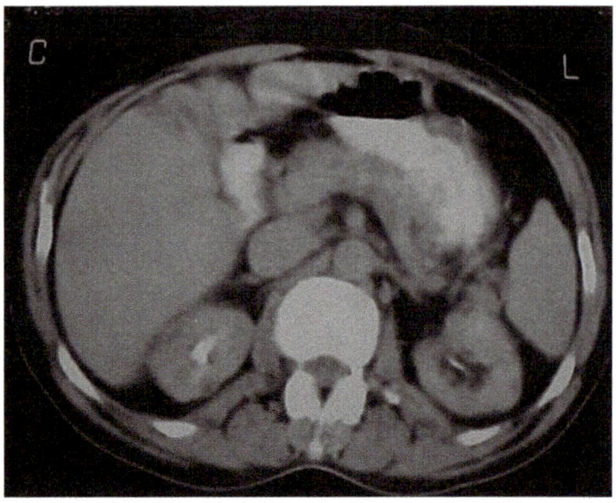


**Fig. 9.43** CT image when patient is in supine position shows 30 degrees tilt of the kidneys due to bulk of psoas muscles

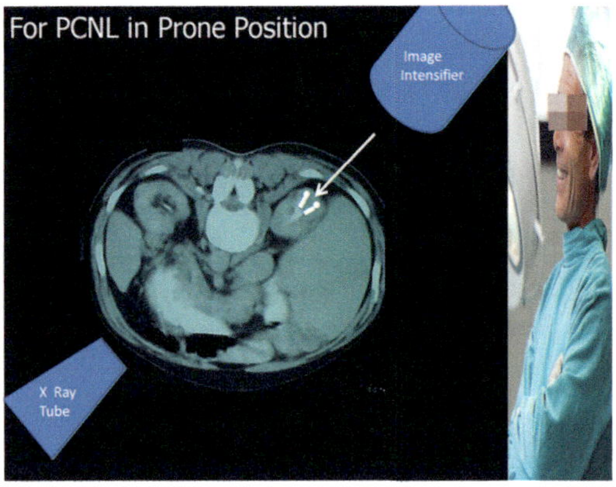


**Fig. 9.42** 30 degrees tilt of C arm allows to visualize target calyx straight head-on for an accurate puncture

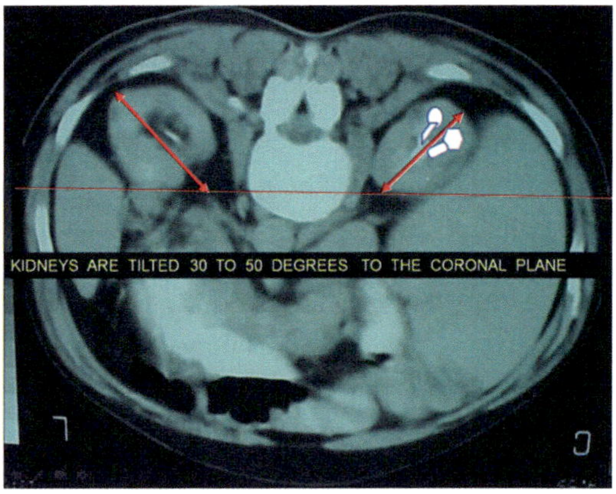


**Fig. 9.44** CT image of same patient when turned prone shows exact anatomical orientation of calyces

as the operating surgeon must visualize his target straight and head-on, in position (Fig. 9.42).

Figure 9.43 shows the CT image of the kidneys when patient is lying in supine position.

When the same patient is turned prone (Fig. 9.44), both the kidneys are seen to be oriented with a 30 degrees tilt to the coronal plane because of presence of bulk of psoas muscles. Since several studies published by Sampaio et al. have demonstrated, that most appropriate place to enter into PCS is through the Brodel's white line, situated 1 cm posterior to the convex border of the kidney and entering PCS through fornix of the chosen calyx, such placement of C arm is the best anatomical orientation to visualize and gain head-on access to the target. It is like visualizing the target straight on its face. Placement of C arm in zero degrees will be showing the straight two-dimensional image of a kidney, actually lying obliquely and not as per the anatomical orientation within the body. In fact, we have become used to seeing straight images of the kidneys, actually oriented obliquely in the body in IVU, but when it comes to visualization of kidneys for the purpose of accurate anatomical access, we should image the kidneys in most perfect anatomical way, as these are.

Now, the tip of the needle is placed on the back in such a way, that it is pointing to the bulk of the stone and well diluted contrast is injected through ureteric catheter very slowly, while continuous monitoring the inflow of contrast into PCS, till the preselected calyx for initial puncture gets adequately opacified. If the filling of target calyx with contrast is very slow, delayed, or obstructed at this time, a very free and fast egress of saline cannot be expected during initial puncture. This happens when bulk and orientation of stone or blood clot, stone matrix or thick pus within PCS does not allow free filling of the target calyx with contrast.

Once the target calyx fills up, some adjustments are made by repositioning of image intensifier so that actual radiological image of this particular calyx on the X-ray monitor gets fixed at 11 o'clock position for the right side (Fig. 9.45) and 1 o'clock position for the left side (Fig. 9.46).

This repositioning allows proper imaging of the maximum length of the needle and the future tract, when it is being advanced towards the target calyx. It also allows to keep a watch on neighbouring organs like colon, if these are coming on the way.

Now, the needle tip is positioned on the back of the patient indicating at the cup of the target calyx and length of the needle is aligned in straight line to the infundibulum of that calyx, so that a straight track can be made advancing up to the renal pelvis. A line may be drawn along the needle track on the skin at this time to guide the direction and alignment of the track.

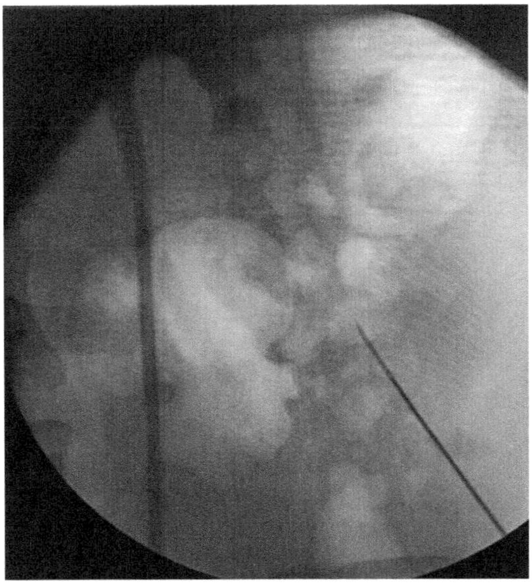

**Fig. 9.45** Target calyx is brought at 11 o'clock position of c arm image for the right side, so that progress, direction, and alignment of maximum length of needle are observed and monitored and colonic gas shadows are continuously observed

If colonic gas shadow starts getting indented or starts moving vigorously with the jerky movements of advancing needle, a colonic puncture must be suspected and needle should be withdrawn immediately (Fig. 9.47) Next, a more medial skin puncture site must be selected on patients body in the same line and another attempt should be made (Fig. 9.48).

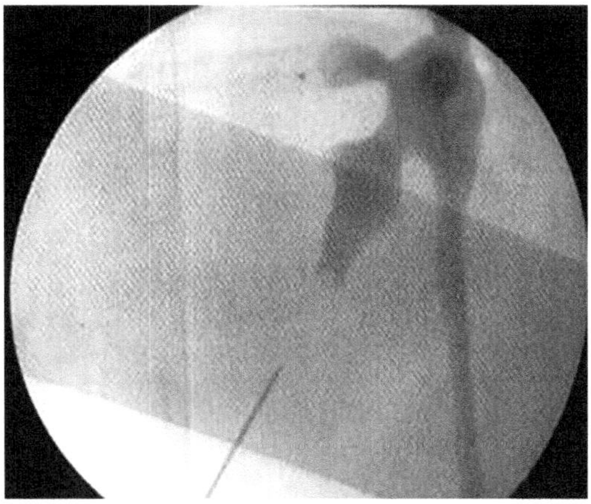

**Fig. 9.46** Target calyx is brought at 1 o'clock position of c arm image for the left side, so that progress, direction, and alignment of maximum length of needle are observed and monitored and colonic gas shadows are continuously observed

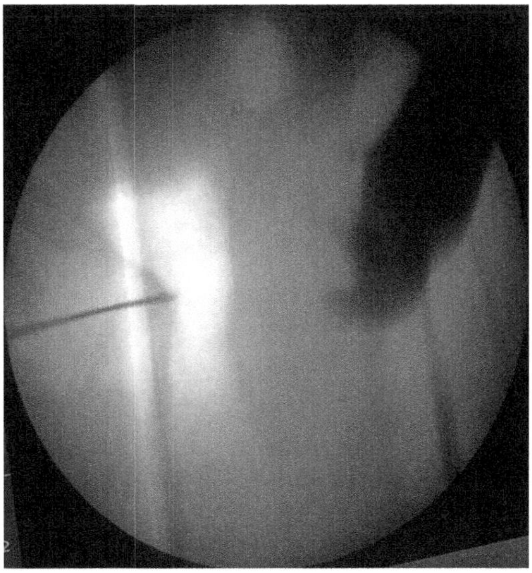

**Fig. 9.47** Needle tip is seen indenting the colonic gas shadow

### 9.7.2 For PCNL in Supine Position

Similar to PCNL in prone position, C arm has to be wheeled in from opposite side only. It has to be tilted 30 degrees in opposite direction, so that image intensifier moves away from the surgeon's head and X-ray tube comes closer to the operating team as shown in Fig. 9.49. This is the ideal way in which kidney will be visualized in accurate anatomical orientation. This positioning has a clear disadvantage of exposing operating team with higher doses of X-ray radiation, because of proximity to the X-ray tube. Due to this significant disadvantage, most of the urosurgeons performing supine PCNL keep the C arm in 0 degree position only and actually visualize the kidney in its oblique orientation.

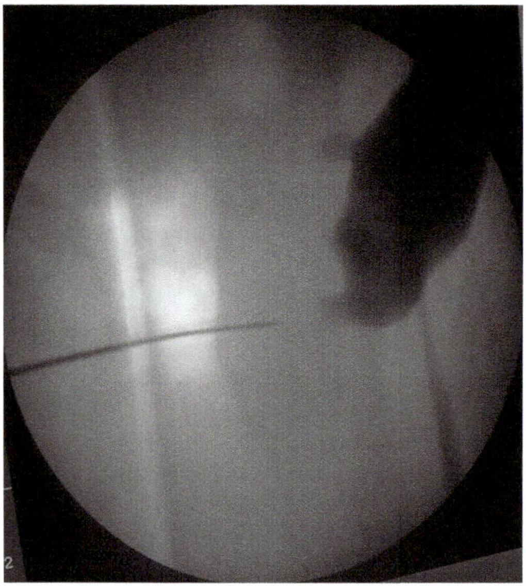

**Fig. 9.48** Needle is positioned on more medial location and advanced

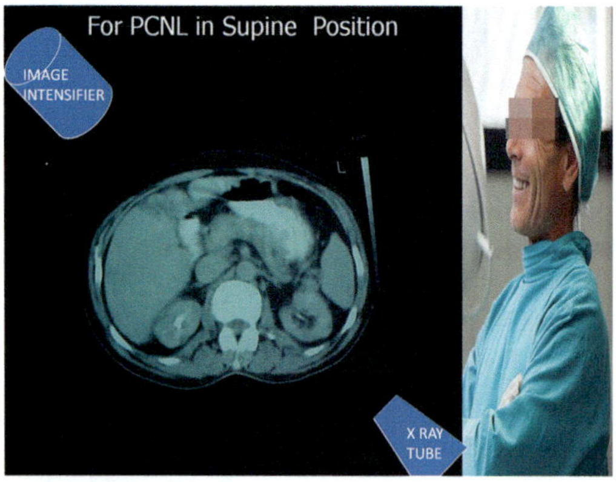


**Fig. 9.49** Showing proper positioning of C arm for supine PCNL, which will help in visualization of kidney in accurate anatomical orientation

## 9.8 What Does Fluoroscopy Show

Mobile C arm X-ray unit is a must for fluoroscopic renal access. There should be a clear minimum distance of 30 inches (76.2 cms.) between the X-ray tube and image intensifier (Fig. 9.50), so that adequate working distance is still available to operate and insert instruments when operating table and overlying patient are brought in this gap. Another important feature in c arm unit, helpful for the beginners is to be able to obtain an image of 9 inches diameter area in one frame, so that good length of approaching needle, as well as neighbouring colonic gas shadow is visualized and alignment with the infundibulum gets well appreciated to create a short straight track safely. After sufficient experience of working under fluoroscopic guidance has been gained, C arm with an image diameter of 6 inches proves adequate and provides better and sharper images of the objects.

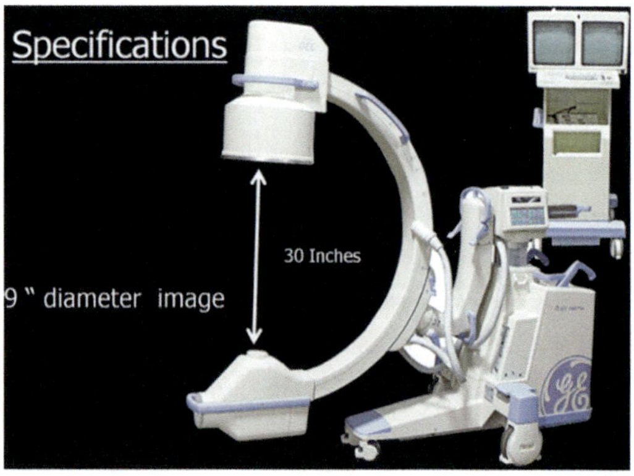


**Fig. 9.50** Showing specifications worth verifying for selection of C arm unit for PCNL. Optimum distance of 76.2 cm between X ray tube and image intensifier leaves just adequate working space between patient's back and image intensifier for urosurgeon to introduce needle and dilators, etc

A fluoroscopic image obtained by the C arm is similar to a picture obtained by a camera. It is a two-dimensional image and lacks in delineation of the third dimension, viz. distance or depth perception between the two objects as becomes clear by analysing following pictures Figs. 9.51 and 9.52.

Although there is a huge distance between the sun and the basket, and moon and the cart or crane, it appears contained within or close by in these pictures. These pictures taken by a camera are not able to demonstrate the real distance (third dimension) between the two objects. We need to take another picture, moving to another nearby location, with both these objects in the same frame, to appreciate the real distance (third dimension) between these two objects. Absolutely, same situation gets repeated when C arm is utilized during fluoroscopic guided access. When the needle tip is just positioned on the skin surface, indicating the target calyx, and C arm is activated, it appears in the obtained image on fluoroscopic monitor that the needle tip has already reached into the target calyx (Fig. 9.53).

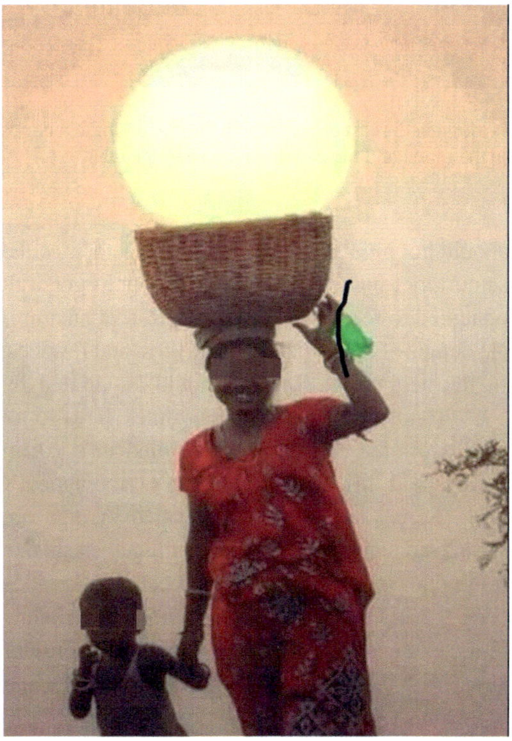

Fig. 9.51 This two-dimensional picture taken with a camera shows sun in the basket. This picture fails to appreciate the third dimension of huge distance between the sun and the basket

It must be appreciated here, that similar image will be obtained on the fluoroscopic monitor, whether the needle tip is on the skin surface (Blue arrow), actually on the target (yellow arrow) or deeper (anterior) to the target (red arrow), but reaching exactly anywhere on the straight imaginary line between the X-ray tube and image intensifier (Fig. 9.54).

Now, C arm has to be positioned at another location, say 0 degree to assess the actual depth or the third dimension. If this relocation of C arm unit to 0 degree is done, leaving the needle at the same position where it was, the needle which was actually superficial or posterior to the targeted calyx will be seen moving lateral to the target in the new image, while the needle which had been positioned deeper (anterior) to the target will be seen moving medial to the target in the new image. If the needle was located exactly on the target calyx, it will be seen at the same point on the target in both the images with locations of C arm at 30 degrees as well as in 0 degree (Fig. 9.55).

Different researchers and urosurgeons have different opinions regarding preferred two locations and movement of the C arm or carrying out whole procedure in one fixed position of the C arm, but this fact must be well appreciated that for true three-dimensional assessment and proper anatomical placement of initial puncture needle and subsequent fluoroscopic renal access, the clinical orientation and situation must be assessed and verified in at least two dimensions. Carrying out whole procedure only in one fixed position of C arm may remain anatomically inaccurate and only guess work.

## 9.9 Use of Contrast

### 9.9.1 Dilution of Contrast

As a basic precaution, the injected contrast for opacification of pelvicalyceal system should be so well diluted, to the extent that once injected, it

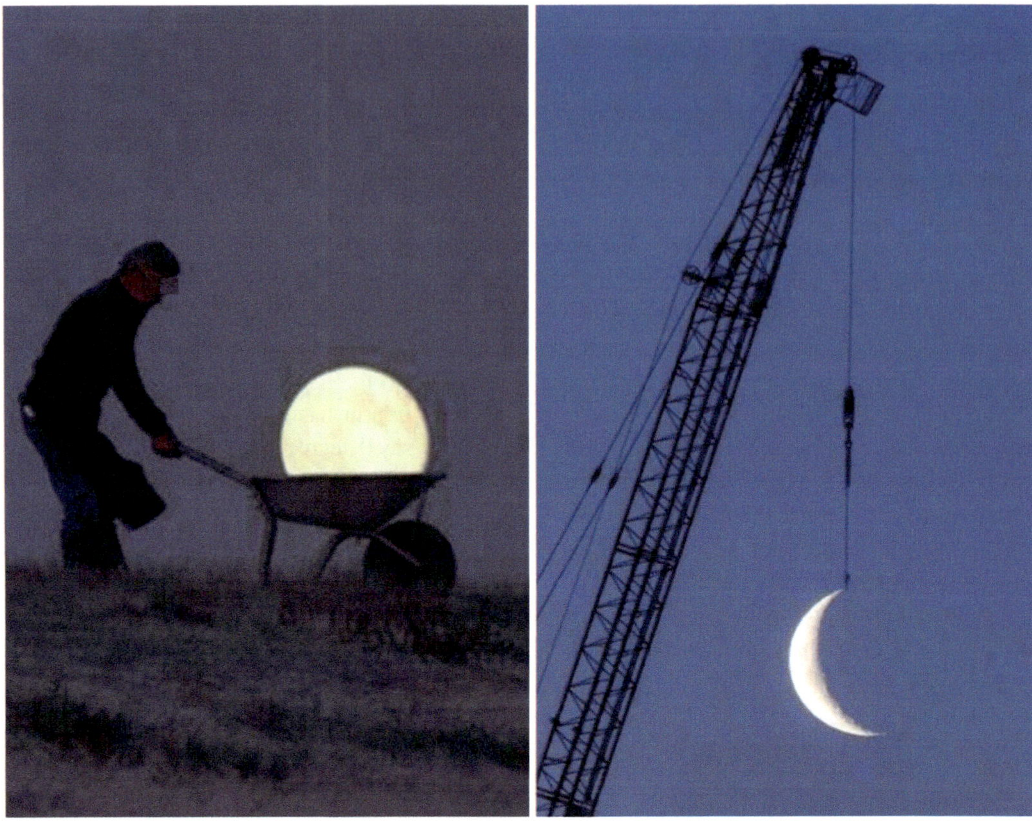

**Fig. 9.52** Two-dimensional picture taken with a camera shows moon in the cart or hanging on the crane. These pictures fail to appreciate the third dimension of huge distance between the moon and the cart and moon and the crane

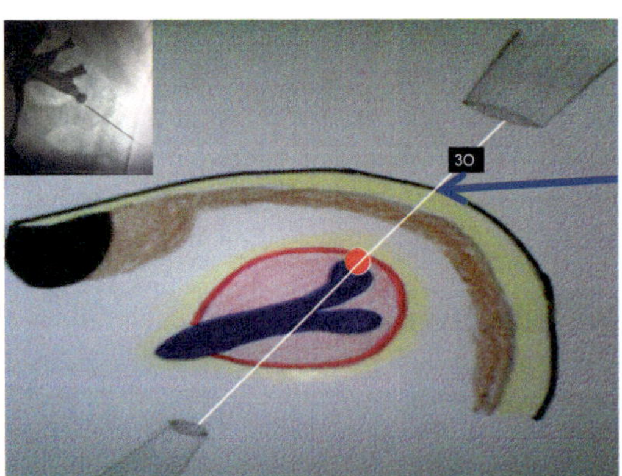


**Fig. 9.53** When the needle tip is just positioned on the skin surface, (Blue arrow) indicating the target calyx, and C arm is activated, it appears in the obtained image on fluoroscopic monitor (inset) as if the needle tip has already reached up to the target calyx. Actual distance between needle tip on the skin and the target calyx (depth) cannot be appreciated in this image. C arm needs to be shifted to another location to appreciate this distance

should not hide away the calculi altogether. At the same time, pelvicalyceal system should get well opacified to render easy identification of anatomical details of the infundibuli, calyces, and fornices. In the beginning, contrast should be diluted by 50% (10 ml contrast and 10 ml saline). 10 to 15 ml of this diluted contrast is then filled in a 20 ml syringe and this syringe is placed on the patient's back. Stone and this contrast filled syringe are visualized under C arm image, together in one frame to compare their respective densities (Fig. 9.56). Contrast is diluted further with saline to the extent that it becomes slightly less dense or at par with the density of the stone, when seen and compared in one frame on fluoroscopic image. This much dilution of contrast, when injected, does not hide away the stone completely.

After proper positioning of the C arm, with 30 degrees tilt, tip of the needle is placed on the

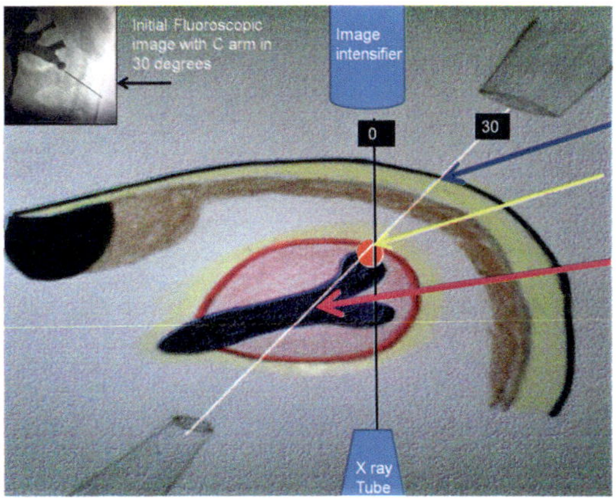


**Fig. 9.54** With the C arm tilted at 30 degrees, if a needle tip gets positioned anywhere on the imaginary line (white) between X-ray tube and image intensifier, it appears in the obtained image on fluoroscopic monitor that the needle tip has exactly reached up to the target calyx (Insert). Now, leaving the needle wherever it is, if the C arm is brought to 0 degree position, and a new image is obtained, the actual superficial or posterior needle (Blue) is seen lateral to the target calyx, while the actual deeper or anterior needle (Red) is seen medial to the target calyx, in the new image. The position of the needle, which is exactly on the target (Yellow), remains absolutely unchanged in both the images, whether C arm is in 30 degrees or 0 degree position

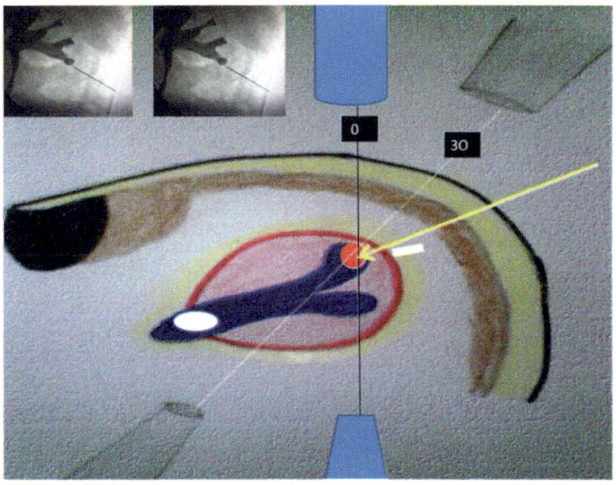


**Fig. 9.55** When an accurate puncture is achieved, the needle tip is noted exactly within the target calyx in both the fluoroscopic images obtained in 30 and 0 degree positions of C arm. If the gradual descent technique is followed, this puncture gets obtained through Brodel's avascular white line and the access falls very well in alignment with the infundibulum, so that the track remains straight and there occurs no torque of the renal parenchyma, while accessing and removing the stones from within pelvicalyceal system

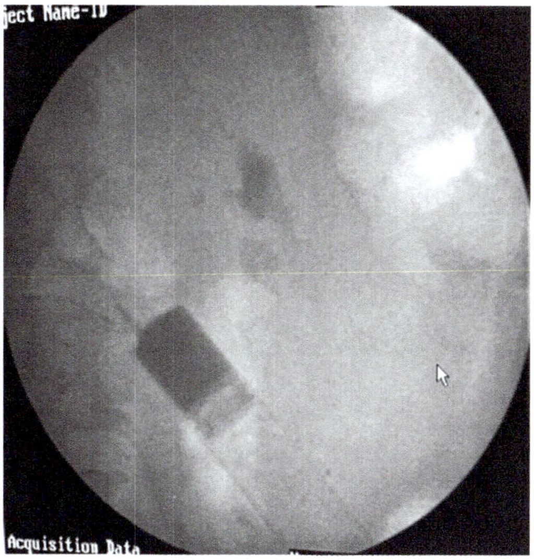


**Fig. 9.56** Contrast filled syringe is brought under fluoroscopy to compare its density with that of stones

patient's back in such a way, that it is pointing to the bulk of the stone (Fig. 9.57). Well diluted contrast is then injected through ureteric catheter very slowly, while continuous monitoring the inflow of contrast into PCS, till the preselected calyx for initial puncture gets adequately opacified. If the filling of target calyx with contrast is very slow, delayed, or obstructed at this time, a very free and fast egress of saline cannot be expected during initial puncture. This happens when bulk and orientation of stone or blood clot, stone matrix or thick pus within PCS does not allow free filling of the target calyx through ureteric catheter, with contrast. In fact, minimum amount of well diluted contrast should be injected in the beginning under direct fluoroscopic control, through already placed ureteric catheter just to adequately opacify the pelvicalyceal system and for orientation for the location of calculi and planning of access. Once PCS gets opacified, needle is adjusted and repositioned on the back of the patient to bring it in direct straight alignment with the infundibulum of the targeted calyx (Fig. 9.58). First passage of the needle is going to dictate the direction and alignment of the track through which fragments of stone are going to be

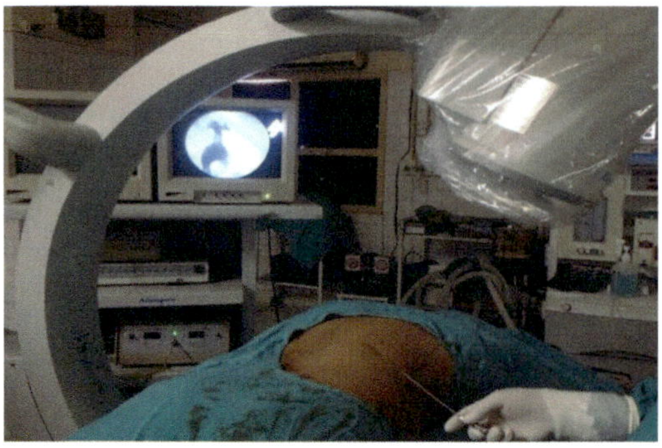

**Fig. 9.57** Tip of the needle is placed on the patient's back in such a way, that it is pointing to the bulk of the stone. Well diluted contrast is then injected through ureteric catheter very slowly

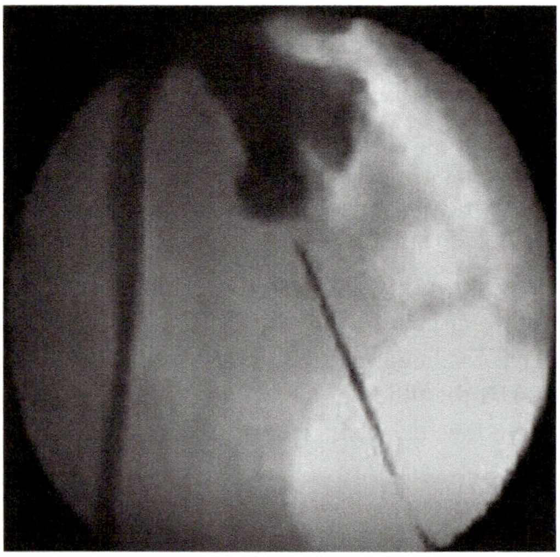

**Fig. 9.58** Correct alignment with the infundibulum will create a straight track for smooth torque free extraction of calculi

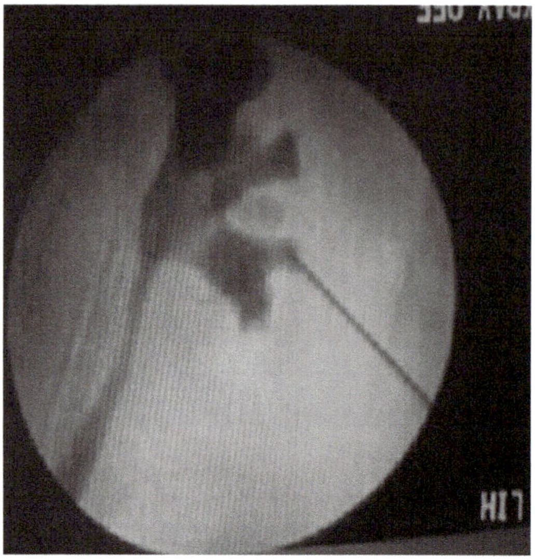

**Fig. 9.59** Needle should be brought in correct alignment with the infundibulum so as to create a straight track. This needle placement needs to be corrected

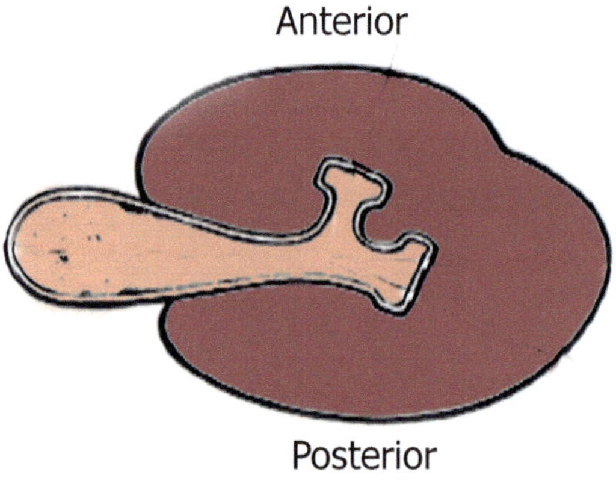


**Fig. 9.60** In Brodel type of kidneys posterior calyces are extending laterally

retrieved throughout the course of PCNL. It should be as straight and aligned to the infundibulum as possible, so that there is no repeated torquing of renal parenchyma and therefore oblique, non-aligned approach to the calyx as shown in Fig. 9.59 should not be accepted.

## 9.10 Which Calyx to Puncture: Anterior or Posterior

This is the most controversial issue during fluoroscopic access. Traditionally since the introduction of PCNL, renal access through posterior calyx has been advocated by most of the researchers [6, 7]. Various techniques have been recommended for confident identification of posterior calyx including injection of air through ureteric catheter. In fact, Brodel had studied corrosion casts of 70 cadaveric kidneys in 1901. He had mentioned that all posterior calyces are lateral calyces (Fig. 9.60) [8]. This concept remained unchallenged for more than 70 years. It was naturally conceived that laterally oriented posterior calyces will be ideal for gaining renal access with patient in prone position and hence all efforts were being made for proper identification of posterior calyces only, for this purpose.

Further, some studies started creating some difference of opinions. Hodson studied calyceal anatomy and classified calyces as anterior and posterior, only on the basis of IVU images in 1972 [9]. He mentioned just the opposite, that all the posterior calyces are medial in location and anterior calyces are located laterally (Fig. 9.61).

In 1984, Kaye and Reinke [10] took the help of CT images, which is the modality of choice to actually identify anterior or posterior calyces. They concluded that Brodel type of kidneys with posterior calyces being lateral (Fig. 9.60) are seen predominantly on the right side (69%), while Hodson type of kidneys with anterior calyces being lateral (Fig. 9.61) are seen predominantly on the left side (70%).

Sampaio FJ studied endocasts and published several articles from 1987 to 2001 [3, 11, 12]. He mentioned that true anterior and posterior orientation of calyces depends upon the region. Superior pole almost always has a compound calyx which drains into pelvis through single midline infundibulum in 98.6% cases. At middle pole, in 96% of cases, calyces are arranged in paired form as anterior and posterior and drain into pelvis independently. At lower pole, only in 58% cases true anterior and posterior orientation of calyces is maintained. In 42% cases at lower pole, calyceal orientation is very variable, superimposed or alternately distributed.

Miller et al. 2013 [13] mentioned that at superior pole, calyces are typically oriented in lateral and medial disposition to each other rather than in anterior and posterior orientation. Hwang TK (2010) advised to access only lateral calyx at superior pole because medial calyceal access is associated with injury to posterior segmental artery [14]. Eisner BH et al. (2009) studied the lower pole anatomy by analysing CT Scans of 101 units. They found out that lower poles are drained either through two or through three calyces. When there are two draining calyces, medial calyx is oriented anteriorly in 95% of cases and lateral calyx is oriented posteriorly in 93% of cases. When three calyces are draining lower pole, the most medial calyx is oriented anteriorly (93%), middle one is oriented posteriorly (70%), and lateral calyx is again oriented anteriorly in 71% of cases. In 31% cases, no calyx was truly posterior [15].

This must be appreciated here that there exists great variation in anterior or posterior orientation of the calyces and nothing can be assumed with certainty in a given case. Moreover, exact anterior or posterior orientation of calyx gets identified in the transverse section of CT image as is evident in Fig. 9.62. This cannot be appreciated in IVU films (Figs. 9.63 and 9.64) or even in coronal sections of CT images (Fig. 9.65).

At present, we do not have availability of CT scan units in operation theatres to guide renal access and we have to depend upon the

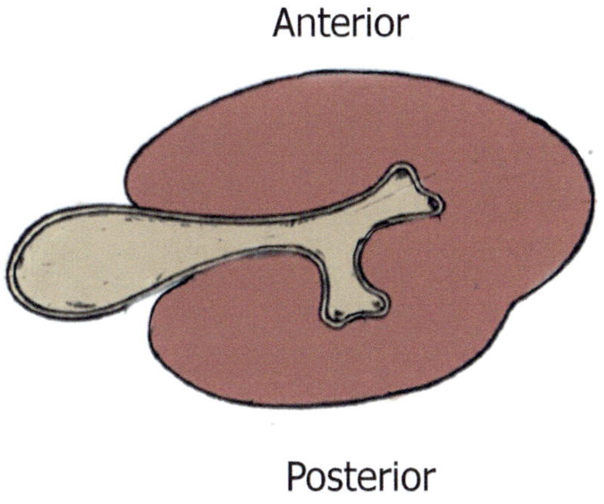


**Fig. 9.61** In Hodson type of kidneys, anterior calyces are extending laterally

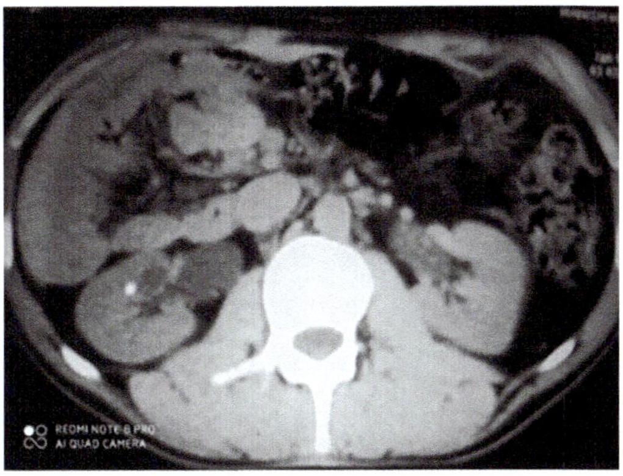

**Fig. 9.62** Only transverse sections of CT images could conclusively demonstrate that this stone is lying in anterior calyx

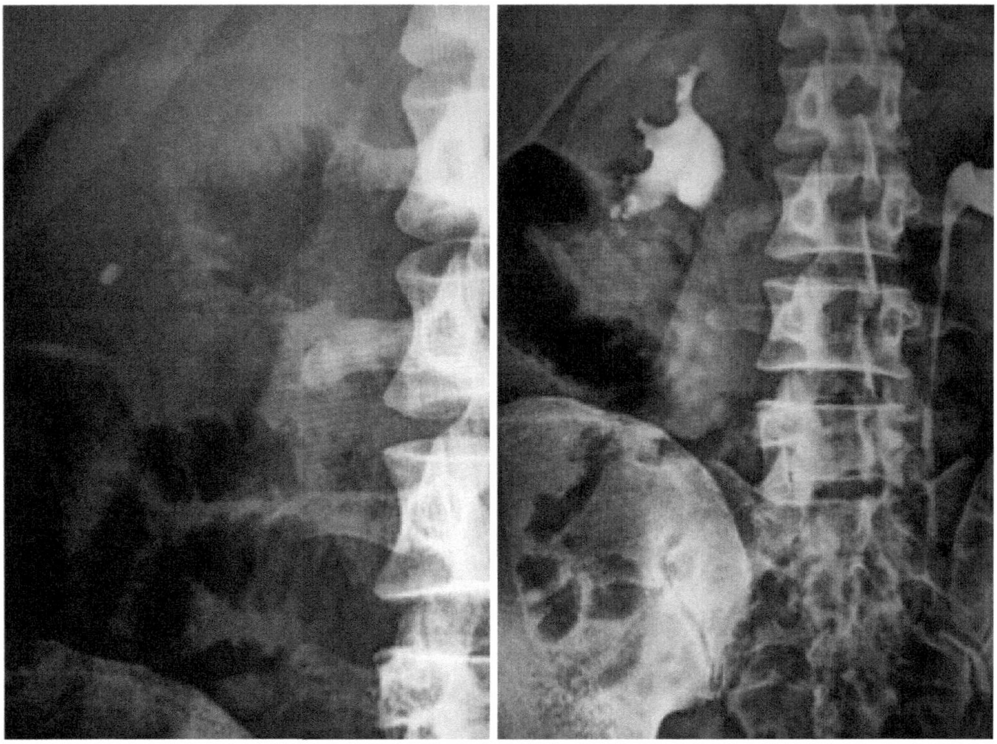

**Fig. 9.63** Presence of stone in anterior or posterior calyx cannot be identified in X-ray KUB and IVU films

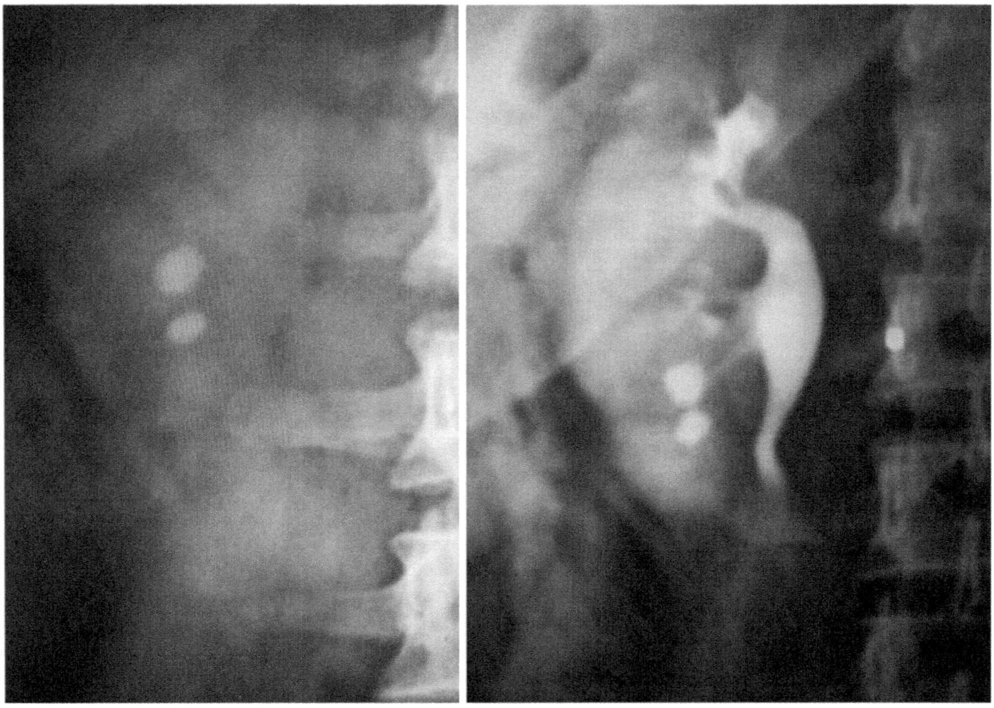

**Fig. 9.64** It is impossible to conclude decisively by studying X-ray KUB and IVU films, as to which calyx is anterior and which one is posterior. Exactly same situation is encountered during PCNL, when only two-dimensional fluoroscopic guidance is available

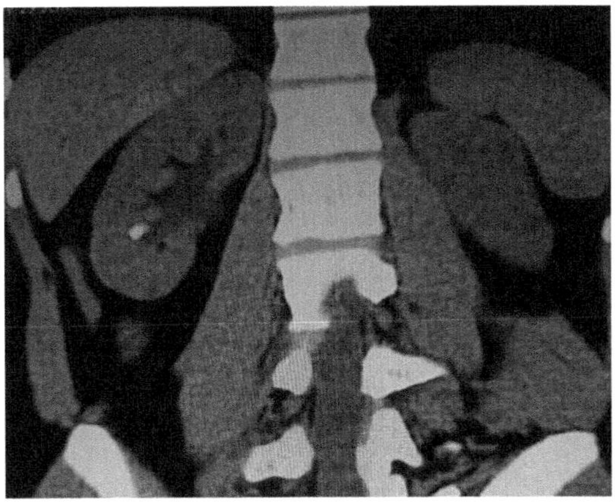

**Fig. 9.65** Presence of stone in anterior or posterior calyx cannot be identified in coronal sections of CT images

two-dimensional fluoroscopic images of C arm radiological units only. Taking all above into consideration, author has always been suggesting, neither to designate any preferred calyx for renal access preoperatively, nor to make any efforts to selectively identify anterior or posterior calyx for renal access. It is advisable to choose *most peripheral calyx* with thinnest renal parenchyma over it, which is leading towards the stone bulk in straight alignment and has a wide infundibulum to work through. In case, there exists an associated calyceal calculus anywhere, the stone bearing calyx must be accessed first, be anterior or posterior to be able to remove all stones through single tract. Proper calyceal puncture of stone bearing calyx has been achieved is confirmed by slight movement of the stone/stones by the needle tip, passage of guide wire or by injecting small quantity of saline and watching slight movement of the stone/stones under fluoroscopy.

## 9.11 Renal Access Techniques

### 9.11.1 Bull's Eye Technique

This is by far the simplest of all techniques for percutaneous renal access. It only requires skills to maintain whole length of initial puncture needle in the same straight line throughout its progress from the skin up to the target calyx. This straight line is an imaginary line (white line in Fig. 9.66) between X-ray tube and the image intensifier passing through the target.

The C arm may be positioned in any way during bull's eye puncture, but the more accurate anatomical position looking straight at the target through convex border of the kidney is achieved, when C arm is positioned with 30 degrees tilt towards the operating surgeon (Fig. 9.67).

In bull's eye technique, the surgeon is expected to maintain the needle tip, whole length of the needle, and the needle hub in same straight line between the X-ray tube and image intensifier and therefore superimposed on each other throughout, till the needle tip hits the target calyx. At no time the longitudinal segment of the needle should appear on the fluoroscopic screen. If the needle is being manipulated and pushed with the hand, there occurs lots of radiation exposure to the hand of the operator, in Bull's eye technique (Fig. 9.66). Most of the surgeons following Bull's eye technique for initial puncture use a sponge forceps, haemostat, or a radiolucent needle holder to avoid undue radiation exposure to their hands.

If C arm remains in the same position throughout (monoplanar approach), it is not possible to assess the depth of the puncture and the needle tip may overshoot and go through and through the target calyx and beyond, without being appreciated. Hence, the C arm should be rotated to another position every now and then (biplanar approach) to assess the depth of the needle achieved so far and the remaining distance between the approaching needle tip and the target calyx.

If renal access is achieved with Bull's eye technique, keeping the C arm in 0 degree position, as shown in Fig. 9.66, this provides a straight vertical entry of the needle and subsequent track into the targeted calyx. This remains the vertical segment of the subsequent track from the skin up to the calyx. The length of this vertical segment depends upon the skin to calyx distance. Further extension of the track into pelvicalyceal system (PCS) through infundibulum and up to the renal pelvis may not be in the same straight line and in alignment. Hence, when a rigid nephroscope is advanced up to the stone in the pelvis, there is a

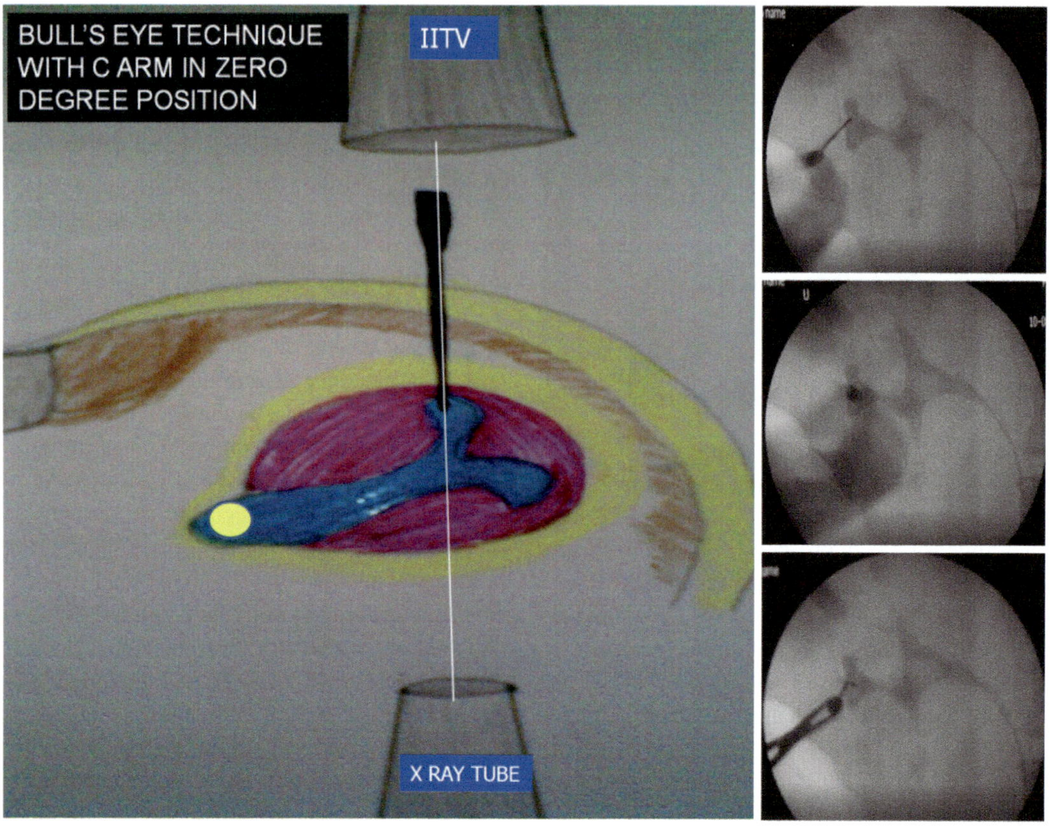


**Fig. 9.66** In bull's eye technique, the surgeon is expected to maintain the needle tip, whole length of the needle, and the needle hub in same straight line between the X-ray tube and image intensifier and therefore superimposed on each other throughout. It is advisable to use some instrument to advance the needle to prevent radiation exposure to hands

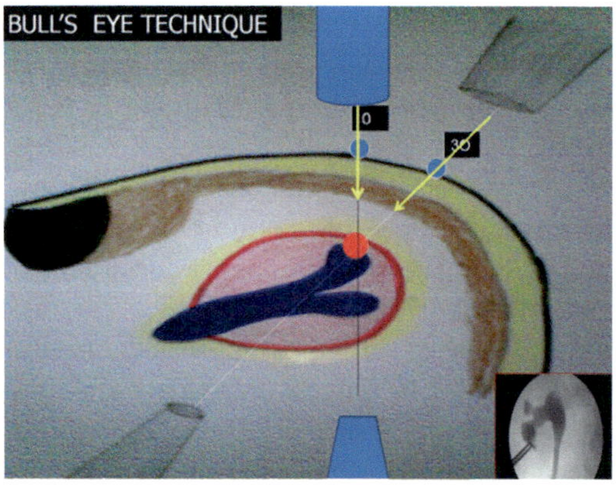


**Fig. 9.67** Renal access with Bull's eye technique can be obtained with C arm either in 0 degree position or in 30 degrees position

point of torque and angulation at the entrance of the calyx, which may result in parenchymal tear and bleeding complication. All tracks made with Bull's eye technique with C arm at 0 degree position tend to enter the renal parenchyma on a more medial location (Fig. 9.68) as compared to the tracks made with gradual descent technique. Medial portion of renal parenchyma tends to be more vascular as compared to the lateral part and hence it is likely to produce more bleeding.

Lastly, these tracks are almost verical tracts (Fig. 9.69) and every stone fragmet has to be picked up and removed with the help of a forceps. Gravity and forceful irrigation are of no help for expulsion of stone fragments through such tracks.

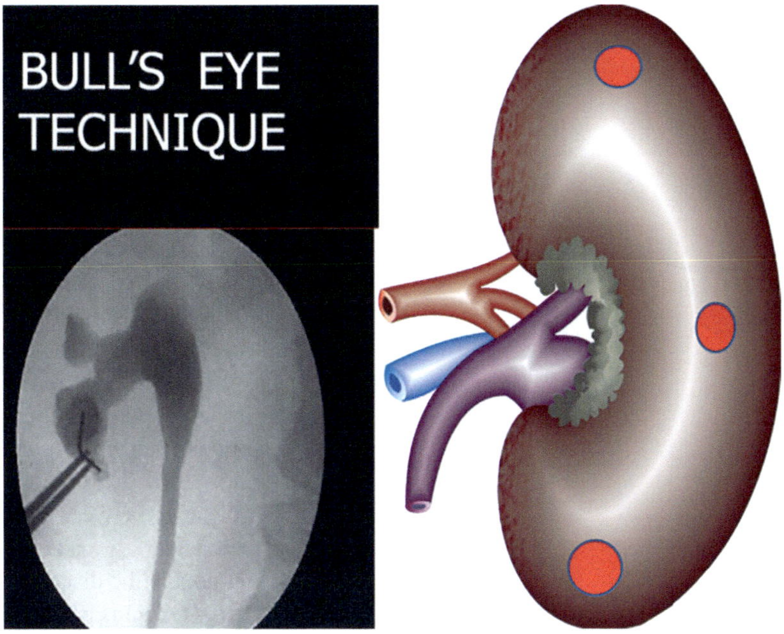


**Fig. 9.68** All tracks made with Bull's eye technique tend to be entering the renal parenchyma on a more medial location

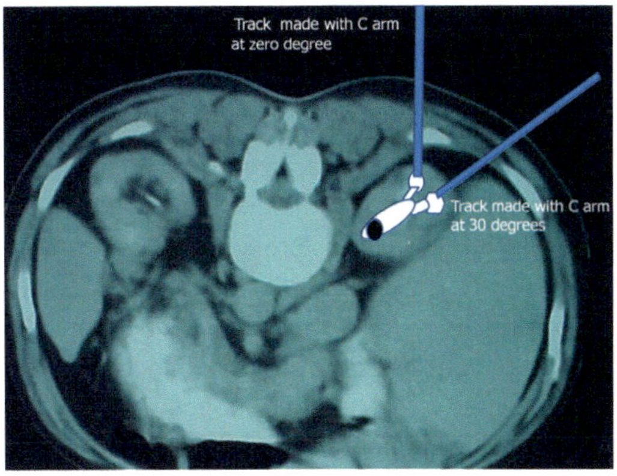


**Fig. 9.69** All tracks made with Bull's eye technique with C arm at 0 degree position tend to be entering the renal parenchyma on a more medial location, as compared to the tracks made with gradual descent technique with C arm at 30 degrees tilted position

### 9.11.2 Triangulation Technique

This technique of gaining access into PCS is based on mathematical trigonometric principles. An imaginary right-angled triangle is created, considering the back of the patient as flat surface. While the patient is in prone position and C arm is in 0 degree position, a mark is made on the skin surface (Point A) corresponding to the target calyx (Fig. 9.70).

Now the C arm is tilted 30 degrees with image intensifier tilting towards the urosurgeon. Another mark is made on the patient's back (point B) corresponding to the target calyx. Target calyx itself is now considered as the third point (point C) of the imaginary triangle (Fig. 9.70). On analysing this triangle, it becomes obvious that angle BAC is of 90 degrees, qualifying it to be considered as a right-angled triangle. Line BC becomes the hypotenuse (line opposite to the right angle and longest line) of this triangle. Another angle ACB is of 30 degrees, because C arm was tilted by an angle of 30 degrees. So, this becomes a 90-30-60 degrees right-angled triangle, in which length of the short arm AB and all the three angles are known. Pythagoras theorem applies on such triangles and exact length of the other two arms AC and BC can easily be calculated. AC is the depth of the target calyx from point A (with C arm in 0 degree position) and BC is the depth of the target calyx from point B (with C arm in 30 degrees tilted position).

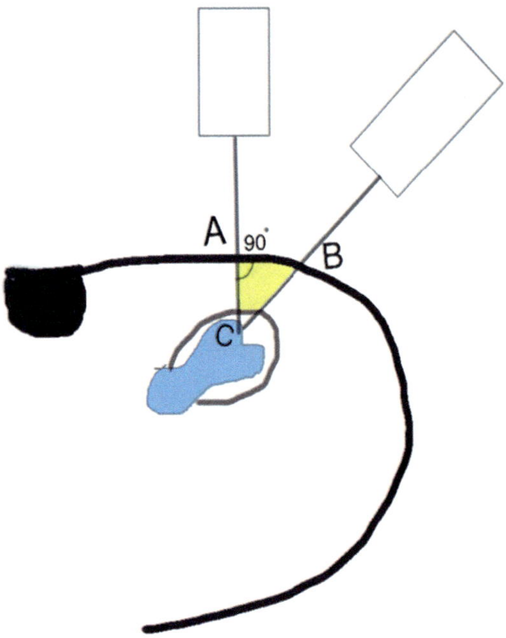


**Fig. 9.70** While the patient is in prone position and C arm is in 0 degree position, a mark is made on the skin surface (Point A) corresponding to the target calyx. Now the C arm is tilted 30 degrees and another mark is made on the patient's back (point B) corresponding to the target calyx. Target calyx itself is now considered as the third point (point C) of the imaginary triangle. On analysing this triangle, it becomes obvious that angle BAC is of 90 degrees, qualifying it to be considered as a right-angled triangle. Line BC becomes the hypotenuse (Line opposite to the right angle and longest line) of this triangle. Another angle ACB is of 30 degrees and as per sine trigonometric function line BC (depth of target) will be twice the length of line AB (difference between two points) in such a triangle

On applying sine trigonometric function

- Sin ACB = sin 30
- = Opposite side of 30 degrees angle (AB)/ Hypotenuse (opposite side of 90 degrees angle (BC) = 1/2
- = AB/BC = 1/2
- Hence BC (Depth of target) = 2 AB

This mathematically calculates the length of line BC (actual depth of the target from the skin) to be twice of the length of line AB (distance between the marks on the patient's back). These mathematical calculations have now predetermined the depth of the target calyx. Now, if the needle is appropriately marked as per calculations and skin puncture is initiated at 30 degrees mark (point B) and needle is continuously maintained at 30 degrees angle on the trajectory as in Bull's eye technique, it should hit the target exactly, when the predetermined depth is reached.

Similar calculations can be made by turning the C arm to 45 degrees (possible in very few C arm units available). If sin ACB = sin 45, then line BC will be 1.414 times of line AB [16].

Practically, most of the urosurgeons following triangulation technique mark two points A and B on the skin, corresponding to target calyx with C arm in 0 degree and 30 degrees, respectively. Distance between these two points is measured and a mark is made on the initial puncture needle at double the distance from the tip of the needle. Now C arm is positioned at 0 degree but the skin puncture is made at previously marked point B, corresponding to target with C arm in 30 degrees position. Needle is advanced strictly at 30 degrees angle with or without the guidance of protractor, till the mark, towards the target calyx, intermittently watching the trajectory under fluoroscopy. If correct angulation is maintained throughout, it hits the target calyx properly. This method requires strict maintenance of exact 30 degrees trajectory throughout the passage of the needle and any slight deviation during the course will not allow the exact hit at the target. This method may not be suitable for supine PCNL.

Significant advantage of triangulation technique over Bull's eye technique is the lower radiation exposure to the hands of the surgeon compared to the Bull's eye technique, which is straightforward and easy to learn by a novice surgeon as per the European Section of Urotechnology [17]. Another salient feature of this technique is that the angle and depth of puncture and thereby the needle trajectory are easily predetermined without the need for sophisticated instrumentation or complex calculations. The theoretical disadvantage of this technique is the fixed angle of puncture, which may not be possible in malrotated kidneys or applicable to all sorts of body contours and habitus.

### 9.11.3 Gradual Descent Technique

This technique is considered similar to landing of an aeroplane onto a runway in a straight and smoothly descending fashion. This technique has been named and popularized by the author. This technique provides minimum bleeding complications as all efforts are made to gain entry through convex border of the kidney into the target calyx through its most lateral aspect, gradually and smoothly traversing the distance from the skin up to the calyx in straight, smoothly descending fashion and in correct alignment with the respective infundibulum ahead, so as not to produce any points of angulation and torque at the renal parenchyma or at the level of infundibulum till the main bulk of the stone. Since the point of puncture into renal parenchyma is at Brodel's avascular line at the convex border of the kidney, it is likely to produce minimum amount of blood loss (Fig. 9.71). Since, hands of the urosurgeon, guiding and pushing the needle do not come in the operative field, there is minimal radiation exposure to the hands.

In this technique, C arm is initially positioned with a 30 degrees tilt towards the operator and image intensifier close to the head of the operator (Fig. 9.72). By such positioning of C arm, X-ray tube shifts far away from the operating team thereby reducing the radiation exposure. This positioning also provides a head-on sighting of the convex border of the kidney for gaining access into PCS. Most peripheral calyx with thinnest overlying renal parenchyma is then identified after slow filling of PCS by diluted contrast. Maximum importance is given to choose that particular calyx, which is leading straight to the

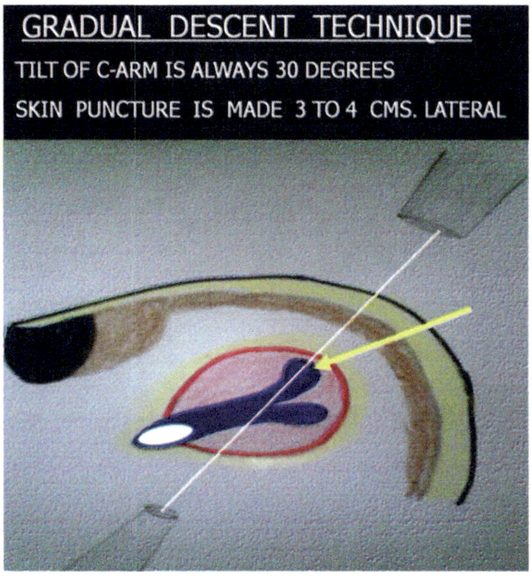


**Fig. 9.72** After positioning C arm at 30 degrees skin puncture is made 3 to 4 cm lateral to the target calyx and needle is gradually advanced towards the cup of the calyx

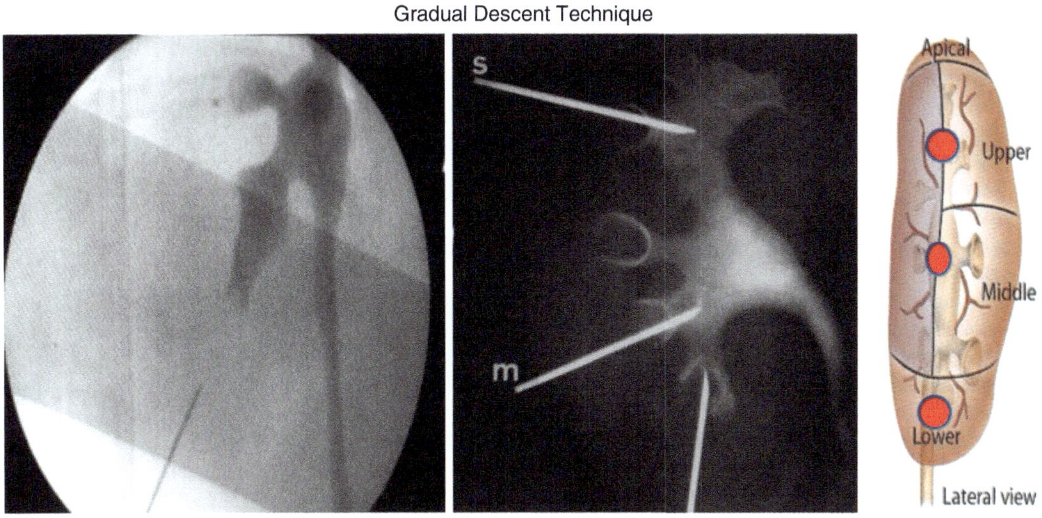


**Fig. 9.71** In gradual descent technique, the needle makes its entry into the renal parenchyma through its most lateral aspect (Brodel's white line), thereby producing minimal bleeding complications

major bulk of the stone and has a wide infundibulum. Now needle tip is positioned on the skin surface at the back at the site of lateral border of the targeted calyx and length of the needle is aligned in direction of straight line to the centre of the infundibulum ahead (Fig. 9.73). This line may be marked on the skin surface.

Now a point of skin puncture is chosen on this line, 3 to 5 cm lateral to the lateral border of targeted calyx, but still medial to the posterior axillary line. Skin puncture is made here and needle is advanced towards the targeted calyx in slow gradual manner. Thus landing into the targeted calyx, from skin surface is begun, 3 to 5 cm lateral and then this distance is utilized in slow gradual descent, straight towards the targeted calyx (Figs. 9.74 and 9.75).

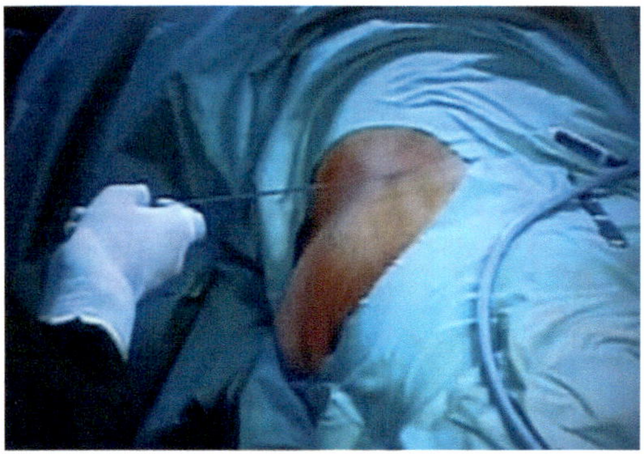

**Fig. 9.73** Needle is placed on the back of the patient in such a way that needle tip is visualized in the cup of the targeted calyx and length of the needle is in correct alignment with the centre of the infundibulum ahead. This line may be marked on the skin surface

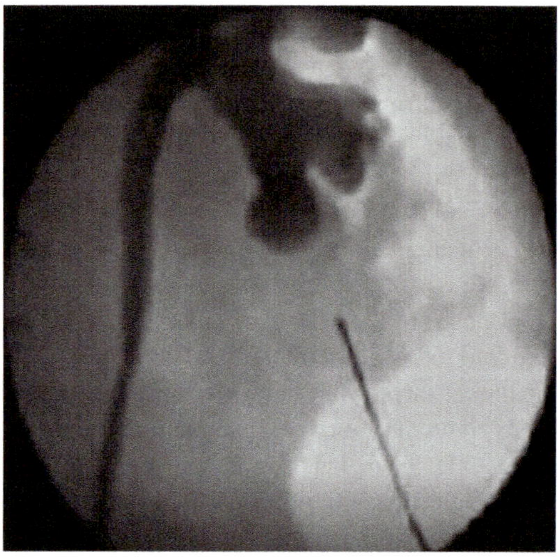

**Fig. 9.75** In gradual descent technique, a point of skin puncture is chosen, 3 to 5 cm. Lateral to the lateral border of targeted calyx. Skin puncture is made here and needle is then advanced in slow gradual manner, descending down towards the targeted calyx

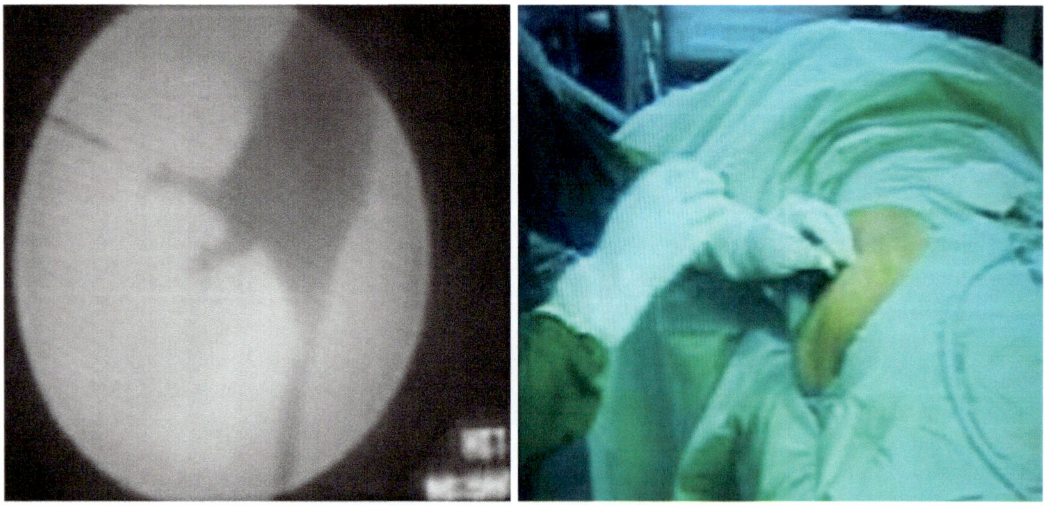

**Fig. 9.74** Now a point of skin puncture is chosen on this line, 3 to 5 cm. Lateral to the lateral border of targeted calyx. Skin puncture is made here and needle is advanced towards the targeted calyx in slow gradual manner with jerky movements

The angle of entry and progress through subcutaneous fat and muscle layers depends upon the built and thickness of individual patient. Female and thick built fatty patients are likely to have thick posterior bulk of Gerota's fascia and kidneys are likely to be situated more deeper from the back. Therefore, the angle of entry will be more (30 to 40 degrees) to reach to the target. In contrast, male patients, thin individuals, and children are likely to have a thin layer of Gerota's fascia and in previously operated patients also, kidneys are likely to be adherent or closer to the posterior abdominal wall. In such cases, the angle of entry will be less (approx. 10 to 25 degrees) to reach to the target. In any case, when the point of skin entry is far lateral, and then the further progress of the needle is also manipulated by holding the needle near its hub at a distance, radiation exposure to the hands of the operator gets minimized. In this technique, since kidney is being approached at its most convex border, special care is taken to avoid injury to the colon in the vicinity. Needle is advanced very gradually towards the kidney in jerky movements, observing the movements of gas shadows outlining the colon, continuously (Fig. 9.75). At any point if colonic gas shadows start moving in unison with the advancing needle, it is removed in toto immediately and skin puncture site is shifted to a more medial location on the same line. Obviously, when skin puncture site gets shifted more medially, the angle of entry needs to be increased to cover the same distance accordingly.

Once the needle tip reaches up to the distance of 1 to 1.5 cm from the target calyx, it is expected to have punctured the overlying renal parenchyma and now the whole kidney should start moving in jerks along with jerky movements of the progressing needle (Fig. 9.76). If the needle is progressing further with absolute accuracy towards the fornix of the target calyx, a clear indentation in the cup of the calyx can be well appreciated. Now, the needle is left in situ with its tip within the target calyx (Fig. 9.77) and C arm is rotated to 0 degree position. Needle tip is constantly observed while the C arm is being repositioned to 0 degree, for its movement.

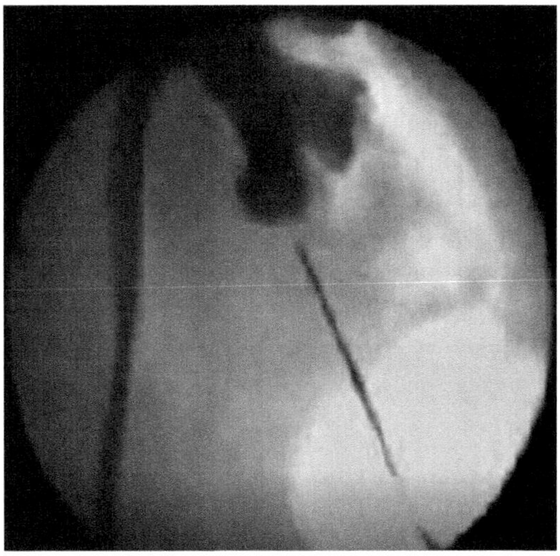

**Fig. 9.76** Once the needle tip reaches up to the distance of 1 to 1.5 cm from the target calyx, it is expected to have punctured the overlying renal parenchyma and now the whole kidney should start moving in jerks along with jerky movements of the progressing needle

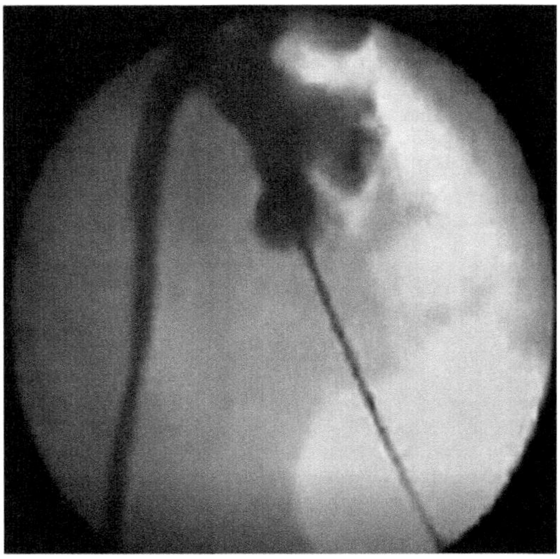

**Fig. 9.77** If the needle is in accurate position, a clear indentation in the cup of the calyx can be well appreciated. Now, the needle is left in situ and C arm is rotated to 0 degree position. If the needle tip constantly remains in the same position accurate puncture has been achieved

If the needle tip, which was seen in the middle of the calyx with C arm in 30 degrees position (Fig. 9.78), now starts moving lateral to the target calyx with the C arm being shifted to 0 degree position (Fig. 9.79), the needle tip is superficial or posterior to the target. The needle needs to be withdrawn up to subcutaneous plane, and angle of entry has to be increased for the next attempt. C arm should be brought back to 30 degrees position and needle should make another straight landing into the target calyx with higher degree of angulation than previous attempt.

If the needle tip, which was seen in the middle of the calyx with C arm in 30 degrees position (Fig. 9.80), now starts moving medial to the target calyx with the C arm being shifted to 0 degree position (Fig. 9.81), the needle tip has gone deeper or anterior to the target. The needle needs to be withdrawn up to subcutaneous plane, and angle of entry has to be decreased for the next attempt. C

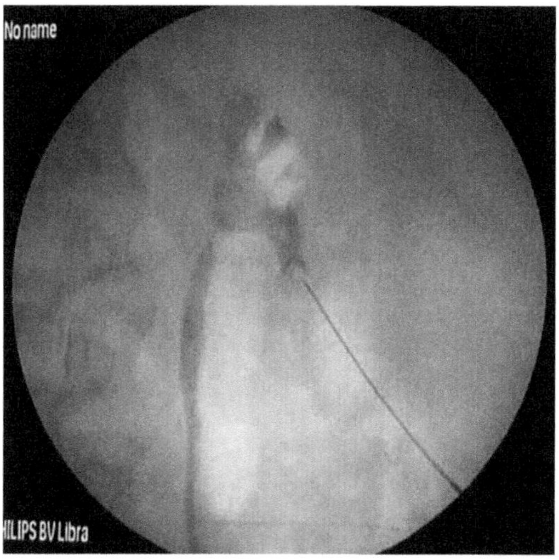


**Fig. 9.78** With C arm in 30 degrees position, needle tip is seen in the cup of the calyx

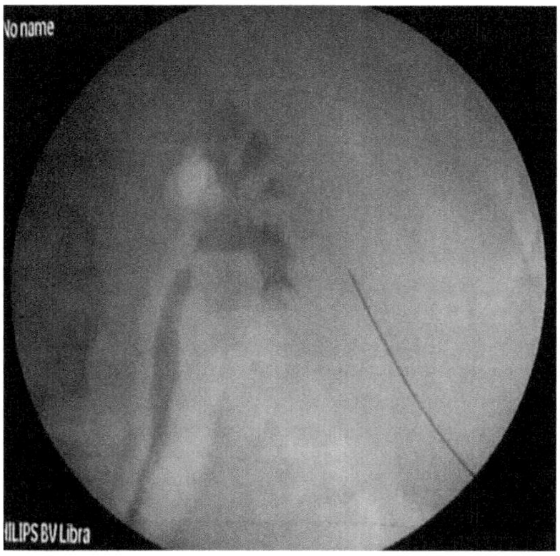


**Fig. 9.79** By shifting C arm to 0 degree position, needle tip is seen moving lateral to the target calyx. It confirms that needle is superficial or posterior to the target

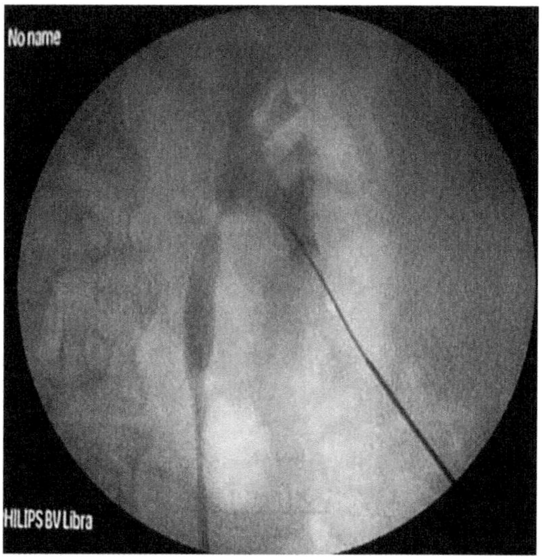


**Fig. 9.80** With C arm in 30 degrees position, needle tip is seen well within the lower calyx

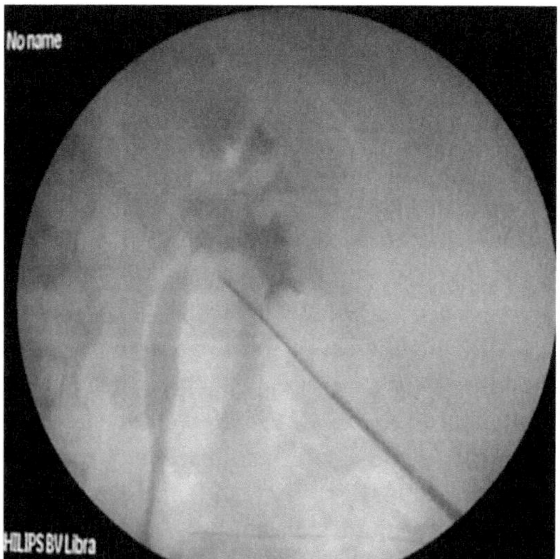


**Fig. 9.81** By shifting C arm to 0 degree position, needle tip is seen shifting medial to the target calyx. It confirms that needle is deeper or anterior to the target

arm should be brought back to 30 degrees position and needle should make another straight landing into the target calyx with corresponding lower degree of angulation.

If the needle tip, which was seen in the middle of the calyx with C arm in 30 degrees position, remains at the same place within the target calyx and does not change its position with the C arm being shifted to 0 degree position, the needle tip is exactly at the target and successful puncture has been achieved. The stylet should be removed and clear efflux of saline can be witnessed.

At times, it needs slight adjustments and corrections in angulation to bring the needle in alignment with the infundibulum so as to get the free efflux of saline injected through ureteric catheter.

At times, needle tip gets slightly advanced across the calyx, through and through and enters the anterior renal parenchyma and small amount of bloody efflux is noted in the beginning. Withdrawl of needle by 1 to 2 mm while simultaneously maintaining gentle suction with 2 ml syringe helps repositioning of needle tip in the space of PCS and smooth flow of saline gets established. Presence of blood clot, thick pus, stone matrix, or tiny stones may not allow a free flow of saline to get established and alternate aspiration and injection of 1 to 2 ml of saline through needle in the same position will solve the problem.

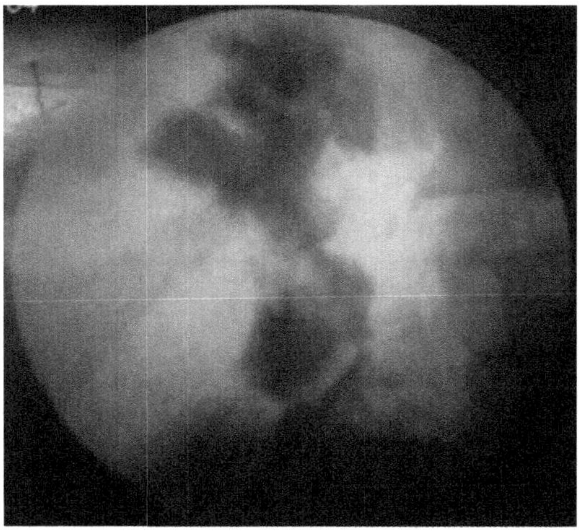

**Fig. 9.82** Contrast extravasation during percutaneous access makes it difficult to identify a selected calyx

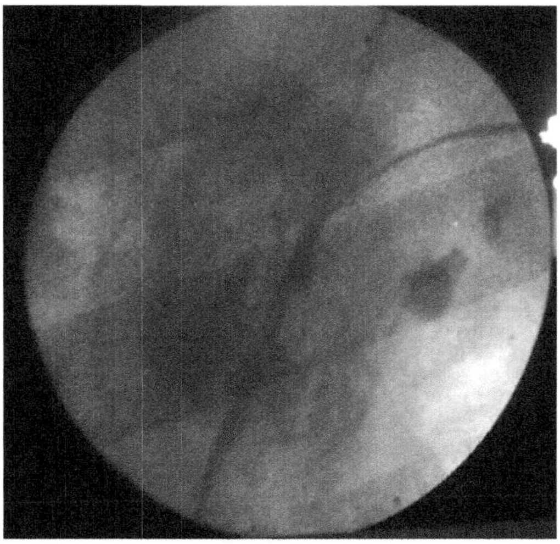

**Fig. 9.83** Accidental contrast extravasation

## 9.12 Troubleshooting during Renal Access

### 9.12.1 Extravasation of Contrast (Figs. 9.82 and 9.83)

**Causes**

1. Rapid injection of high volume of contrast with higher pressure in PCS (Normal capacity of undilated PCS is 5 to 8 ml only).
2. Improper placement of ureteric catheter may happen in cases where impacted calculus at PUJ does not allow free passage of guide wire or ureteric catheter and manipulations are undertaken with an oedematous mucosa around. Ureteric catheter or guide wire may raise a submucosal tunnel (Fig. 9.84). At times even straight tip guide wire may cause perforation and go beyond the confines of PCS (Fig. 9.85). If ureteric catheter is threaded over such a guide wire, extravasation is bound to happen. This will go unrecognized till contrast is instilled.
3. During several attempts of initial puncture, if PCS was accessed and punctured successfully in one or more attempts but needle was removed from PCS due to any reason, further injection of contrast will lead to extravasation.

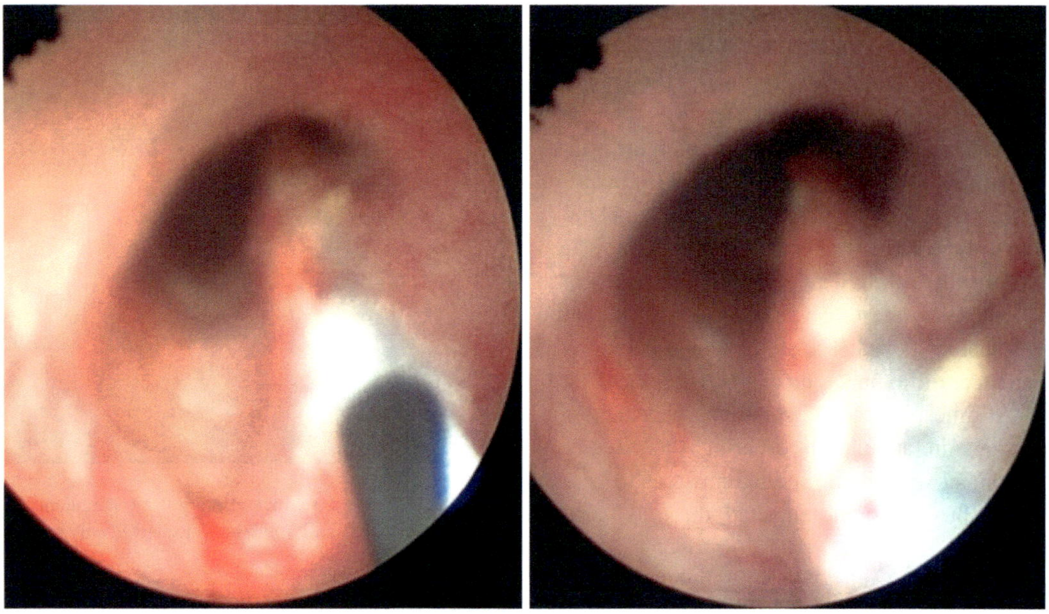

**Fig. 9.84** Creation of submucosal tunnel during passage of Cobra guide wire

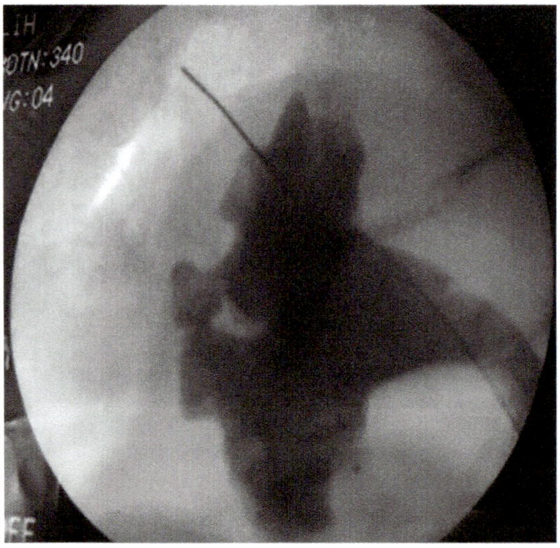

**Fig. 9.85** Perforation and passage of proximal 3 cm length of Cobra guide wire, outside the pelvicalyceal system

**Remedial Measures**

1. In case, contrast is found to be extravasating, further injection must be stopped immediately. Small quantity of saline should be injected. Waiting for 5 to 15 min dilutes the extravasated contrast to some extent. Giving diuretics during this time may also be of some help. Now, ureteric catheter should be withdrawn very slowly under fluoroscopic guidance to pull it down to bring it back within PCS, at PUJ, just below the probable site of perforation, distal to the stone or in upper ureter as the situation may be. Further, saline should be injected in small aliquots and return dripping of saline should be observed from ureteric catheter. Return dripping of saline is a good indicator of presence of tip of ureteric catheter within PCS. Once, reasonable surety of tip of ureteric catheter within upper ureter or PCS gets established, slightly higher concentration of contrast is injected this time, just to adequately opacify the target calyx within already extravasated contrast. Thus, this manoeuvre of injecting much diluted contrast in the beginning and higher concentration of contrast subsequently gives a second chance to the operating surgeon to identify and access the target calyx.
2. If extravasated contrast is not disappearing and remains dark enough to obscure the anatomy of PCS, ureteric catheter must be pulled down by 2 to 6 cm, to the level, where one feels confident that, it must be within PCS or may be in upper ureter. Then first bolus of 5 to

15 ml of saline is injected so as to distend the PCS, and then immediately a new Terumo glide wire is passed. Progress of guide wire is watched. It should reach up to superior or middle calyx and then should coil and take a turn backwards. If this happens, it should be left in situ.

Now a Bull's eye puncture is made *in the coil of guide wire*, while saline is being injected freely through ureteric catheter. Once, reasonably free outflow of saline from puncturing needle is obtained, contrast is injected through this needle and PCS gets opacified adequately.

3. At times stone guided punctures are helpful in such situation.
4. Ultrasound guided puncture is another good alternative.
5. Air pyelogram may also be considered for obtaining access in such situation.
6. Abandoning the procedure and postponing for 48 hours or more is the last option.

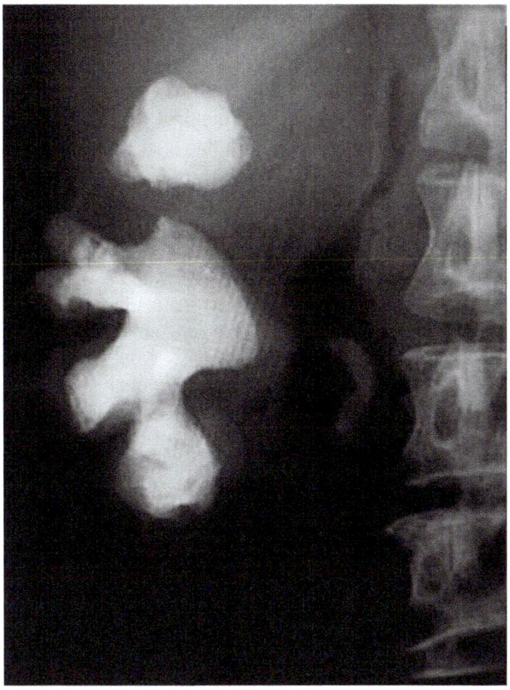

**Fig. 9.86** Staghorn stone filling up all the calyces, rendering placement of guide wire difficult

### 9.12.2 Inability to Pass Guide Wire

**Causes**

At times it becomes impossible to introduce and park a guide wire in PCS in cases where calyx is completely filled up with the bulk of the stone and no free space is available (Fig. 9.86).

**Remedial Measures**

1. Terumo hydrophilic guide wires are supposed to be very slippery and flexible. It is possible that these guide wires may prove to be of some help in these situations.
2. Pelvicalyceal system should be distended adequately with retrograde injection of saline so as to create some space between the mucosa and the filling stone. Now the needle hub is bent downwards, while the needle tip is maintained at the same place, thereby giving the direction to the guide wire to slide over the back of the stone and enter the PCS. This manoeuvre has proved to be extremely useful for successful placement of guide wire in PCS (Fig. 9.87).

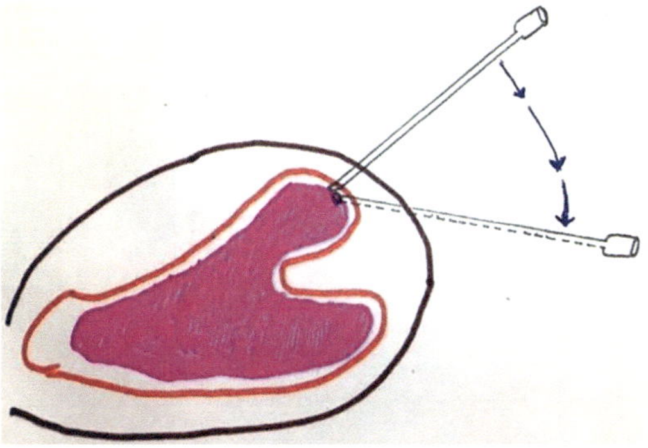

**Fig. 9.87** Tilting the initial puncture needle downwards and directing the guide wire to slide over the back of the stone to advance within pelvicalyceal system may solve the problem

## References


1. Fernstrom I, Johansson B. Percutaneous pyelolithotomy. A new extraction technique. Scand J Urol Nephrol. 1976;10:257–9.
2. Hwang TK, Seo SI. Percutaneous access for urological disease. In: Baba S, Ono Y, editors. Recent advances in endourology. 8th ed. Japan: Springer; 2006. p. 25–39.

3. Sampaio FJ, Mandarim-De-Lacerda CA, De Aragão AH. [The collector system of the kidney. Applied anatomy based on the analysis of 3-dimensional casts]. J Urol (Paris). 1987;93:183–5 (PMID: 3680967).
4. Hopper KD, Sherman JL, Luethke JM, Ghaed N. The retrorenal colon in the supine and prone patient. Radiology. 1987;162:443–6.
5. Sagalovich D, Besa C, Tran TY, Thummar H, Le Grand B, Taouli B, Gupta M. Prone percutaneous nephrolithotomy: does bolster orientation matter? Urology. 2017;108:46–51. https://doi.org/10.1016/j.urology.2017.07.005. Epub 2017 Jul 18
6. Miller NL, Matlaga BR, Lingemann JE. Technique for fluoroscopic percutaneous renal access. J Urol. 2007;178:15–23. https://doi.org/10.1016/j.juro.2007.03.01. (PMID: 17574053)
7. Ko R, Soucy F, Denstedt JD, Razvi H. Percutaneous nephrolithotomy made easier: a practical guide, tips and tricks. BJU Int. 2008;101:535–9. https://doi.org/10.1111/J1464-410X.2007.07259.x. (PMID: 17922862)
8. Schultheiss D, Engel RM, Crosby RW, Lees GP, Truss MC, Jonas U. Max Brodel (1870–1941) and medical illustration in urology. J Urol. 2000;164:1137–42. https://doi.org/10.1016/S0022-5347(05)67128-5. (PMID: 10992353)
9. Settlage J. Derek Hodson: teaching and learning about science: language, theories, methods, history, traditions and value. Sci & Educ. 2011;20:393–6. https://doi.org/10.1007/s11191-010-9266-7.
10. Kaye KW, Reinke DB. Detailed caliceal anatomy for endourology. J Urol. 1984;132:1085–8. (PMID: 6502793)
11. Sampaio FJ. Renal anatomy. Endourologic considerations. Urol Clin North Am. 2000;27:585–607. https://doi.org/10.1016/S0094-0143(05)70109-9.
12. Sampaio FJ. Renal collecting system anatomy: its possible role in the effectiveness of renal stone treatment. Curr Opin Urol. 2001;11:359–66. https://doi.org/10.1097/00042307-200107000-00004. (PMID: 11429494)
13. Miller J, Durack JC, Sorensen MD, Wang JH, Stoller ML. Renal calyceal anatomy characterization with 3-dimensional in vivo computerized tomography imaging. J Urol. 2013;189:562–7. https://doi.org/10.1016/j.juro.2012.09.040. (PMID: 23260557)
14. Hwang TK. Percutaneous nephroscopic surgery. Korean J Urol. 2010;51:298–307. https://doi.org/10.4111/kju.2010.51.5.298. (PMID: 20495691)
15. Eisner BH, Cloyd J, Stoller ML. Lower-pole fluoroscopy-guided percutaneous renal access: which calix is posterior? J Endourol. 2009;23:1621–5.
16. Darlington D, Chinnathambi J, Jamburaj A, et al. Trigonometric concept of fluoroscopy-guided percutaneous renal access. Cureus. 2020 June 25;12(6):e8817. https://doi.org/10.7759/cureus.8817.
17. Kyriazis I, Liatsikos E, Sopilidis O, Kallidonis P, Skolarikos A. European section of urotechnology educational video on fluoroscopic guided puncture in percutaneous nephrolithotomy: all techniques step by step. BJU Int. 2017;120:739–41. https://doi.org/10.1111/bju.13894.

# 10 USG-guided Puncture in Mini-PCNL

Thomas Knoll and Nabil Atassi

## 10.1 Introduction

Establishment of the renal access is one, if not the key point in the success of a PCNL [1]. It is achieved by an exact and proper puncture of the collecting system of the kidney. Once established, the success of the procedure in terms of Stone-Free Rate (SFR) and safety can be significantly increased [2]. The use of ultrasonography for access in PCNL was first described in the 1970s. Since then, its efficacy, safety, and feasibility were demonstrated with sufficient literature-based data [3]. Ultrasonography-guided access alone as well as an intraoperative combined ultrasonography–fluoroscopy-guided access implicates the advantage of a more adequate puncture and fewer access-related complications [4]. Regarding ultrasound-guided access, Stone-Free Rates are comparable with the positive effect of a lower complication rate [5–7]. The identification of surrounding organs is possible and nearby eliminates the risk of inadvertent organ injuries [8]. Ultrasonography guidance of the renal puncture has various advantages: It is real time, safe, and rapid in experienced hands, suitable in case of renal failure, as the use of nephrotoxic contrast medium is unnecessary. It is free of radiation for patients including children and pregnant women and operating personnel [9–11]. Ultrasonography-guided access is safe for the experienced surgeon, SFR, and safety increases significantly after a learning curve of a minimum of 20 interventions [12, 13]. During that learning curve of younger surgeons, Ultrasonography-guided access showed to be as well safe and feasible [14]. So, there are a lot of good reasons to perform the puncture of the collecting system as the first step during the intervention by the surgeon itself instead of leaving it to the radiologist as it is common in some countries, considering that there is no significant difference in success between access obtained by either an interventional radiologist or a urologist [15]. Regarding dilatation of the renal tract, few data is available showing that it can be safely performed by ultrasound guidance with equal efficacy and safety compared to fluoroscopic guidance [16]. Disadvantages in ultrasonography-alone guided puncture can be the difficulty to puncture non-dilated collecting systems and sometimes poor visualization of the guidewire and even the puncture needle itself [17]. This problem can be resolved by the placement of a ureteral catheter and injection of saline solution with or without a contrast agent [8, 18]. Latest studies assessed the feasibility of contrast-enhanced ultrasound for non-dilated kidneys in percutaneous nephrolithotomy with promising results that need to be further validated.

T. Knoll (✉) · N. Atassi
Department of Urology, Klinikum Sindelfingen, Böblingen, Germany
e-mail: T.Knoll@klinikverbund-suedwest.de; N.Atassi@klinikverbund-suedwest.de


M. S. Agrawal et al. (eds.), *Minimally Invasive Percutaneous Nephrolithotomy*,
https://doi.org/10.1007/978-981-16-6001-6_10

## 10.2 Principles of Ultrasound for Renal Access

Ultrasonography-guided access can be performed safely both in prone and supine positions [19–21]. The safest access to the renal collecting system is a long and posterior lower calyx, as it is at the closest distance to the skin and has less risk of interference with other structures such as surrounding organs [18, 22]. In some cases, due to the location of the stone, an upper-pole puncture might be needed and can also be safely performed by ultrasonography guidance [23]. The first step in preoperative planning of the procedure is to identify the ideal target calyx and to obtain three-dimensional knowledge of the kidney and the stone. It is essential to understand the anatomical location of the kidney: It is located anterior to the psoas muscle, between the 12th thoracic vertebral body and the second/third lumbar vertebral body. Both kidneys are within the retroperitoneum at approximately 30° posterior to the frontal plane of the body (Figs. 10.1 and 10.2). Access to the kidney is always established individually according to the particular anatomy. Frequently, the ribs or the iliac crest limit the space for access. In these cases, the area has to be shifted a few degrees (caudally or cranially 10–20°) [24]. The ideal puncture passes through the extension of a renal

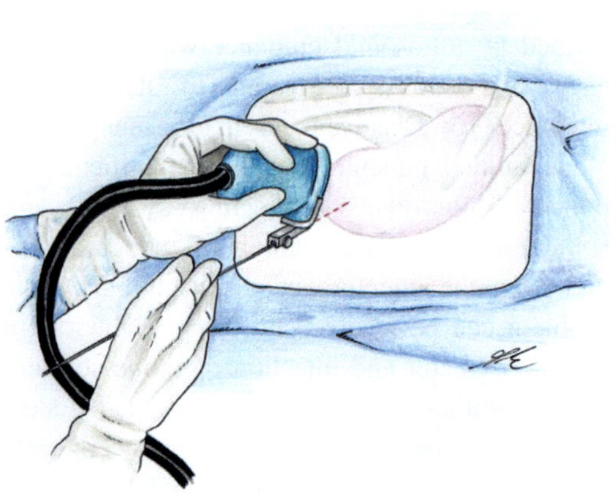

**Fig. 10.1** Determination of the puncture site and direction

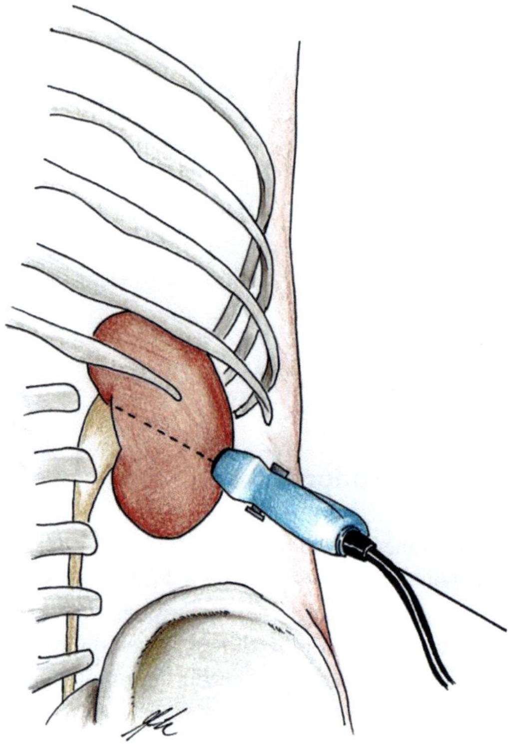

**Fig. 10.2** Positioning of the US probe for puncture of the lower calyx

calyceal papilla (Fig. 10.1). The puncture site direction is determined to be as close as possible from the calyx to the skin. The procedure may be facilitated by using a diuretic to dilate the calyx [25]. The ultrasonography scanner has to be moved laterally within the defined puncture plane until the access calyx points directly toward the scanner (Fig. 10.3). An electronically generated puncture line (depends on the device used) that indicates in the longer axis of the needle guidance adapter helps find the right puncturing line and angle. It is intended to puncture the avascular zone in the center of the calyx. This is achieved by moving the scanner head laterally on the predefined puncture plane while keeping the scanning plane within the predefined puncture plane (Fig. 10.1). The image will change until the access calyx points directly toward the scanner head (Fig. 10.4). This is the least traumatic and nearly avascular path through

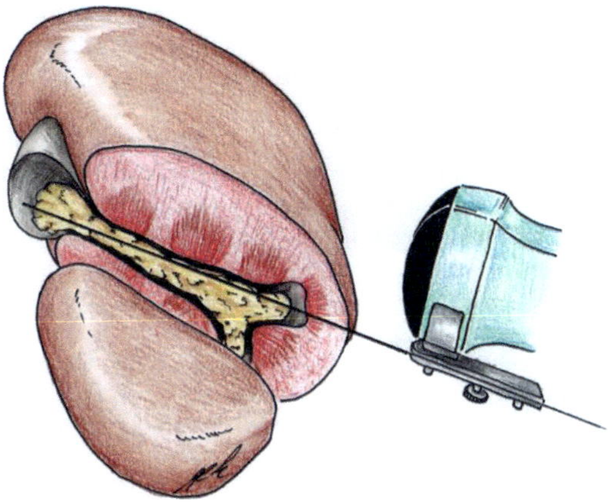

**Fig. 10.3** Puncture direction of the needle

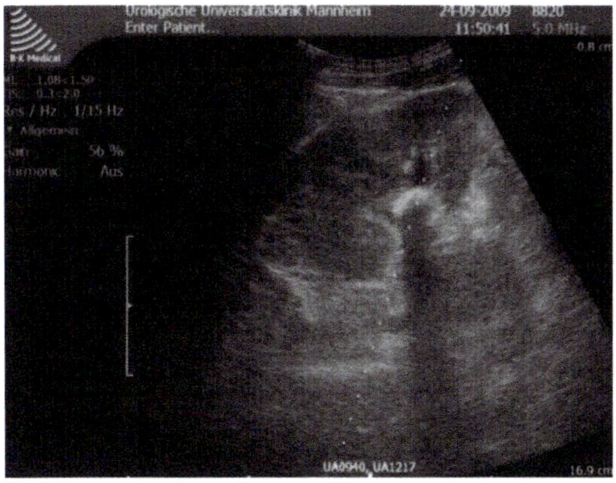

**Fig. 10.4** Ultrasound picture: Puncture direction of the needle

the kidney parenchyma and the calyx to the renal pelvis [Knoll/Michel et al.]. The use of a needle guidance adapter is not mandatory, a freehand puncture can also be performed. Using the needle guidance adapter may be advantageous for the beginner, but one has to consider, that the needle can be deflected from the predefined path due to different tissue consistencies. Freehand puncture allows easier detection and correction of the needle's direction. To correct the needle's direction, it has to be moved outside the kidney, sometimes even out of the skin. Once the direction of the puncture inside the kidney is defined, it should be finished. The needle can be followed until it reaches the calyx by ultrasound. The success of the puncture can be verified by urine flow through the inner part of the hollow needle. In those the stone completely fills the target calyx, this effect will not appear. The direction of the puncture will then directly target the stone [24]. Haptic confirmation of stone contact can be useful to assure the optimal position of the needle tip. Ultrasonography also allows the use of Doppler Mode to visualize renal vasculature. It can facilitate the needle puncture without causing injury to significant vessels [26]. There also is first data indicating that contrast-enhanced ultrasound (CEUS) could be valuable for percutaneous nephrolithotomy in a non-dilated kidney improving visibility and facilitating the selection of suitable calyx for puncture [27].

## 10.3 Technique of Combined Ultrasound-fluoroscopy Guided Access

Regarding and interpreting the recent status-quo of available data, the ideal imaging technique in percutaneous access for (Mini-)PCNL seems to be a combination of ultrasonography and fluoroscopic guidance, especially for more complex stones [6, 18]. While simpler stones seem to be accessible with ultrasound-alone guidance with no radiation at all, more complex stone treatment shows better outcomes using a combined access [28]. The combined approach increases the accuracy of the puncture and decreases the radiation exposure for patients, surgeons, and nurses [29]. Practically, determination of the target calyx and puncture plane, puncture site, and puncture direction moves in the long axis of the target calyx: The best way to identify is by fluoroscopy. In particular, an initial puncture under ultrasound guidance in a fluoroscopy suite appears to be the best modality for percutaneous access in percutaneous nephrolithotomy [30]. Especially for inexperienced surgeons during the learning curve, the combined access surely is an additional safeguard to visualize the collecting system with the help of fluoroscopic guidance. The surgeon's experience in any way is fundamental in choosing the best modality for percutaneous access.

## References


1. Knoll T, Daels F, Desai J, Hoznek A, et al. Percutaneous nephrolithotomy: technique. World J Urol. 2017;35:1361–8. https://doi.org/10.1007/s00345-017-2001-0.
2. Iordache A, Baston C, Guler-Margaritis SS, et al. Ultrasound for kidney access in percutaneous nephrolithotomy: a contemporary review. Med Ultrason. 2018;20(4):508–14. https://doi.org/10.11152/mu-1618.
3. Basiri A, Ziaee AM, Kianian HR, Mehrabi S, Karami H, Moghaddam SM. Ultrasonographic versus fluoroscopic access for percutaneous nephrolithotomy: a randomized clinical trial. J Endourol. 2008;22:281–4.
4. Hudnall M, Usawachintachit M, Metzler I, et al. Ultrasound guidance reduces percutaneous nephrolithotomy cost compared to fluoroscopy. Urology. 2017;103:52–8. https://doi.org/10.1016/j.urology.2016.12.030.
5. Yang YH, Wen YC, Chen KC, Chen C. Ultrasound-guided versus fluoroscopy-guided percutaneous nephrolithotomy: a systematic review and meta-analysis. World J Urol. 2019;37(5):777–88. https://doi.org/10.1007/s00345-018-2443-z.
6. Andonian S, Scoffone CM, Louie MK, et al. Does imaging modality used for percutaneous renal access make a difference? A matched case analysis. J Endourol. 2013;27(1):24–8. https://doi.org/10.1089/end.2012.0347.
7. Corrales M, Doizi S, Barghouthy Y, Kamkoum H, Somani BK, Traxer O. Ultrasound or fluoroscopy for PCNL access, is there really a difference? J Endourol. 2020;35(3):241–8. https://doi.org/10.1089/end.2020.0672.
8. Ng FC, Yam WL, Lim TYB, Teo JK, Ng KK, Lim SK. Ultrasound-guided percutaneous nephrolithotomy: advantages and limitations. Investig Clin Urol. 2017;58(5):346–52. https://doi.org/10.4111/icu.2017.58.5.346.
9. Osman M, Wendt-Nordahl G, Heger K, et al. Percutaneous nephrolithotomy with ultrasonography-guided renal access: experience from over 300 cases. BJU Int. 2005;96:875–8.
10. Falahatkar S, Allahkhah A, Kazemzadeh M, Enshaei A, Shakiba M, Moghaddas F. Complete supine PCNL: ultrasound vs. fluoroscopic guided: a randomized clinical trial. Int Braz J Urol. 2016;42(4):710–6.
11. Hong Y, Ye H, Yang B, et al. Ultrasound-guided minimally invasive percutaneous nephrolithotomy is effective in the management of pediatric upper ureteral and renal stones. J Investig Surg. 2020;34(10):1078–82.
12. Usawachintachit M, Masic S, Allen IE, Li J, Chi T. Adopting ultrasound guidance for prone percutaneous nephrolithotomy: evaluating the learning curve for the experienced surgeon. J Endourol. 2016;30(8):856–63. https://doi.org/10.1089/end.2016.0241.
13. Song Y, Ma Y, Song Y, Fei X. Evaluating the learning curve for percutaneous nephrolithotomy under total ultrasound guidance. Hills RK, editor. PLoS One. 2015;10(8):e0132986.
14. Jessen JP, Honeck P, Knoll T, Wendt-Nordahl G. Percutaneous nephrolithotomy under combined sonographic/radiologic guided puncture: results of a learning curve using the modified Clavien grading system. World J Urol. 2013;31(6):1599–603. https://doi.org/10.1007/s00345-012-1016-9.
15. Armitage JN, Withington J, Fowler S, et al. Percutaneous nephrolithotomy access by urologist or interventional radiologist: practice and outcomes in the UK. BJU Int. 2017;119(6):913–8. https://doi.org/10.1111/bju.13817.
16. Armas-Phan M, Tzou DT, Bayne DB, Wiener SV, Stoller ML, Chi T. Ultrasound guidance can be used safely for renal tract dilatation during percutaneous nephrolithotomy. BJU Int. 2020;125(2):284–91. https://doi.org/10.1111/bju.14737.
17. Chu C, Masic S, Usawachintachit M, et al. Ultrasound guided renal access for percutaneous nephrolithotomy: a description of three novel ultrasound-guided needle techniques. J Endourol. 2016;30:153–8.
18. Agarwal M, Agrawal MS, Jaiswal A, Kumar D, Yadav H, Lavania P. Safety and efficacy of ultrasonography as an adjunct to fluoroscopy for renal access in percutaneous nephrolithotomy (PCNL). BJU Int. 2011;108(8):1346–9.
19. Birowo P, Raharja PAR, Putra HWK, Rustandi R, Atmoko W, Rasyid N. X-ray-free ultrasound-guided percutaneous nephrolithotomy in supine position using Alken metal telescoping dilators in a large kidney stone: a case report. Res Rep Urol. 2020;12:287–93.
20. Karami H, Rezaei A, Mohammadhosseini M, Javanmard B, Mazloomfard M, Lotfi B. Ultrasonography-guided percutaneous nephrolithotomy in the flank position versus fluoroscopy-guided percutaneous nephrolithotomy in the prone position: a comparative study. J Endourol. 2010;24(8):1357–61.
21. El-Shaer W, Kandeel W, Abdel-Lateef S, Torky A, Elshaer A. Complete ultrasound-guided percutaneous nephrolithotomy in prone and supine positions: a randomized controlled study. Urology. 2019;128:31–7. https://doi.org/10.1016/j.urology.2019.03.004.
22. Desai M. Ultrasonography-guided punctures-with and without puncture guide. J Endourol. 2009;23(10):1641–3.
23. Sahan A, Cubuk A, Ozkaptan O, et al. Safety of upper pole puncture in percutaneous nephrolithotomy with the guidance of ultrasonography versus fluoroscopy: a comparative study. Urol Int. 2020;104(9–10):769–74. https://doi.org/10.1159/000509448.
24. Knoll T, Michel MS, Alken P. Percutaneous nephrolithotomy: the Mannheim technique. BJU Int. 2007;99:213–31.

25. Gupta S, Gulati M, Suri S. Ultrasound-guided percutaneous nephrostomy in non-dilated pelvicaliceal system. J Clin Ultrasound. 2016;26(3):177–9.
26. Tzeng BC, Wang CJ, Huang SW, Chang CH. Doppler ultrasound-guided percutaneous nephrolithotomy: a prospective randomized study. Urology. 2011;78:535–9.
27. Guo X, Zhang Z, Liu Z, et al. Assessment of the contrast-enhanced ultrasound in percutaneous nephrolithotomy for the treatment of patients with non-dilated collecting system [published online ahead of print, 2020 Sep 16]. J Endourol. 2020; https://doi.org/10.1089/end.2020.0564.
28. Zhu W, Li J, Yuan J, et al. A prospective and randomised trial comparing fluoroscopic, total ultrasonographic, and combined guidance for renal access in mini-percutaneous nephrolithotomy. BJU Int. 2017;119(4):612–8. https://doi.org/10.1111/bju.13703.
29. Baralo B, Samson P, Hoenig D, Smith A. Percutaneous kidney stone surgery and radiation exposure: a review. Asian J Urol. 2020;7(1):10–7. https://doi.org/10.1016/j.ajur.2019.03.007.
30. Wang Y, Jiang F, Hou Y, et al. Doppler ultrasound and X-ray-guided percutaneous nephrolithotomy with one-step balloon dilation for complex renal stones. Urol Int. 2013;91(3):326–30. https://doi.org/10.1159/000350522.

# 11 Newer Advances in Access

Jean de la Rosette, Amir H. Kashi, and Saman Farshid

Percutaneous nephrolithotomy (PCNL) was introduced almost four decades ago by Fernstrom and Johansson [1] and revolutionized the treatment for renal stones. While PCNL has undergone significant developments in instrumentation and technique during the past decade it still maintains to follow the same principles initially laid down. PCNL can be categorized into three phases of access, dilation, and nephroscopy. The access phase has been repeatedly declared as the most important and difficult phase of PCNL and in the opinion of many urologists, a key step in operation success [2–4]. Therefore, many studies have focused on the improvement of the access phase to be quicker, more accurate, and with fewer complications. Fluoroscopy has been used for more than four decades as the main guidance modality in PCNL and its advantages of disadvantages have been extensively explored and disclosed. The CROES study revealed that fluoroscopy is the major imaging modality in 87% of patients [5]. Modern c-ARM devices produce more accurate images with relatively less irradiation resulting in better functionality in the operating room. Nevertheless, fluoroscopy imaging is associated with some inherent disadvantages not yet resolved by technology improvements.

Radiation is a key concern for physicians and personnel. Several studies have evaluated radiation dose in PCNL and most studies have revealed a total yearly radiation dose less than the maximum allowed doses [6]. However, there are concerns about non-dose-dependent adverse effects of radiation and there are also concerns on radiation for high-risk patients including children and pregnant women in whom radiation should be minimized and optimally excluded at all [7]. The adverse effects of radiation received in the diagnosis, treatment, and follow-up are cumulative and every attempt to reduce radiation dose in each phase is valuable [8]. The quality of the image in radiation-based systems is dependent on the amount of radiation emitted [9] and for better image quality, more radiation should be emitted. Another disadvantage of conventional fluoroscopy is the failure to reveal soft tissue information including organs in the access tract [10]. Kidneys are in proximity to the liver, spleen, and pleura at their posterior surface and bowels at the lateral borders. Therefore, posterior access to kidneys risks injury to the aforementioned organs. Retro-renal colon is a recognized

J. de la Rosette (✉)
Department of Urology, Medipol Mega University Hospital, Istanbul Medipol University, Istanbul, Turkey

A. H. Kashi
Urology and Nephrology Research Center (UNRC), Shahid Labbafinejad Hospital, Shahid Beheshti University of Medical Sciences (SBMU), Tehran, Iran

S. Farshid
Clinical Research Development Unit, Imam Khomeini Hospital, Urumieh University of Medical Sciences, Urumieh, Iran


M. S. Agrawal et al. (eds.), *Minimally Invasive Percutaneous Nephrolithotomy*,
https://doi.org/10.1007/978-981-16-6001-6_11

anatomic variation in a small percentage of patients and failure of its preoperative diagnosis can result in considerable complications [11]. Conventional fluoroscopy fails to reveal any of these organs in the access tract and hence historically, the diagnosis of injury to these organs had been made postoperatively losing precious time for their management.

Opacification of the pelvicalyceal system by radio-opaque media is required for fluoroscopy-guided access and is performed by retrograde insertion of a ureteral catheter which is sometimes difficult due to neobladder, edema of the ureteral orifice, or bladder trabeculation with severe diverticula formation. Also, in the case of contrast extravasation, fluoroscopy-guided access will be faced with difficulties. Supine, prone, lateral, or a combination of these positions has been described for patient positioning in PCNL; however, in patients with skeletal deformities resulting in overlap of renal stone with vertebrae, fluoroscopy access will be difficult in many of these positions. In addition, fluoroscopy produces 2D images and estimation of needle depth is based on additional fluoroscopy by rotating the c-ARM to caudal, cranial, or lateral positions. This maneuver is less able to reveal the depth of the needle in relation to target the calyx in case of a dilated caliceal system or multiple calices as a result of caliceal overlapping. Identification of the posterior calyx is not perfect with fluoroscopy imaging.

These shortages have caused fluoroscopy to be recognized as a suboptimal guidance modality for percutaneous renal access (PRA) and a continuous search to find better guidance methods to quicken access with more accuracy and fewer complications.

The importance of these becomes greater as PCNL is confronting powerful rivals in recent years like retrograde intrarenal surgery. If the accuracy and safety of PCNL are not improved and its complications are not significantly minimized, PCNL is doomed to the same destiny as we have witnessed for shock wave lithotripsy.

One of the oldest substitutes for fluoroscopy-guided PCNL has been the use of ultrasonography for only the access obtaining phase or the total process of percutaneous access and tract dilation. The experience with ultrasonography-guided access is more than two decades and its safety and efficacy in comparison with fluoroscopy have been established in several studies. A recent meta-analysis of randomized clinical trials comparing fluoroscopy versus ultrasonography showed encouraging results. This meta-analysis revealed that ultrasonography-guided PCNL was comparable with fluoroscopy-guided PCNL in all studied parameters except for Clavien grade II complications which were higher in the fluoroscopy-guided access [12].

The advantages of ultrasonography include disclosing organs in the access tract, absence of radiation, demonstration of posterior and anterior calices, and identification of some renal pathologies like renal cyst and obstructed calyx. Besides, ultrasonography is a continuous real-time imaging modality that reveals renal parenchyma and pelvicalyceal system and their adjacent organs in the access tract and can be continuously used until successful access is achieved without any concern for imaging time. Nonetheless, the adoption of ultrasonography has been slow and gradual due to several disadvantages. In obese patients and patients with a high skin-to-stone distance, the accuracy and precision of ultrasonography drops. Ultrasonography-guided access is more difficult with atrophic kidneys, and in patients with a history of renal surgery, there is the possibility of less accuracy in visualization of needle path and adjacent organs. The presence of gas, bone, and air in access pathway or pelvicalyceal system will result in the drop in image quality [13]. The resolution and spatial contrast of ultrasonography are limited. Ultrasound machines are not present in every operating room and working with them needs extensive education. Ultrasonography-guided puncture is sometimes difficult as the operator needs to visualize the needle path in the 2D ultrasound image which scans a limited width of tissue. A slight deviation of needle path due to tissue resistance can result in extrusion of the needle from the ultrasound screen or failure to access the target calyx [14].

The current gold standard in percutaneous renal access is a combination of fluoroscopy and ultrasonography guidance modalities to be able to reduce radiation dose and visualize access tract organs. Nevertheless, in addition to the above-mentioned disadvantages for ultrasonography and fluoroscopy, their learning curve is steep causing morbidity and complications during the learning phase [4].

There is still a constant search to find novel percutaneous guidance methods with higher precision and lower complications. It comes as no surprise that in recent years, various methods have been reported on. Some of these methods have only been examined in laboratory settings/scaffolds, and some in human or animal phantom models or in living animals. Only a few numbers have been examined on human subjects with renal stones. In the following sections, the most noticeable methods are presented.

## 11.1 Integrated Optical System in the Needle

An important consideration in percutaneous renal access is to be assured of proper entry into the pelvicalyceal system before dilation of the access tract. Perhaps the most secure method to ensure entry to the renal caliceal system and appropriateness of the entry site is direct visual inspection. Endoscopic control of the needle entry and access dilation has been described a long time ago and can be in an antegrade or retrograde fashion. The retrograde approach requires two surgeons for an operation and is performed most often in the supine position. This method will be explained in detail in the ECIRS section and will not be discussed here.

The antegrade approach was first reported by Bader and colleagues [15]. This approach consists of combined integrated optical and irrigation systems in a 1.6-mm needle (4.8F). This device is only slightly larger than a standard 18G needle (1.3 mm). They first evaluated the performance of this optical needle in 18 patients. Access was guided by ultrasonography and dilation with fluoroscopy. In 4/15 patients a second puncture was needed and in one patient the puncture failed to enter the target calyx. In 3/15 patients with entry into renal calyx, the guidewire could not be passed into another calyx or the ureter due to an inappropriate entry angle. The advantage of this method is that upon entry to the kidney, the appropriateness of entry site can be evaluated prior to dilation and to avoid dilation in case of suboptimal access. Besides, with the help of the optical needle, more expertise can be acquired in performing the percutaneous access since the needle path can be directly viewed. Nonetheless, the results of clinical studies did not yield ideal outcomes and primary access was successful only in 66% of instances. One of the main problems with this method is that the guidance modality is ultrasonography (or less commonly fluoroscopy) with their inherent inadequacies previously described. In addition, only after entry to the renal system the accuracy of entry can be evaluated and not in the planning phase. However, this modality has the potential to determine possible retrorenal colon violation during the access as visual inspection of the colon is possible [11].

To enhance fluoroscopy-based access also innovative avenues have been explored in this field. Novel radiation-based technologies use the 3D reconstruction of kidney and organs to optimize access tract selection and avoidance of organ injury. They will be discussed in the next sections.

## 11.2 UroDyna-CT

One of the disadvantages of fluoroscopy previously described is its inability to visualize soft tissues and the 2D nature of fluoroscopy images. 3D soft tissue imaging can overcome these shortcomings. UroDyna-CT (Siemens Healthcare Solutions, Erlangen, Germany) is a ceiling-mounted fluoroscopy unit with cone-beamed imaging [9]. This unit takes 396 images during 8 sec with its 240° rotatable arms and then reconstructs 3D images of the kidney and adjacent organs. The appropriate access tract is chosen and by use of a laser guide planning tool (SyngoiGuide) a laser cross is projected on the patient's body indicating entry site and angle. Access is then obtained by the bull's eye method and depth of entry is determined by additional fluoroscopy at 0°. This technology was initially evaluated on 12 patients with complex punctures including patients with unclear ultrasound images, or suspicion of bowel adjacent to kidneys, or failed prior conventional access. The radiation dose was reported very high with a median (range) of 6113 (1081–7957) $\mu Gym^2$. Nine (75%) of punctures were successful. UroDyna-CT imaging duration was 8 sec, 3D image reconstruction was completed in less than 2 min and planning time was on average 6 min (range: 4–15 min). In three patients, the puncture was unsuccessful: In two cases, inadequate visualization occurred due to extravasation and in one case access failed due to kidney excessive movement. In these cases, ultrasonography guidance was used to establish access. UroDyna-CT use is possible in operating rooms that are fitted with cone beam imaging technology. UroDyna-CT is associated with a steep learning curve and in a significant percentage of patients (25%), access failed.

Imaging in UroDyna-CT is not real time and for evaluation of the depth of needle entry, conventional fluoroscopy is required. Adjustment and correction of the needle path is possible with this technology. The developers of this technology advise its usage ONLY in complex access cases or failure of conventional percutaneous access methods which includes a small percentage of PCNL cases. With this in mind and considering the steep learning curve of this technology, it seems that the usage of this method should ideally be restricted to designated referral centers for the treatment of selected patients.

## 11.3 iPAD-Assisted PCNL

The only method that uses augmented reality to visualize organs in the access tract is iPAD-assisted puncture method [16]. The sequence of procedures can be divided into a preoperative and an intraoperative phase.

In the preoperative phase, a CT scan is acquired in the same position of the surgery with placing the necessary cushions during surgery and at the end of the inspiration phase. Five radio-opaque markers are placed on the patient body. MITK software reconstructs important organs like kidneys, bowels, stone, and bones and it is possible to reconstruct other important organs like liver and spleen if needed. Excretory images are used to reconstruct the pelvicalyceal system and ureter if necessary. The reconstructed organs will be displayed semi-transparently on images of the patient's body taken by the iPAD camera with control of radio-opaque markers. During the intraoperative phase, the patient is positioned on the operation table in the same position and with the same cushions used during preoperative imaging. Radio-opaque markers are placed in their previous locations. iPAD is then used as camera and screen, information is relayed through WLAN to the server and visualization models are created and displayed on the iPAD screen. The kidney is stabilized with the help of the anesthesiology team and its movements are prevented and confirmed by fluoroscopy. Access is made in inspiration. This technology has been evaluated in a clinical trial enrolling 22 patients and comparing them with 22 similar patients matched for age, gender, stone size, and location. The stone volume in the control group was higher; however, researchers did not present a statistical comparison of this difference (312 (36–2750) versus 153 (19–2856)). The results of this study disclosed a shorter puncture and fluoroscopy time in the control group relative to the iPAD group ($2.14 \pm 1.22$ versus $6.17 \pm 5.13$ min for puncture time ($P = 0.01$) and 52.5 (11–208) versus 378 (33–1100) for radiation ($P < 0.01$)). There was no failure for percutaneous renal access in the patients studied, however, in the iPAD group, three patients needed 3 or 4 needling attempts while in the control group all accesses were established by ≤2 needling attempts.

The authors reported software problems resulting in an inaccurate overlay of segmentated organs in ten patients as markers were not appropriately recognized by the software in these patients. In the other 12 patients, puncture time was not different from the control group. The iPAD technology is in the research and development phase, especially for software.

The iPAD method is the only technology that employs augmented reality on images to reconstruct organs in the access tract. Robotic technologies only use augmented reality to determine site and angle of entry and do not disclose access tract organs. A main problem with this technology is target organ movement that results in target loss. Imaging in the same position and fixing respiration by the help of the anesthesia team were used to mitigate organ movements, however, these strategies have not adequately addressed the organ movements. The last points are that displayed images in the iPAD technology are 2D images that are based on 3D reconstruction of the anatomy. Perhaps it would have been better to construct the puncture on a 3D image. Obviously, organ reconstruction is not real time and is based on the preoperative CT scan and the possibility of access correction is minimal. Besides, kidney deformation due to respiration is not demonstrated when using this technology.

## 11.4 Other Radiation-Based Methods

Some other technologies used radiation-based improvements to optimize renal access. One of these technologies is Sabre Source [17] which has been examined in a phantom model of human kidneys. Sabre Source (Minrad International Inc.; New York; USA) is a real-time image guidance that is mounted on a c-ARM and indicates access site and angle by crosshair. The c-ARM is rotated for a bull's eye access technique and the laser beam demonstrates the entry site for renal access. In this technique, the needle collimator has a small hole in its back allowing entry of a laser beam. When the needle location and angle are both appropriate, the needle lights up by the emitted laser beam. A locator is then used to stabilize the needle. In a phantom model, this technique was associated with a 70% reduction in fluoroscopy for percutaneous renal access. The performance of this technique in patients with kidney movement due to respiration needs to be evaluated in clinical studies yet.

## 11.5 Polaris Technology

Polaris ® is an infrared camera that detects reflective markers on various instruments [18]. Under fluoroscopy, several images are taken at 30°, 0°, and −30°. Then c-ARM is moved aside and ultrasonography is used for percutaneous access. Real-time ultrasonography images are displayed on an ultrasound monitor and a reconstructed virtual 3D image is displayed on the Polaris monitor which illustrates the access tract on fluoroscopy images. This technique has also been evaluated in human phantom models.

The so far discussed techniques, apart from optical technique use fluoroscopy for access guidance during renal access, bear the previously mentioned disadvantages of fluoroscopy. Development of ultrasonography-guided percutaneous renal access technologies have been presented in recent years and various ultrasound-guided technologies have been introduced including modification of ultrasound technology (3D or 4D) or combination of ultrasound with other technologies including magnetic navigation. These will be discussed in the following sections.

## 11.6 3D Ultrasonography

In 3D ultrasonography, parallel images obtained from 2D ultrasonography are received by a computer that reconstructs volume-rendered images or multiplanar images displayed simultaneously on a computer screen. Few studies have been performed on the performance of 3D ultrasonography and it seems that multiplanar images are superior to volume-rendered images regarding percutaneous access [19].

## 11.7 Ureteroscopic Doppler Ultrasonography

In this technology, a Doppler transducer is mounted on the tip of a 120-cm-long 3F wide catheter which is introduced into the kidney by flexible ureteroscopy. The Doppler probe investigates the renal blood flow in its calices to find the best location for the renal access with the least blood flow [20]. This technology has been evaluated in pigs but needs further studies in human subjects.

One of the problems of ultrasound previously mentioned is its 2D image nature and that needle navigation to target calyx is based on 2D images which is less accurate than a 3D technology. The combination of ultrasound with electromagnetic navigation has recently been studied in a few technologies which are discussed next.

## 11.8 Real-Time Virtual Sonography (RVS)

In this technology, real-time ultrasonography is merged with CT and MRI (through magnetic navigation) and volume location images are produced. This technology has been used for prostate biopsy and focal therapy [21]. For percutaneous renal access, an electromagnetic sensor is mounted on an ultrasound probe and 3D images are produced showing the location and direction of the ultrasound probe in the formed magnetic field [13]. Software then displays ultrasound images side to side to reconstructed images on one screen. Clinical evaluation of this technology was performed in 15 patients and compared to 15 control patients who underwent conventional sonography-guided renal access. Study results revealed a lower frequency of needling attempts and hemoglobin drop in the RVS group. Additionally, no Clavien grade III complication was observed in the RVS group versus three cases in the conventional ultrasonography group. One of the problems of this technology in synchronizing ultrasound images with CT is kidney movement. To minimize this concern, the CT position is similar to the operation position (similar to the iPAD technology) and access is performed at the end of expiration. Nonetheless, patients undergo radiation in the preoperative CT scan, and synchronizing images causes increasing operation duration.

## 11.9 SonixGPS

SonixGPS [22] is an ultrasound guidance technology employing time navigation technology. In this technology, position sensors are mounted on an ultrasound transducer, and access needle. This technology has previously been used for neural block and vascular access [23]. One of the advantages of this technology is that it is possible to track needle trajectory through electromagnetic (EM) navigation even when the needle is not in the ultrasound plan resulting in a more accurate puncture and reducing the possibility of adjacent organ injury. This method has been compared with conventional ultrasound-guided renal access in a retrospective study on 74 patients (37 in each arm). Hydronephrosis severity was more pronounced in the control group in comparison with the SonixGPS group rendering the control group an easier target for percutaneous renal access by ultrasound guidance. Nevertheless. Access duration was shorter in the SonixGPS group (6.62 (2–13) versus 11.53 (4–26) min). Also, success upon first entry was 84% (31/37) in the SonixGPS group versus 51% (19/37) in the conventional ultrasound group. Bleeding was reported less in the SonixGPS group (median (range) of hemoglobin drop in SonixGPS: 13.79 (7–33) versus 20.97 (8–41) in the ultrasound group) and complications were also less frequent as no complication was observed in 25/37 patients in the SonixGPS group versus 15/37 patients in the conventional ultrasound group. One of the key successes of this study was that all accesses were successfully made to the target calyx in the SonixGPS group. One of the reasons for this increased success rate is enhanced accuracy of targeting by adding EM navigation so that access can be established even when the needle is not observable in the ultrasound image.

In another study, the first entry success rate of SonixGPS was reported as high as 100% which is interestingly high. A similar technology to SonixGPS was described by Chau et al. [24] using magnetic field-based ultrasound navigation to track needle trajectory real time to the target calyx. The needle puncture was guided freehand by ultrasound and no needle guide was used resulting in an 83% success rate on the first entry.

## 11.10 Electromagnetic Tracking (EMT)

The use of an Electromagnetic sensor in the SonixGPS was associated with an astonishingly high success rate. Thereafter, several researchers have focused integration of EM navigation with guidance systems of percutaneous access. One of the innovations is the use of EM sensors in the target calyx resulting in the use of three sensors in ultrasound probe, needle tip, and target calyx with a presumably higher precision for EM navigation. A group of researchers in Portugal have evaluated the performance of this technology in laboratory scaffolds, animal models, and then in a clinical trial on human subjects.

The results of the scaffold laboratory study [25] revealed a precision of 1.35 mm for location and 0.51° for an angle which is similar to results obtained in other studies for location (0.79–1.40 mm) and angle (1.0–1.57°). It was also discovered that EM navigation was not distorted by 2D ultrasound probes and analog or digital ureteroscopes while 3D and 4D ultrasound probes caused significant interference with signal reception of EM sensors. EM navigation was then studied for kidney and ureteral access in 12 pigs. All 12 kidney punctures were successfully made in an average duration of 19 sec and all ureteral punctures were successfully made in an average duration of 51 sec. Lastly, this technology was evaluated in ten patients with renal pelvis stones. Relatively easy patients for percutaneous renal access with pelvis stones of 1.5–2.5 cm with Guy stone score of 1 (90%) or 2 (10%) were included. Patients with obesity, bilateral stones, solitary kidney, chronic kidney disease, or abnormal anatomy were excluded. The authors did not report hydronephrosis severity of patients which is an important consideration in ultrasound-guided renal access. Necessary equipment include an EM producing unit, two sensor interface units that decrease EM interference in the operation room and send spatial data to a computer for analysis, 18G access needle and 1.1 mm ureteral catheter both with Aurora EMT sensors with 5° of freedom in their tips and 3D puncture software [3].

Patients are positioned in the modified Galdako-Valvidia position and a ureteral catheter is placed in the fornix of the target calyx by a flexible ureteroscope. Ultrasound is used to ensure the absence of organs in the access tract. Real-time ultrasound and EM navigation produced 3D images to help navigate the needle to the target calyx. Needle entry is confirmed by visual ureteroscopy and slight modifications are made in case necessary. Other steps of guidewire insertion and dilation and sheath entry are controlled by visual endoscopy. Study results on ten patients revealed a median (range) access time of 20 (15–35) seconds. All accesses were successful on the first entry with no need for fluoroscopy.

One of the reasons for the considerable success of this technology is the illustration of the virtual access pathway by 3D software so that continuity of needle trajectory to the ureteral catheter tip can be evaluated before needle entry. In addition, the access path can be continuously projected after the needle insertion and modifications made if necessary. The advantages of this technology were absence of radiation, real-time 3D illustration of needle trajectory, real-time determination of needle entrance and angle and its modification, easier learning, continuous monitoring by EMT sensors and ureteroscopy and the possibility of slight modifications in access tract, real-time control of anatomical changes in access tract and performance of surgery in supine position with no wasting of time for a change of position.

Disadvantages include not a perfect investigation of organs in the access tract due to the absence of CT investigation and difficulty in the introduction of ureteral catheter into target calyx when it is loaded with stones. It should also be notified that this clinical study was a limited clinical study on relatively simple patients for percutaneous renal access. Furthermore, patients with difficult ultrasound investigation including obese with a less quality ultrasound image and less precise EM navigation due to higher distance of stone with EM source generator were excluded from the study. Also, patients in whom flexible ureteroscopy is not possible can be ideally treated with another EM-based technology like SonixGPS.

## 11.11 Robots

Studies on the use of robotics in percutaneous renal access date back to two decades ago. Nevertheless, no commercially available master-slave systems are available for renal access and research and development are necessary for the improvement of robotic instruments.

The PACKY-RCM robot has been evaluated on human subjects two decades ago. No statistically significant difference was observed in needling attempts, and access duration with the manual method. Besides, in 13% of cases, the robot was unable to obtain access after six needling attempts and a manual method was used to establish renal access resulting in no improvement of percutaneous renal access in the robotic arm of the study [26].

AccuBot robot has been used for renal biopsy in human phantom models resulting in improved access time and precision relative to the manual method. However, this technology has not been investigated in human subjects and kidney movement may cause a significant difference in clinical application relative to a phantom model [27].

The current role of robots is in laparoscopy-assisted PCNL which can obviously be performed by robots instead of conventional laparoscopy instruments [28]. This technique is applicable for kidneys in which retroperitoneal access is not possible and anterior access is needed to be made through an anterior abdominal wall like pelvic kidneys.

## 11.12 Comparison of New Access Methods and Conclusion

The important factors upon which it is possible to compare novel percutaneous renal access methods are precision, learning curve, radiation dosage, success rate, morbidity, and cost.

EMT technique and SonixGPS were associated with 100% success rendering them as promising technologies. High success rates of these procedures are due to their real-time identification of the needle and the target calyx in 3D images and the possibility of pathway modification based on ultrasound and EMT data. First entry success rates were 73% for optical method [15], 58% for UroDyna-CT [9] and 64–68% [16, 29] for iPAD technologies. The success rates of other technologies were also lower than EMT and Sonix GPS.

In terms of the learning curve, EMT and Sonix GPS are easier to learn than conventional fluoroscopy or ultrasound-guided PCNL as control of needle can be made by real-time EMT in addition to ultrasound guidance and that 3D images help to improve navigation of needle to the target calyx with less error and easier learning. Learning curve is declared to be only 12 cases for the EMT technology [30, 31] which is considerably less than 40–60 cases for conventional fluoroscopy-guided PCNL [32]. The learning curve of UroDyna-CT is steep as indicated in its relevant section. In the case of iPAD-assisted PCNL, learning of in-training surgeons was shorter compared with expert surgeons.

Regarding radiation, SonixGPS and EMT technologies are radiation-free technologies. Optical methods can be guided by ultrasonography or fluoroscopy. UroDyna-CT and iPAD-assisted methods are radiation-based technologies.

In some novel technologies, fixation of respiration with the help of the anesthesia team is required for percutaneous renal access. Recently, the use of spinal anesthesia has increased in PCNL and in some centers, spinal anesthesia is the main modality for anesthesia in PCNL [33]. In these patients, patient cooperation is required for respiratory fixation which may not be as easy as the control of respiration by the anesthesia team.

Table 11.1 summarizes a comparison of the most important novel percutaneous renal access technologies.

**Table 11.1** Comparision of different novel technologies to obtain percutaneous access to perform PCNL

| Technology | Reference | Advantages | Disadvantages |
|---|---|---|---|
| Optical system in the needle | [15] | Secure identification of the needle<br>Real-time needle visualization via ultrasound easy handling and learning curve<br>No ionizing radiation<br>Most secure way of needle identification in renal pelvicalyceal system | Needle redirection not possible in the case of error trajectory<br>2D imaging<br>Difficult visualization in obese patients<br>Examiner dependence |
| UroDyna-CT | [9] | 3D anatomy imaging<br>Quick, safe, and highly accurate puncture<br>Applicable in complex cases<br>Trajectory visualization in real time and possibility of trajectory change | Higher ionizing radiation dose than conventional technique<br>Technique hampered by excessive renal motility<br>Steep learning curve<br>High installation cost<br>Advised only for complex cases |
| iPad-assisted puncture | [16] | Correct selection of the needle location, angle, and trajectory<br>3D imaging<br>Correct visualization of anatomy<br>Minimal spatial errors<br>Short learning curve for in-training surgeons | Use of ionizing radiation<br>No real-time 3D image<br>Only minimal adjustments of the path allowed<br>Patient in prone position<br>Software problems<br>Longer learning curve of expert surgeons |
| Ultrasonography using Sonix GPS navigation | [22] | No ionizing radiation<br>Needle trajectory prediction<br>Operator can keep track of the needle during the procedure with 3D display<br>Allows adjustment of the trajectory during the procedure<br>Easier to perform than conventional puncture | In obese patients, the ultrasound image is highly impaired, and use of fluoroscopy is recommended<br>2D imaging |
| EMT | [3] | No ionizing radiation<br>3D image of the needle trajectory in real time position and orientation of the needle in real time<br>Easy handling and technical learning<br>Shorter execution time<br>Ability to redefine the trajectory<br>Procedure done in supine position. | Lack of visualization of anatomical structures in the puncture path<br>Difficult to insert a ureteral catheter with an electromagnetic sensor in the desired calyx in situations in which the calyx is fully occupied by stones |

## References


1. Fernström I, Johansson B. Percutaneous pyelolithotomy. A new extraction technique. Scand J Urol Nephrol. 1976;10(3):257–9.
2. Basiri A, Kashi AH, Zeinali M, Nasiri M, Sarhangnejad R, Valipour R. Ultrasound—guided access during percutaneous nephrolithotomy: entering desired calyx with appropriate entry site and angle. Int Braz J Urol. 2016;42(6):1160–7.
3. Lima E, Rodrigues PL, Mota P, Carvalho N, Dias E, Correia-Pinto J, Autorino R, Vilaça JL. Ureteroscopy-assisted percutaneous kidney access made easy: first clinical experience with a novel navigation system using electromagnetic guidance (IDEAL stage 1). Eur Urol. 2017;72(4):610–6.
4. Rassweiler-Seyfried MC, Lima E, Ritter M, Klein JT, Michel MS. [Navigation systems for the percutaneous access to the kidney]. Urologe A. 2020;59(9):1017–25.
5. de la Rosette J, Assimos D, Desai M, Gutierrez J, Lingeman J, Scarpa R, Tefekli A. The Clinical Research Office of the Endourological Society percutaneous nephrolithotomy global study: indications, complications, and outcomes in 5803 patients. J Endourol. 2011;25(1):11–7.
6. Basiri A, Mohammadi Sichani M, Hosseini SR, Moradi Vadjargah A, Shakhssalim N, Kashi AH, Kamranmanesh M, Nasseh H. X-ray-free percutaneous nephrolithotomy in supine position with ultrasound guidance. World J Urol. 2010;28(2):239–44.
7. Basiri A, Nouralizadeh A, Kashi AH, Radfar MH, Nasiri MR, Zeinali M, Sarhangnejad R, Hosseini-Sharifi SH. X-ray free minimally invasive surgery for urolithiasis in pregnancy. Urol J. 2016;13(1):2496–501.
8. Mahesh M. Fluoroscopy: patient radiation exposure issues. Radiographics. 2001;21(4):1033–45.
9. Ritter M, Rassweiler MC, Michel MS. The Uro dyna-CT enables three-dimensional planned laser-guided complex punctures. Eur Urol. 2015;68(5):880–4.
10. Andonian S, Scoffone CM, Louie MK, Gross AJ, Grabe M, Daels FP, Shah HN, de la Rosette JJ. Does imaging modality used for percutaneous renal access make a difference? A matched case analysis. J Endourol. 2013;27(1):24–8.
11. Maghsoudi R, Etemadian M, Kashi AH, Mehravaran K. Management of colon perforation during percutaneous nephrolithotomy: 12 years of experience in a referral center. J Endourol. 2017;31(10):1032–6.
12. Yang YH, Wen YC, Chen KC, Chen C. Ultrasound-guided versus fluoroscopy-guided percutaneous nephrolithotomy: a systematic review and meta-analysis. World J Urol. 2019;37(5):777–88.
13. Hamamoto S, Unno R, Taguchi K, Ando R, Hamakawa T, Naiki T, Okada S, Inoue T, Okada A, Kohri K, et al. A new navigation system of renal puncture for endoscopic combined intrarenal surgery: real-time virtual sonography-guided renal access. Urology. 2017;109:44–50.
14. Wang Y, Jiang F, Wang Y, Hou Y, Zhang H, Chen Q, Xu N, Lu Z, Hu J, Lu J, et al. Post-percutaneous nephrolithotomy septic shock and severe hemorrhage: a study of risk factors. Urol Int. 2012;88(3):307–10.
15. Bader MJ, Gratzke C, Seitz M, Sharma R, Stief CG, Desai M. The "all-seeing needle": initial results of an optical puncture system confirming access in percutaneous nephrolithotomy. Eur Urol. 2011;59(6):1054–9.
16. Rassweiler-Seyfried MC, Rassweiler JJ, Weiss C, Müller M, Meinzer HP, Maier-Hein L, Klein JT. iPad-assisted percutaneous nephrolithotomy (PCNL): a matched pair analysis compared to standard PCNL. World J Urol. 2020;38(2):447–53.
17. Howlett J, Lazarus J, Kaestner L. SabreSource™: a novel percutaneous nephrolithotomy apparatus to aid collecting system puncture—a preliminary report. S Afr J Surg. 2020;58(2):105.
18. Mozer P, Conort P, Leroy A, Baumann M, Payan Y, Troccaz J, Chartier-Kastler E, Richard F. Aid to percutaneous renal access by virtual projection of the ultrasound puncture tract onto fluoroscopic images. J Endourol. 2007;21(5):460–5.
19. Rose SC, Nelson TR, Deutsch R. Display of 3-dimensional ultrasonographic images for interventional procedures: volume-rendered versus multiplanar display. J Ultrasound Med. 2004;23(11):1465–73.
20. Patel RM, Limfueco L, Tapiero S, O'Leary M, Cooper V, Parkhomenko E, Kaler KS, Okhunov Z, Regan D, Landman J, et al. Ureteroscopic Doppler ultrasonography: mapping renal blood flow from within the collecting system. J Endourol. 2020;34(6):687–91.
21. Miyagawa T, Ishikawa S, Kimura T, Suetomi T, Tsutsumi M, Irie T, Kondoh M, Mitake T. Real-time virtual sonography for navigation during targeted prostate biopsy using magnetic resonance imaging data. Int J Urol. 2010;17(10):855–60.
22. Li X, Long Q, Chen X, He D, He H. Assessment of the SonixGPS system for its application in real-time ultrasonography navigation-guided percutaneous nephrolithotomy for the treatment of complex kidney stones. Urolithiasis. 2017;45(2):221–7.
23. Brinkmann S, Tang R, Sawka A, Vaghadia H. Single-operator real-time ultrasound-guided spinal injection using SonixGPS™: a case series. Can J Anaesth. 2013;60(9):896–901.
24. Chau HL, Chan HC, Li TB, Cheung MH, Lam KM, So HS. An innovative free-hand puncture technique to reduce radiation in percutaneous nephrolithotomy using ultrasound with navigation system under magnetic field: a single-center experience in Hong Kong. J Endourol. 2016;30(2):160–4.
25. Gomes-Fonseca J, Veloso F, Queirós S, Morais P, Pinho ACM, Fonseca JC, Correia-Pinto J, Lima E, Vilaça JL. Technical note: assessment of electromagnetic tracking systems in a surgical environment using ultrasonography and ureteroscopy instruments for percutaneous renal access. Med Phys. 2020;47(1):19–26.
26. Su LM, Stoianovici D, Jarrett TW, Patriciu A, Roberts WW, Cadeddu JA, Ramakumar S, Solomon SB, Kavoussi LR. Robotic percutaneous access to the

kidney: comparison with standard manual access. J Endourol. 2002;16(7):471–5.
27. Pollock R, Mozer P, Guzzo TJ, Marx J, Matlaga B, Petrisor D, Vigaru B, Badaan S, Stoianovici D, Allaf ME. Prospects in percutaneous ablative targeting: comparison of a computer-assisted navigation system and the AcuBot robotic system. J Endourol. 2010;24(8):1269–72.
28. Simforoosh N, Radfar MH, Valipour R, Dadpour M, Kashi AH. Laparoscopic pyelolithotomy for the management of large renal stones with intrarenal pelvis anatomy. Urol J. 2020;18:40–4.
29. Rassweiler JJ, Müller M, Fangerau M, Klein J, Goezen AS, Pereira P, Meinzer HP, Teber D. iPad-assisted percutaneous access to the kidney using marker-based navigation: initial clinical experience. Eur Urol. 2012;61(3):628–31.
30. Huber J, Wegner I, Garg Y, Singh V, Sankhwar SN. Re: collecting system percutaneous access using real-time tracking sensors: first pig model in vivo experience: P. L. Rodrigues, J. L. Vilaça, C. Oliveira, A. Cicione, J. Rassweiler, J. Fonseca, N. F. Rodrigues, J. Correia-Pinto and E. Lima J Urol 2013;190:1932–1937. J Urol. 2014;191(5):1476–8.
31. Rodrigues PL, Vilaça JL, Oliveira C, Cicione A, Rassweiler J, Fonseca J, Rodrigues NF, Correia-Pinto J, Lima E. Collecting system percutaneous access using real-time tracking sensors: first pig model in vivo experience. J Urol. 2013;190(5):1932–7.
32. Ziaee SA, Sichani MM, Kashi AH, Samzadeh M. Evaluation of the learning curve for percutaneous nephrolithotomy. Urol J. 2010;7(4):226–31.
33. Basiri A, Kashi AH, Zeinali M, Nasiri MR, Valipour R, Sarhangnejad R. Limitations of spinal anesthesia for patient and surgeon during percutaneous nephrolithotomy. Urol J. 2018;15(4):164–7.

# 12 Access in Supine Position

Guido Giusti, Mario Basulto-Martínez, Silvia Proietti, Giuseppe Saitta, and Yuyi Yeow

## 12.1 Introduction

The most remarkable and constantly debated modifications that percutaneous nephrolithotomy (PCNL) has undergone are the tract miniaturization and the patient's position. Despite safety and effectiveness between the prone and supine positions being comparable, and the fact that surgeons should be familiar with both approaches, many advantages favor supine. Hence, several centers worldwide have set supine position as their standard practice. Moreover, mini-perc has proved better outcomes for small-medium size stones when compared to retrograde intrarenal surgery (RIRS), especially for lower pole ones. Similarly, smaller tracts have proved lower hemoglobin drop and transfusion rate when compared to standard size while maintaining the stone-free rates (SFR) [1–3].

When compared to prone, the supine position makes anesthesia administration and patient positioning easier and faster, improves ergonomics and upper calyx approachability from a lower pole access, makes it easier switching to an endoscopic combined approach when needed, and also might decrease intrarenal pressure and radiation exposure [2, 4].

When percutaneous renal access was first described and then largely adopted, it was performed in a prone position as surgeons theorized it was less likely to injure the colon [5]. However, thanks to cross-sectional imaging now, we can be aware of any retro renal structures in advance and evidence suggests these injuries are uncommon in a supine position as they are in prone. Colonic injuries occur in ~0.5% of cases, and the retro renal colon is the major risk factor. Retro renal colon can be defined as the presence of colon behind a line traced from the anterolateral aspect of the vertebral bodies to the renal hilum on computed tomography (CT) scan, as reported by Prassopoulus et al. [6]. However, Hopper et al. [7], found 4.7% of the significant retro renal colon in subjects in prone whereas only 1.9% in supine due to organs' displacement by gravity. Valdivia-Uría was the first to describe supine PCNL in 1987 and since then, many advantages for supine PCNL have been reported [6–10].

Thus, urologists adopting a supine approach must acknowledge these features and be minded with the anatomical orientation to feel comfortable with it. Furthermore, the decision of miniaturizing the tracts must rely upon proper patient selection to enhance success.

G. Giusti (✉) · M. Basulto-Martínez · S. Proietti
G. Saitta
European Training Center in Endourology, Department of Urology, IRCCS Ospedale San Raffaele, Milan, Italy

Y. Yeow
Department of Urology, Tan Tock Seng Hospital, Singapore, Singapore
e-mail: yuyi_yeow@ttsh.com.sg


M. S. Agrawal et al. (eds.), *Minimally Invasive Percutaneous Nephrolithotomy*,
https://doi.org/10.1007/978-981-16-6001-6_12

## 12.2 Evolution of Percutaneous Renal Access

Creating a renal access was originally an open procedure aimed at urinary diversion; however, in 1955 the first percutaneous approach was reported, and 20 years later, the first percutaneous treatment of a stone [5, 11]. Currently, minimally invasive techniques have displaced old practices with image guidance, whether fluoroscopy, ultrasound, or endoscopic-assisted view; or a combination thereof. Moreover, the created tract can be safely used either for nephroscopy, lithotripsy, tumor treatment, among others [11, 12].

Percutaneous renal access techniques were mainly established in a prone position, under fluoroscopy and using standard size PCNL (i.e., 30F), but the constant refinements to these concepts have brought a wide variety of approaches. Two major techniques are commonly spread, from which many variations and simplifications have arisen: the bull's eye and triangulation technique.

Bull's eye is performed aligning the calyx, the needle, and the fluoroscopy's intensifier (rotated 30°) obtaining a bull's eye-like image on the monitor. Then, a needle is advanced, and its trajectory is continuously traced by fluoroscopy. The major drawbacks of this technique are the higher radiation exposure and its complexity; therefore, several modifications have been communicated.

In the triangulation technique basically, the mediolateral orientation is set in the monoplanar anteroposterior view (0°) and the depth is controlled with an oblique cephalad view (30°), implying less radiation but still facing some complexity, thus simplifications and refinements have been developed as well.

Currently, there is a wide variety of modifications and mixes of these techniques and are conducted with help of US and whether in prone and supine positions. Many centers have adapted their own approach; however, for learning and academic proposes, it is important to set a standardized and reproducible technique [13, 14].

Regardless, a recent preliminary study supports the feasibility of a non-papillary puncture [15], evidence points the safest way to access is through the papilla regardless of the positioning and imaging guidance. Furthermore, most surgeons gain their own access under fluoroscopy guidance or sometimes combined with US. Nonetheless, there is a current growing awareness to prevent ionizing radiation exposure; therefore, US-guided access and endoscopically assisted puncture have attracted interest [16, 17].

## 12.3 Access Guidance Methods

Fluoroscopy has played a major role in renal image-guided access as it provides surgeons many advantages that might not be replaced with US. New techniques have sought to decrease radiation exposure but going totally fluoroscopy-free is still risky especially for inexperienced surgeons, as the fluoroscopy images provide important information for collecting system anatomy, orientation, stones characteristics, and location, and are paramount when complications arise, as surgeons might detect contrast extravasation, opacification of surrounding organs, and it turns easier to go back into the urinary tract when accidentally slipping out or going through a false passage. On the other hand, US has the strength to identify organs interposed in the planned tract avoiding injures, and also can detect perirenal collections, along with the key feature of preventing radiation. To date, regardless of that X-ray-free PCNL has widely been described, the safest way is to always have both image modalities available [18–22].

## 12.4 Position and Technique Description

In the supine position, after intubation and anesthesia administration, the patient is pulled down toward the edge of the surgical table as if placed for standard lithotomy position. However, the stone side remains straight on half of the table and the contralateral leg on the stirrup. With this, we avoid the stirrup holder bumping with our instruments especially when trying to reach an upper calyx from a low pole access when some alignment of the scope onto the patient's body. Contralateral arm also remains straight and the stone sidearm is placed over the patient's chest high enough to avoid conflict with the C-arm of mobile fluoroscopy. The patient is slightly rotated from stone side toward the opposite side, and a tubular cushion is placed below the patient from the scapula to the gluteus. A good option is using a swimming noodle (about 7 cm in diameter). The patient is then pulled laterally toward the stone side and left 5 cm inside the metallic edge of the table in order to avoid interpose with fluoroscopy [2]. Figure 12.1 displays the final supine position. Once the patient has been properly positioned and landmarks are drawn, skin prepping and draping are then carried out, a flexible cystoscope is inserted via the urethra into the bladder and the respective ureteral orifice is identified and cannulated with a guidewire, over which an occlusion balloon is placed and inflated after performing a pyelogram. In our center, we still place an occlusion balloon at the ureteropelvic junction (UPJ) in the majority of cases as we consider it very useful to facilitate the puncture by dilating the collecting system.

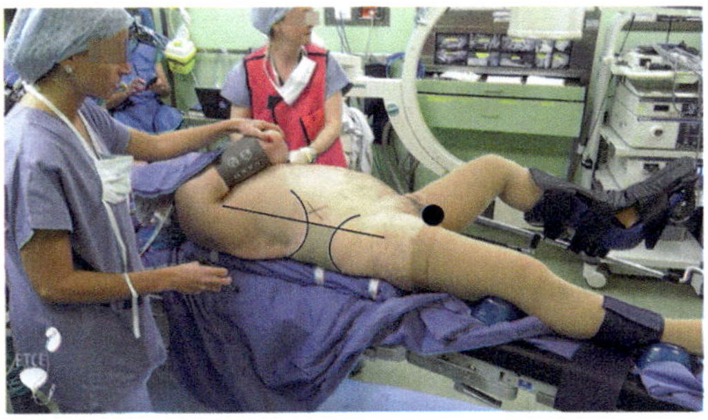

**Fig. 12.1** Giusti's supine position for percutaneous nephrolithotomy. The stone side remains straight with the patient near the edge of the table (about 5 cm inside) with a cushion roll (about 7 cm in diameter) positioned below the flank and the contralateral leg on stirrup. The safe zone for puncture (shown in green) is comprised between the safety landmarks of the posterior axillary line, costal flange, and iliac crest

### 12.4.1 Choosing the Best Calyx

The proper selection of a calyx must ensure the best chances to treat the whole stone(s), and this is mostly where the bigger part of the stone is located. However, other factors are important as well, such as ruling out organ interposition, ensuring going through the parenchyma and through the papilla, and puncturing within security zone. The proper assessment of a preoperative computed tomography scan is key when planning the access. The features to be assessed are kidney anatomy and location, stone characteristics with special regards to HU density, stone-to-skin distance, surrounding fat thick and surrounding organs, hydronephrosis and obstruction, retrorenal structures, and parenchymal thickness.

For stones located in the lower calyx and renal pelvis is always easier to access from the lower pole; for stones located in the middle calyx and ureteropelvic junction, the middle calyx might be the best option; and stones located in the upper pole are mostly reachable from the lower pole in supine unlike prone (Fig. 12.2), but in some cases and upper calyx puncture might be needed (Fig. 12.3).

Nonetheless, a thorough evaluation of the anatomy must be carried out in order to decide where the puncture would be best at. However, when stones are located in parallel calyces, it is unlikely to reach them from a single access; therefore, an extra access should be considered, otherwise using flexible equipment (i.e., mini-Endoscopic Combined Intrarenal Surgery) (Fig. 12.2d).

### 12.4.2 Choosing the Instruments

Mini-perc instruments are available from different companies, each with its own advantages and drawbacks. Usually, mini-perc set comes with two lengths: if supine position is supposed to be adopted, longer access sheaths and dilators are suggested in order to overcome the longer tract faced in this position.

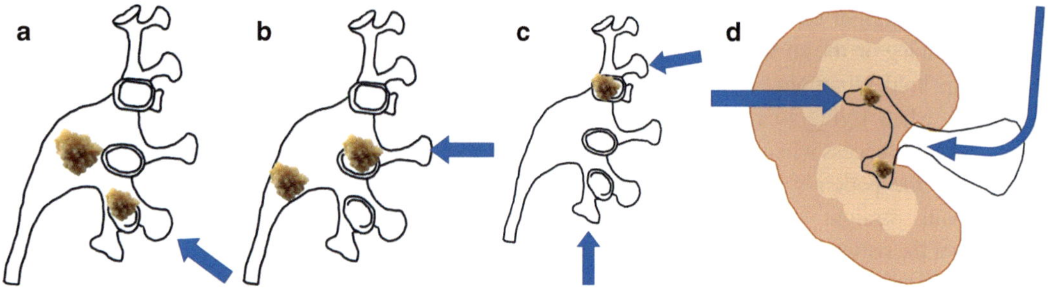


**Fig. 12.2** Best approaches for different stone locations in mini-perc. (**a**), stones located in the lower pole and/or renal pelvis are better reached through a lower pole access; (**b**), stones located in the middle calyx and/or the ureteropelvic junction are better reached through a middle calyx access; (**c**), stones located and the upper pole are mostly reached through the lower pole or through an upper pole access; and (**d**), when facing stones in parallel calyx either a combined approach or additional access are needed to reach all the stones

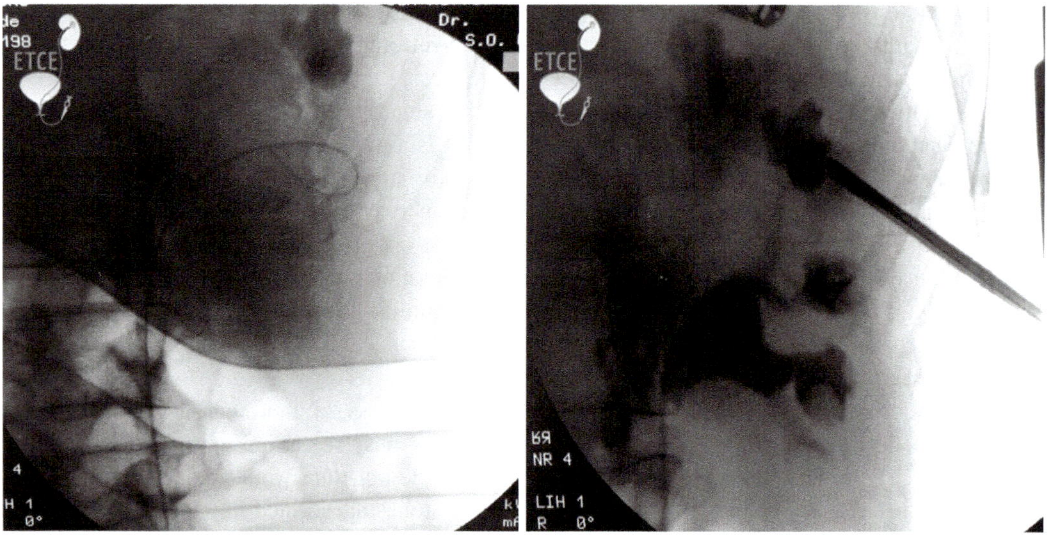

**Fig. 12.3** Upper pole access for supine mini-perc

An important factor is having a difference between the access sheath and scope size of at least 3–4 Fr, in order to ensure low pressure in the kidney. Besides, bearing in mind that not all access sheath sizes fit flexible nephroscope, which are 16Fr, and can be very useful in rendering a patient stone-free. However, if the surgeon decides it is necessary to use a flexible nephroscope, it is always feasible to upsize the access. In Table 12.1, the most commonly manufactured mini-perc sets are enlisted.

### 12.4.3 Puncture

The wanted calyx is targeted by placing the needle over the patient by fluoroscopic biplanar view (0°) so the direction is set. Once achieved, the surgeon should back off with the needle toward the security zone and puncture the skin toward the previously set directions and with the needle in line with the infundibulum and parallel to the ground. While advancing the needle slowly and constantly checking fluoroscopically, as we

**Table 12.1** Commonly manufactured mini-perc sets

| Name | Company, Country | Access sheath (size × length) | Nephroscope (size × length) | Working channel* (Fr) |
|---|---|---|---|---|
| MIP-M | Karl Storz, Germany | 15/16 Fr × 18 cm<br>16.5/15. Fr × 18 cm<br>21/22 Fr × 18 cm | 12 Fr × 22 cm | 6.7 (up to 5 Fr) |
| MIP-S | Karl Storz, Germany | (XS) 8.5/9.5 Fr × 18 cm<br>(S) 11/12 Fr × 18 cm | 7.5 Fr × 24 cm | 2 |
| Miniature Nephroscope | Richard Wolf, Germany | Continuous irrigation:<br>15 Fr × 20.5 cm<br>18 Fr × 20.5 cm<br>Amplatz sheath:<br>18 Fr × 15 cm | 12 Fr × 22.5 | 6 |
| Mini Nephroscope | Olympus, Japan | NA | 15 Fr × 23 cm | 7.5 (up to 6 Fr) |
| Ultra mini nephroscope | SchöllyFliberoptic GMBH, Germany | 11 Fr × 22 cm<br>13 Fr × 22 cm<br>Inner sheaths 6 Fr and 7.5 Fr | 3 Fr | NA |
| Micro Perc | Guangdong Key Laboratory of Urology, China | 7 Fr × 25.2 cm | 3 Fr | 3.3 |

*Some scopes have a combined irrigation/working channel and can accommodate instruments of different sizes, which are presented in parenthesis in the column
Information retrieved from manufacture's product brochure

are nearing the desired calyx, the kidney should move and the tip of the papilla should flatten, both signs of a proper depth and correct targeting. This may be easier to visualize by doing gentle push movements with the needle. Once the collecting systems have been reached, the inner part of the needle is removed to verify if urine comes out spontaneously. Conversely to prone, in supine position there is no need to aspirate with a syringe: if the needle is in, spontaneous dropping out of urine is determined by gravity. If urine does not come out spontaneously, puncture is not correct and the needle should be redirected. We suggest using an instillation mix with indigo carmine + contrast medium diluted at 50% with saline so that we ensure being inside the tract and, in case of a concomitant cyst, discriminating when puncturing it instead of collecting system. Moreover, in case of accidental loss of access, retrograde injection of the colored solution may highlight the previous path to get back into the collecting system avoiding a second challenging puncture.

If the needle is in the correct position in two-dimension fluoroscopic view but urine does not come out, it means that the correct depth is missing, and the needle must be redirected. Sometimes, when the puncture attempt fails the depth by just a few milliliters, minor direction adjustments are needed, by backing out of the kidney with the needle and advancing again with the adjusted directions. Otherwise, we can rotate the C-arm 30° toward the patient's head to see whether the needle is above the papilla, meaning the puncture is too posterior; or alternatively, the needle is below the papilla, meaning puncture is too anterior. Hence, the surgeon must back out of the kidney with the needle and safely readjust the directions by tilling down the hands to reach anteriorly or rising them up to reach posteriorly, as needed according to fluoroscopy vision (Fig. 12.4).

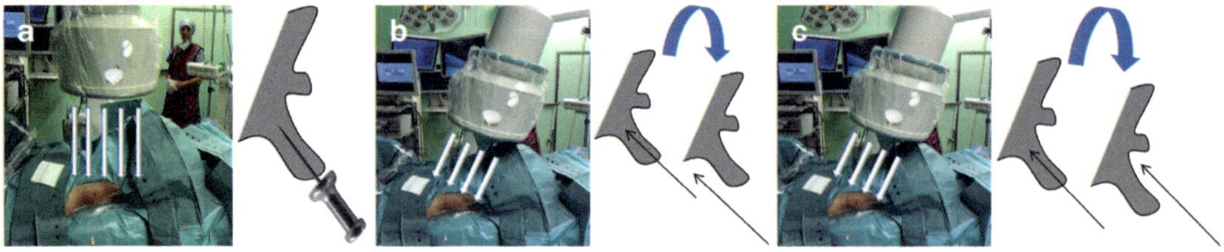


**Fig. 12.4** In the monoplanar view (**a**) the needle might be aligned with the wanted calyx but missing proper depth. Thus, rotate the C-arm 30° toward the patient's head to notice whether the needle is displaced (**b**) below the papilla, meaning that the puncture was too anterior; or (**c**) above the papilla, meaning that the puncture was too posterior. Therefore, surgeons can realign the needle respectively with the C-arm back again at 0°

### 12.4.4 Dilation

With the needle properly positioned into the collecting system, a 0.038′ guide wire is inserted and advanced down to the ureter and a small skin and fascial incision are made with the scalpel. When facing difficulties cannulating the ureter, place a cobra catheter over the guidewire, remove the guidewire so that the cobra catheter can be twisted to negotiate the UPJ, and reinsert the guidewire down to the ureter. Then, an 8/10 Fr dilator is inserted, and a second guidewire must be placed for safety. Hence, one guidewire is placed into the dispenser coil and attached to the draping for safety, and the remaining guidewire is used to dilate the tract. After these steps, we are safely inside the urinary tract through the planned calyx, and therefore, the metallic dilator is placed over the guidewire by a gentle push and twist movements until inside the collecting system, always under fluoroscopic control.

Then, the metallic access sheath is placed over the dilator bearing in mind that it should be firmly held by the non-dominant hand and then removed, as the access has been safely and successfully created. Then, lithotripsy can be started (Fig. 12.5).

When facing a difficult access, a stepwise dilation is suggested. After having gained access into the collecting system with the guidewire, dilate the tract using a 9-Fr diameter set (i.e., MIP-S set) and commence nephroscopy including exploration of the entire tract to rule out eventual adjacent organ injuries and/or false passages or wrong tracts, making the needed adjustments under vision. Once assured the access is correct and injuries are ruled out, the tract size can be uneventfully increased to mini-perc or even standard PCNL.

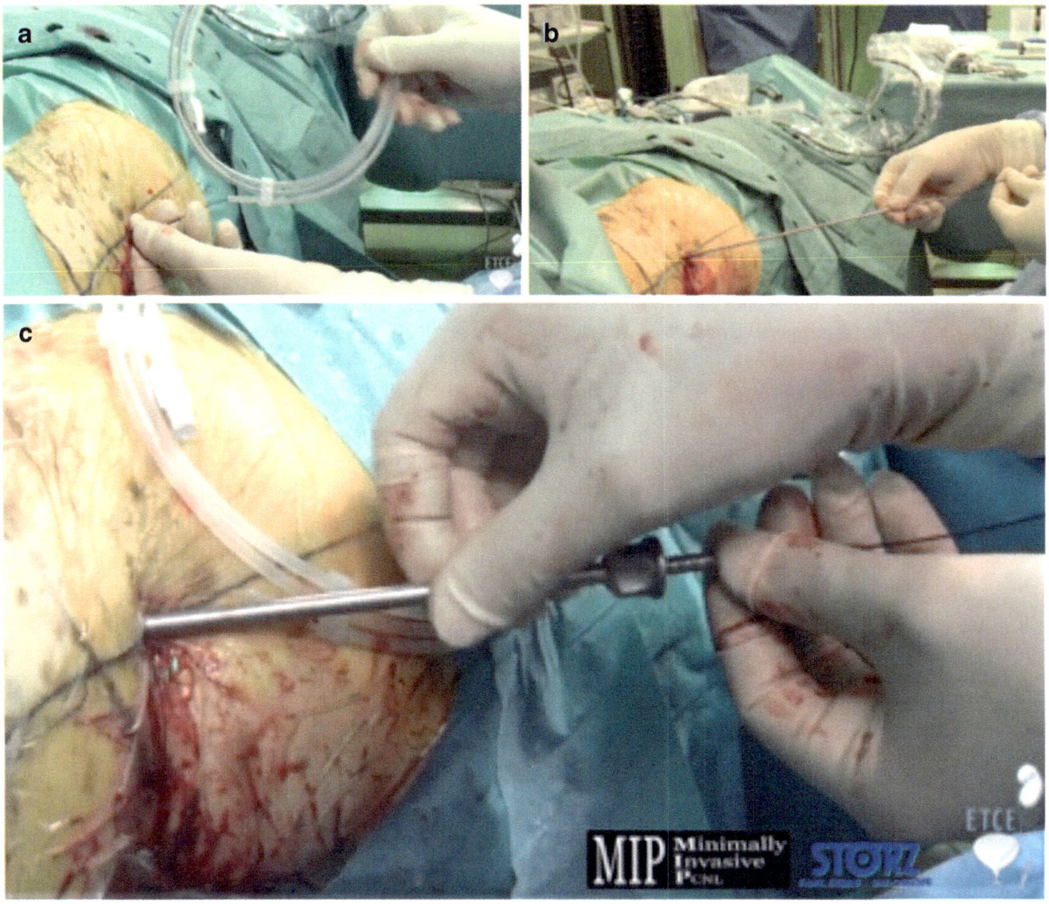


**Fig. 12.5** Dilation of the tract. (**a**) once the guidewire is in, a second guidewire is placed and kept for safety in the dispenser coil attached to the drapes. (**b**) The metallic dilator is inserted into the collecting system over the guidewire, and then, (**c**) while firmly holding the metallic dilator with the non-dominant hand, the access sheath is placed over pushing and twisting forward

## References


1. Yuri P, Hariwibowo R, Soeroharjo I, Danarto R, Hendri AZ, Brodjonegoro SR, et al. Meta-analysis of optimal Management of Lower Pole Stone of 10-20 mm: flexible ureteroscopy (FURS) versus extracorporeal shock wave lithotripsy (ESWL) versus Percutaneus Nephrolithotomy (PCNL). Acta Med Indones. 2018;50(1):18–25.
2. Proietti S, Rodríguez-Socarrás ME, Eisner B, De Coninck V, Sofer M, Saitta G, et al. Supine percutaneous nephrolithotomy: tips and tricks. Transl Androl Urol [Internet]. 2019;8(S4):S381–8. Available from: http://tau.amegroups.com/article/view/27817/25575
3. Proietti S, Giusti G, Desai M, Ganpule A. A critical review of miniaturised percutaneous nephrolithotomy: is smaller better? Eur Urol Focus. 2017;3(1):56–61.
4. Sofer M, Giusti G, Proietti S, Mintz I, Kabha M, Matzkin H, et al. Upper calyx approachability through a lower calyx access for prone versus supine percutaneous nephrolithotomy. J Urol [Internet]. 2016;195(2):377–82. Available from: http://www.jurology.com/doi/10.1016/j.juro.2015.07.101
5. Fernström I, Johansson B. Percutaneous pyelolithotomy. A new extraction technique. Scand J Urol Nephrol. 1976;10(3):257–9.
6. Sharma G, Jangid DK, Yadav SS, Mathur R, Tomar V. Retro-renal colon: role in percutaneous access. Urolithiasis. 2015;43(2):171–5.
7. Hopper KD, Sherman JL, Luethke JM, Ghaed N. The retrorenal colon in the supine and prone patient. Radiology [Internet]. 1987;162(2):443–6. Available from: http://www.ncbi.nlm.nih.gov/pubmed/3797658
8. Valdivia Uría J, Lachares Santamaría E, Villarroya Rodríguez S, Llop Tabemer J, Abril Baquero G,

Aranda Lassa JM. Percutaneous nephrolithectomy: simplified technic (preliminary report). Arch Esp Urol. 1987;3(40):177–80.
9. Valdivia JG, Scarpa RM, Duvdevani M, Gross AJ, Nadler RB, Nutahara K, et al. Supine versus prone position during percutaneous nephrolithotomy: a report from the clinical research Office of the Endourological Society Percutaneous Nephrolithotomy Global Study. J Endourol. 2011;25(10):1619–25.
10. Quaresima L, Conti A, Vici A, Tiroli M, Cantoro D, Rreshketa A, et al. Safety and efficacy of percutaneous nephrolithotomy in the Galdakao-modified supine Valdivia position: a prospective analysis. Arch Ital di Urol e Androl. 2016;88(2):93–6.
11. Patel SR, Nakada SY. The modern history and evolution of percutaneous nephrolithotomy. J Endourol [Internet]. 2015;29(2):153–7. Available from: http://www.ncbi.nlm.nih.gov/pubmed/25093997
12. Türk C, Knoll T, Petrik A, Sarika K, Skolarikos A, Straub M, et al. European Association of Urology Guidelines on Urolithiasis [Internet]. 2015. Available from: http://uroweb.org/wp-content/uploads/EAU-Guidelines-Urolithiasis-2015-v2.pdf
13. Miller NL, Matlaga BR, Lingeman JE. Techniques for fluoroscopic percutaneous renal access. J Urol [Internet]. 2007;178(1):15–23. https://doi.org/10.1016/j.juro.2007.03.014.
14. Negrete-Pulido O, Molina-Torres M, Eduardo Castaño-Tostado AML, JG-A. Percutaneous renal access: the learning curve of a simplified approach. J Endourol. 2010;24(3):457–60.
15. Kyriazis I, Kallidonis P, Vasilas M, Panagopoulos V, Kamal W, Liatsikos E. Challenging the wisdom of puncture at the calyceal fornix in percutaneous nephrolithotripsy: feasibility and safety study with 137 patients operated via a non-calyceal percutaneous track. World J Urol. 2016;35:1–7.
16. Iordache A, Baston C, Silviu-Stelian G-M, Angelescu E, Cerempei V, Olivier T, et al. Ultrasound for kidney access in percutaneous nephrolithotomy: a contemporary review. Med Ultrason [Internet]. 2018;20(4):508. Available from: https://www.medultrason.ro/medultrason/index.php/medultrason/article/view/1618
17. Armas-Phan M, Tzou DT, Bayne DB, Wiener SV, Stoller ML, Chi T. Ultrasound guidance can be used safely for renal tract dilatation during percutaneous nephrolithotomy. BJU Int [Internet]. 2020;125(2):284–91. https://doi.org/10.1111/bju.14737.
18. Manzo BO, Gómez F, Figueroa A, Sánchez HM, Leal M, Emiliani E, et al. A new simplified biplanar (0-90°) fluoroscopic puncture technique for percutaneous nephrolithotomy. Reducing fluoroscopy without ultrasound. Initial experience and outcomes. Urology [Internet]. 2020;140:165–70. https://doi.org/10.1016/j.urology.2020.03.002.
19. Beiko D, Razvi H, Bhojani N, Bjazevic J, Bayne DB, Tzou DT, et al. Techniques-ultrasound-guided percutaneous nephrolithotomy: how we do it. Can Urol Assoc J. 2020;14(3):104–10.
20. Basiri A, Mohammadi Sichani M, Hosseini SR, Moradi Vadjargah A, Shakhssalim N, Kashi AH, et al. X-ray-free percutaneous nephrolithotomy in supine position with ultrasound guidance. World J Urol [Internet]. 2010;28(2):239–44. https://doi.org/10.1007/s00345-009-0451-8.
21. Birowo P, PAR R, HWK P, Rustandi R, Atmoko W, Rasyid N. X-ray-free ultrasound-guided versus fluoroscopy-guided percutaneous nephrolithotomy: a comparative study with historical control. Int Urol Nephrol [Internet]. 2020; https://doi.org/10.1007/s11255-020-02577-w.
22. Hudnall M, Usawachintachit M, Metzler I, Tzou DT, Harrison B, Lobo E, et al. Ultrasound guidance reduces percutaneous nephrolithotomy cost compared to fluoroscopy. Urology [Internet]. 2017;103:52–8. Available from: https://linkinghub.elsevier.com/retrieve/pii/S0090429516310172

# 13 Simulation-Based Training for Access

Ashish V. Rawandale-Patil and Lokesh G. Patni

## 13.1 Introduction

Percutaneous renal access (PRA) is the key to minimally invasive renal surgeries. Initial puncture, tract dilatation and sheath placement remain the crucial steps that determine outcome of the surgery.

It has been reported that 24 cases are required for the trainee to obtain a good proficiency for percutaneous nephrolithotomy (PCNL), they become competent after 60 cases and excellence is obtained at more than 100 cases [1].

Halsted approach of "see one, do one, teach one" has been the conventional approach to surgical training. Nowadays with increasing complexity of cases, rapid development in the technology and medico legal pressures have contracted the training opportunities for the younger surgeons. At the same time operative skill evaluation of the trainees by the mentor is also a difficult task due to lack of objective parameters and varied spectra of clinical cases. As a solution to surgical training, animal or simulation labs are now being organised to train the young surgeons and overcome their learning curve of various essential surgical skills.

## 13.2 Training for Percutaneous Renal Access

Acquiring a new surgical skill is a process and not an event. In order to acquire the surgical skill a novice surgeon has to go through three phases which may be described as under.

***Cognitive phase:*** It includes education on topics like anatomy, operating room arrangement, instrument armamentarium and more. This is the mandatory foundation required prior to performing a new psychomotor skill. This phase of training is achieved by book readings, didactic lectures, instructional courses, illustrations and group discussions.

***Integrative phase:*** This phase includes application of learned skills to acquire the ability to perform a task. Ideally this is best possible in an operative room set-up, but the lack of opportunities makes simulators a better tool for learning. This step helps transferring the acquired knowledge to learn psychomotor skills [2, 3].

***Autonomic phase:*** This includes sufficient repetitive practice to enhance the proficiency to perform the learned art, so that the motor skills are executed automatically with little cognitive input.

A. V. Rawandale-Patil (✉) · L. G. Patni
Institute of Urology, Dhule, Maharashtra, India


M. S. Agrawal et al. (eds.), *Minimally Invasive Percutaneous Nephrolithotomy*,
https://doi.org/10.1007/978-981-16-6001-6_13

Simulators are now being widely used to train the residents. Any teaching module should be able to provide the trainee and the mentor with the following:

(A) A basic three-dimensional (3-D) orientation of the retroperitoneum, kidney and pelvicalyceal system.
(B) Ability to allow the mentor to provide instructions on the steps of percutaneous renal access.
(C) Ability of the mentor to deliver knowledge of common mistakes during the procedure, the ways to identify and correct them.
(D) Ability to train and enhance the skills.
(E) To allow post training evaluation to assess the improvement in the trainee.
(F) Formulation of tailored simulation sessions for the candidate according to their level of performance.

Global attempts are underway to create a wholesome simulator which could help to reproduce all these essentials of renal access.

## 13.3 Available Avenues for Training

### 13.3.1 Animal Laboratories

Wet animal laboratories are being used for a long time to develop new surgical skills and techniques. Live animals like pigs and goats have been employed for training. The porcine kidney anatomically resembles the human kidney. It is more friable and has a less capacious pelvicalyceal system. Animal labs have an advantage in terms of near human anatomy with natural tissue haptics, bleeding, respiratory movements, etc., but the major disadvantages include ethical issues, availability, specimen/animal preparation time, limited practice sessions due to lack of reusability, permission issues, biological borne diseases, animal rights issues and so on. These restraints have led to development of non-animal dry labs worldwide for training of young surgeons.

### 13.3.2 Dry Labs

Dry simulation labs using non-animal models are being established worldwide for training of novices. They consist of various fidelity bench models, using various targets or artificial models resembling human kidney.

Various levels of simulation models have been developed over the years ranging from low fidelity models to high fidelity software based complex models. As the fidelity of the simulator improves it gives more real experience of operating room.

### 13.3.3 Hybrid Labs

Apart from mannequin-based non-biological models, hybrid models using harvested animal organs as a target for practicing PRA are also being practised. This helps to improve the tissue haptics and realism. The models overcome various issues associated with use of live anaesthetised animals but availability, storage, preparation time, biological borne diseases recurring cost and reusability for these models are still a concern.

## 13.4 Simulators Available for Dry Labs

### 13.4.1 Radiation Free Training Modules

These are the training modules where actual X-rays are not used with a simulator, during training. It has been studied that the mean radiation time during a percutaneous puncture is 7 minutes and expose the surgeon to a mean entrance skin dose of 110 mGy [4]. The exposure is more when considered for the complete PCNL procedure. To avoid the radiation exposure during the training of percutaneous renal procedures virtual fluoroscopy (virtual reality) simulators were developed. They produce fluoroscopy like images on the screen using computer-based software or visible light optics.

#### 13.4.1.1 Puncture Logic Bench (Fig. 13.1)

The authors have devised a teaching aid for the novices to help them understand the logic behind the percutaneous renal access. It is a simple low fidelity device made up of plastic sheets demonstrating the horizontal and vertical planes of puncture. The target is then approached via a fixed entry point. The movements including the planar directional changes are learnt by the student which helps him understand the 3-D orientation of the calyx with respect to the skin entry point. This also reveals the geometrical concept of puncture technique.

#### 13.4.1.2 Rawandale's Virtual Fluoroscopy Simulator (Fig. 13.2a & b)

It is a mid-fidelity simulator designed and fabricated by the authors. The simulator based upon the principle of visible light optics and shadows. It has a C-arm replica with the lower end replaced with a visible light source. The camera on the top captures the image casted by a target onto a translucent sheet. The image is transmitted to a monitor. A mannequin with vertebra and lower ribs resembles the human torso in prone position. The trainee punctures through the translucent fascia placed in the flank region of the torso.

The surgeon activates the foot switch and reproduces the fluoroscopy like image. The image mimics the real fluoroscopy image of the pelvicalyceal system. Any puncture technique can be used. Once the initial puncture needle reaches the targeted calyx, an electronic beep indicates completion of the task. An internal camera visually confirms the position of the needle below the fascia in case of successful/unsuccessful puncture. This view can be used as an added aid for learning. The respiratory excursions are managed with help of a motorised cam arrangement. Various shapes of targets (pelvicalyceal system) are available to change the difficulty level of the tasks.

In a phase I study conducted by the authors, the simulators demonstrated a favourable face and content validity as evaluated by the experts. It is a low-cost alternative for the available virtual reality simulators [5, 6].

The model lacks objective electronic feedback and scoring like the computerised surgical simulators, but it allows the trainee to practise all of the steps of the percutaneous renal access in a radiation free environment, at home or office-based laboratory.

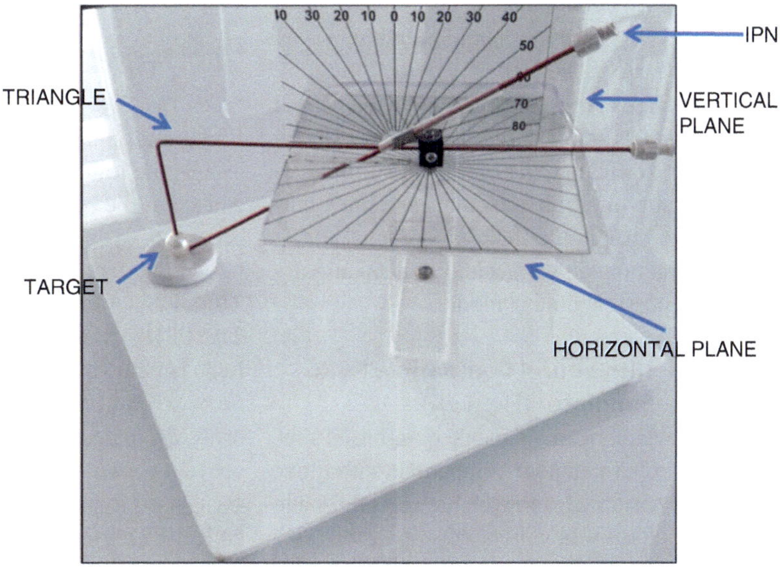


**Fig. 13.1** Puncture logic bench

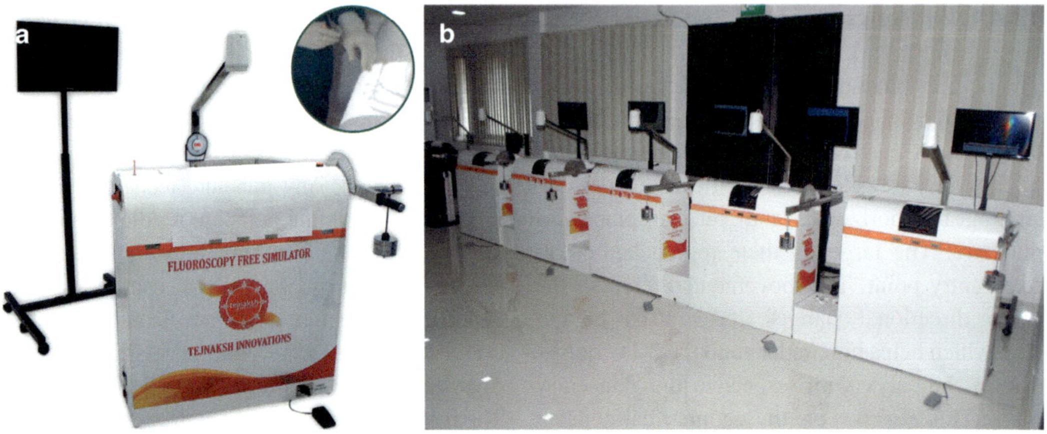


**Fig. 13.2** (**a**) Rawandale's virtual fluoroscopy simulator. (**b**) simulation room

#### 13.4.1.3 SimPORTAL C-arm Trainer (CAT) Simulation Model (Fig. 13.3) [7]

Veneziano and co-workers designed a C-arm training model for performing PRA. The model consists of a replica of C-arm mounted with two video cameras. The flank is simulated with a silicon model containing replica of human kidney with pelvicalyceal system, ureter, ribs and vertebra. The camera captures the images of the kidney and pelvicalyceal system and projects it on the monitor that mimics images produced on a C-arm. The authors claim that the fluoroscopy-free CAT is an economically feasible and accurate model for training parallax without any radiation hazard to the learner.

SimPORTAL is available commercially but it has hard haptics and puncture through the silicon slab is very difficult. The clarity of the images decreases after multiple punctures and the recurring cost to change the flank model may not be cheap. Dilatation of the tract and stone manipulation is not possible on this model.

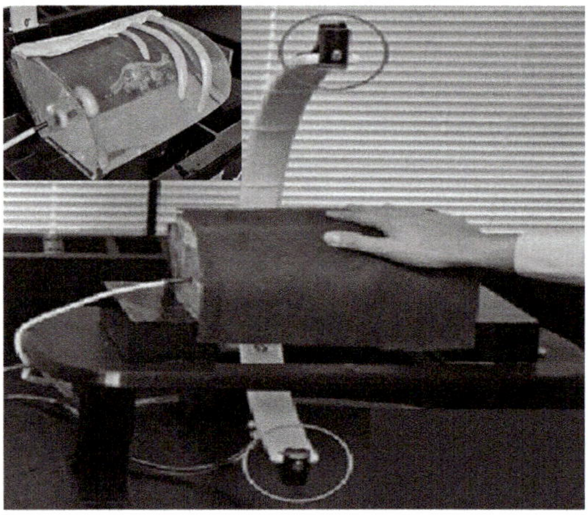

**Fig. 13.3** Sim portal

#### 13.4.1.4 Ultrasound Compatible PERC Simulator (Fig. 13.4)

Authors have fabricated a mannequin-based simulator for initial puncture compatible with ultrasound. It consists of a recyclable cassette made up of specialised wax with targets of various size filled with liquid to simulate the target calyx. It orients the trainee to use the ultrasound machine and learn the concept of ultrasound based renal access [6, 8].

#### 13.4.1.5 PERC Mentor™

The PERC Mentor™ developed by Simbionix; Lod, Israel (Fig. 13.5) is one of the high fidelity fluoroscopy-free simulator. It gives real-time fluoroscopy images using a virtual C-arm controlled via foot pedal. A metal needle with a spatial sensor is used to puncture a digitally projected renal collecting system. A retrograde ureteric catheter

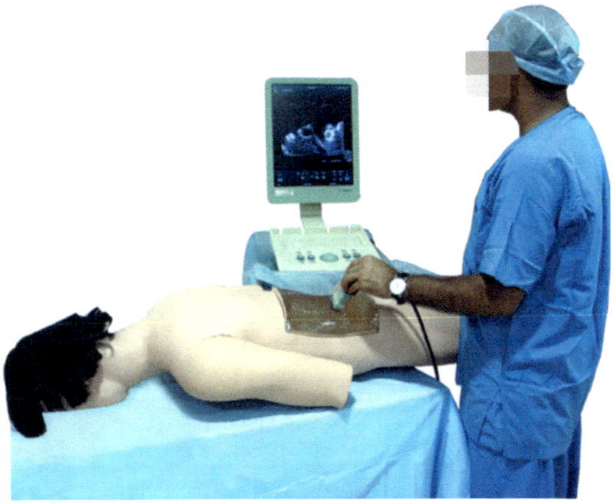

**Fig. 13.4** Rawandale's ultrasound guided simulator

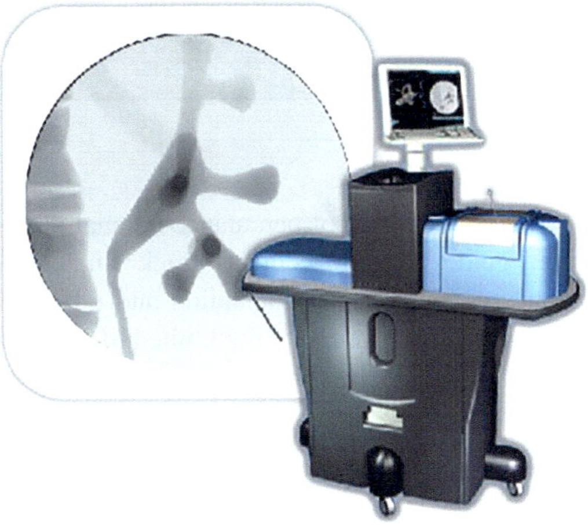

**Fig. 13.5** PERC mentor

can be used to instil contrast medium if required. Special ports are available to place the guide wire and initial track dilators into the fictitious collecting system. Various database case scenarios with different difficulty levels to improve the skills of the trainee are preloaded onto the console. It also provides an orientation of 3-D anatomy of kidney and perirenal structures to the trainee. Objective parameters such as overall procedure time, number of punctures, fluoroscopy time, rib collisions, collecting-system perforations, and blood-vessel injuries are recorded by the simulator. This allows for continuous real-time monitoring of the trainee and can be utilised to device a tailored programme based on individual performance.

Phase I and II studies [9, 10] conducted by Knudsen et al. demonstrated a statistically significant improvement in the baseline performance of the participants and favourable results using the task of performing percutaneous renal access in an anesthetised pig.

PERC Mentor is one of the most high-end simulator produced till date but still it also has its own pitfalls. The simulator lacks the natural tissue haptics, and the needle used for initial puncture does not resemble the usual initial puncture needle. The needle is thick and contains a wire attached to the hub which interferes with movement of the needle. There are separate slots for introduction of wires and catheters and available armamentarium for practice is also limited. The image on the monitor often pixelates and the instrument movement may not be exactly replicated by the software. Occasional glitches are known with the software.

#### 13.4.1.6 Virtual Reality Simulator (Marion Surgical K181) (Fig. 13.6)

The mechanical simulators use physical objects (such as mannequins or kidney models) to provide haptics while in virtual reality simulators the physical interactions are rendered by a robotic haptic system, while the visuals are shown using either a screen or a head-mounted display.

Marion Surgical K181 is a virtual reality surgical simulator for PCNL training that allows the users to interact with a virtual patient in a virtual operating room. The system consists of the virtual reality visual headset which simulates a virtual operating room. The virtual room includes a C-Arm that can be operated manually or over voice command or through a motion controller provided. The screen displays the images from the endoscope. The user can physically interact with various instruments like endoscopes, needles and graspers. The instruments are attached to a haptic robotic device which provides various degrees of freedom. Tissue force is provided by a tissue simulation software which is a feedback from the various movements of the instruments attached to the robotic arm and the video feed from the endoscopes. The surgeon can perform

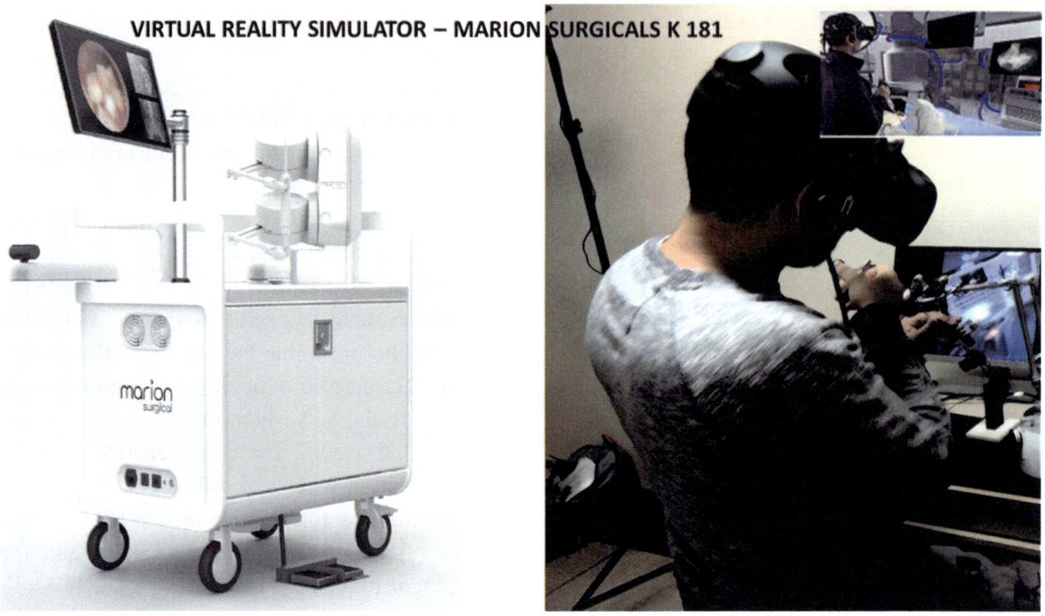


**Fig. 13.6** Marion surgical's K181

initial puncture as well as stone fragmentation and extraction using the instruments.

The authors evaluated the face and construct validity of the simulator in the study and concluded that the simulator is an effective tool for practice, hand-eye coordination training and it can be added as another tool available to residents aiding in their skill development [11].

### 13.4.2 Radiation-based Training Modules

Radiation-based simulators allow the trainee to learn in a near natural OR environment. They help to learn the optimum use of fluoroscopy during PRA.

#### 13.4.2.1 PERC Trainer™

Developed by Mediskills Limited (United Kingdom), PERC trainer™ is a low fidelity trainer (Fig. 13.7) available commercially. It is fluoroscopy and ultrasound compatible and allows performance of percutaneous renal puncture, guide wire placement, track dilatation, nephroscopy, stone fragmentation and retrieval. The major disadvantage is the limited life span if tract is dilated many times. Cost may be a limiting factor as once damaged the whole bench has to be replaced. When used with a fluoroscopy machine the simulator carries the hazards associated with radiation.

#### 13.4.2.2 Vegetable Model (Fig. 13.8)

A bench model using a vegetable substrate was described by Sinha et al. [12]. This low fidelity model was used to orient the trainee to depth and distance perception during a PCNL puncture. A small study concluded that this model was easily replicable, inexpensive and can be used for training PCNL puncture.

#### 13.4.2.3 Sponge Trainer (Fig. 13.9) [13]

Ahmad M. Tawfik and colleagues designed and validated a sponge trainer for percutaneous renal access. They used simple sponge blocks of vari-

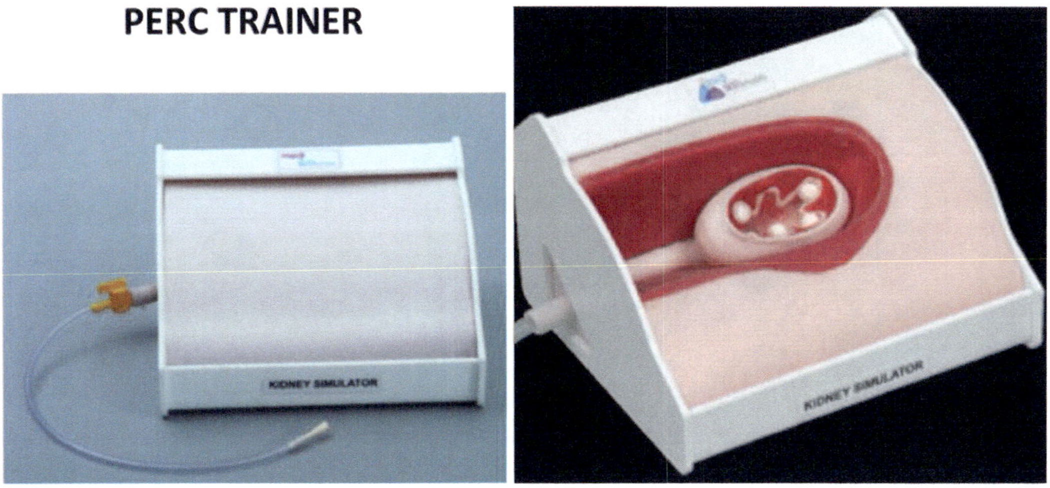


**Fig. 13.7** PERC trainer

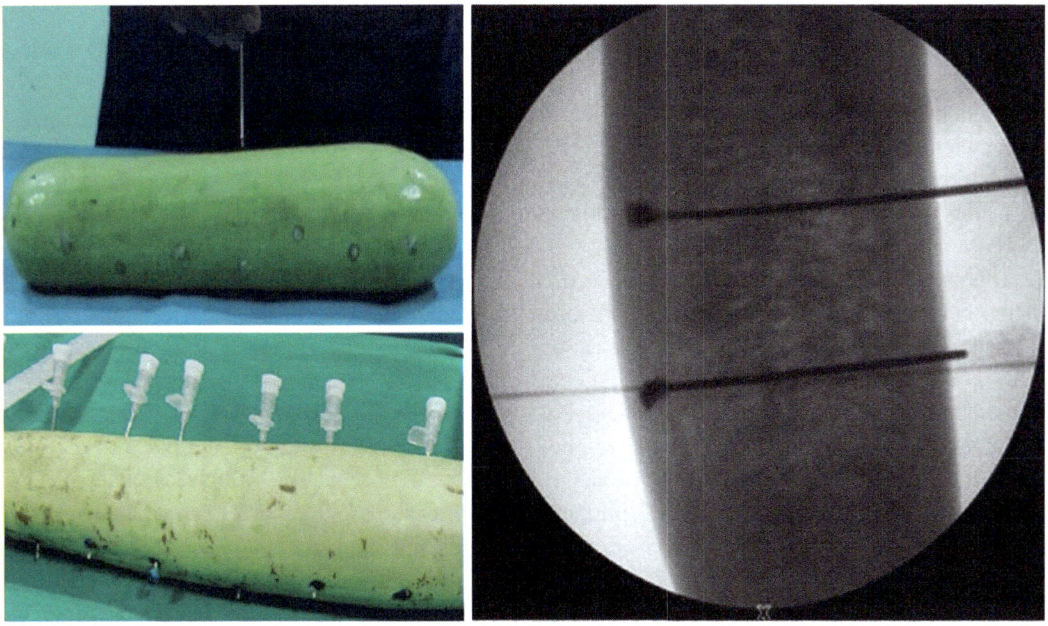

**Fig. 13.8** Vegetable model for PRA

ous sizes to simulate the human torso. Trainees were asked to perform various tasks during the study. They performed PRA under guidance of their mentors in the operating room and the results were compared. The authors concluded that the model is a good tool to train the novices in percutaneous renal access. It is an inexpensive, low fidelity, easily available and reproducible model for practice of PRA, but it lacked tactile feedback and tissue haptics.

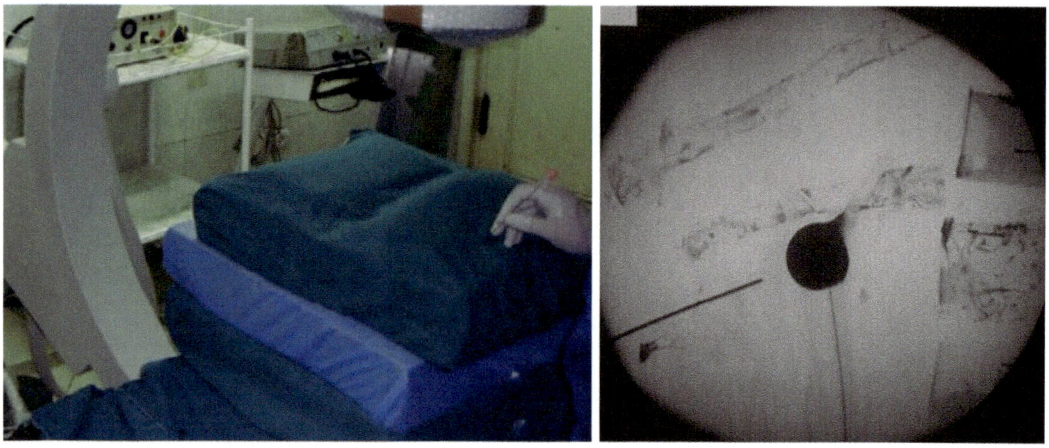

**Fig. 13.9** Sponge trainer

#### 13.4.2.4 Rawandale's Fluoroscopy-based Percutaneous Nephrolithotomy Simulator (Fig. 13.10) [6, 14]

The authors designed, patented and fabricated their own novel fluoroscopy-based PCNL simulator to overcome the availability, cost and reusability factors associated with commercially available PCNL simulators.

This mid-fidelity simulator was designed using the computer-assisted designing software, fabricated using plastic and metal sheets along with a mass-produced silicone kidney model housed in a mannequin. A cassette made up of polyvinyl foams/rubber of variable density simulates the parietal wall and retroperitoneum. Placed on the operating table the model simulates a patient torso. Fluoroscopy can be used at the lowest settings 50 kVA and 0.6 mA to reduce trainee radiation exposure. Any access technique can be used with the model. A successful puncture is confirmed by returning fluid which can be instilled through the ureter of the silicon kidney. On successful puncture, a wire is then parked into the system. After dilatation of the tract the amplatz sheath is placed. If the initial puncture needle hits the metallic spine and/or ribs, it activates an alarm thus providing a real-time feedback to the trainee. Respiratory excursions are being replicated by a motorised mechanism.

It is a low-cost, mid-fidelity simulator. It is reusable. The kidney model can be used for up to 800 punctures. It weighs around 6 kilogrammes and can be easily shifted from place to place. It gives a 3-D orientation of the renal and perirenal anatomy and provides near natural haptics. Being fluoroscopy compatible it is used in the OR environment. Fluoroscopy training can be done on the simulator in a controlled environment. Routine instruments used during PCNL such as initial puncture needle, wires, scopes, etc., can be used with this model. A primary study has provided positive evidence for the simulator as a training and evaluation tool.

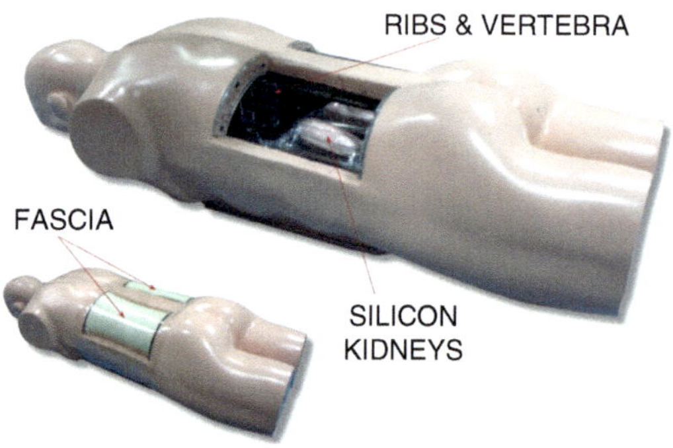


**Fig. 13.10** Rawandale's fluoroscopy-based simulator

#### 13.4.2.5 3-D Printed Kidney Replica Bench (Fig. 13.11) [15–17]

Phantom kidney models made up of water-soluble plastic or wax embedded in silicon were fabricated using 3-D printing technology, for practising initial puncture and planning for per-

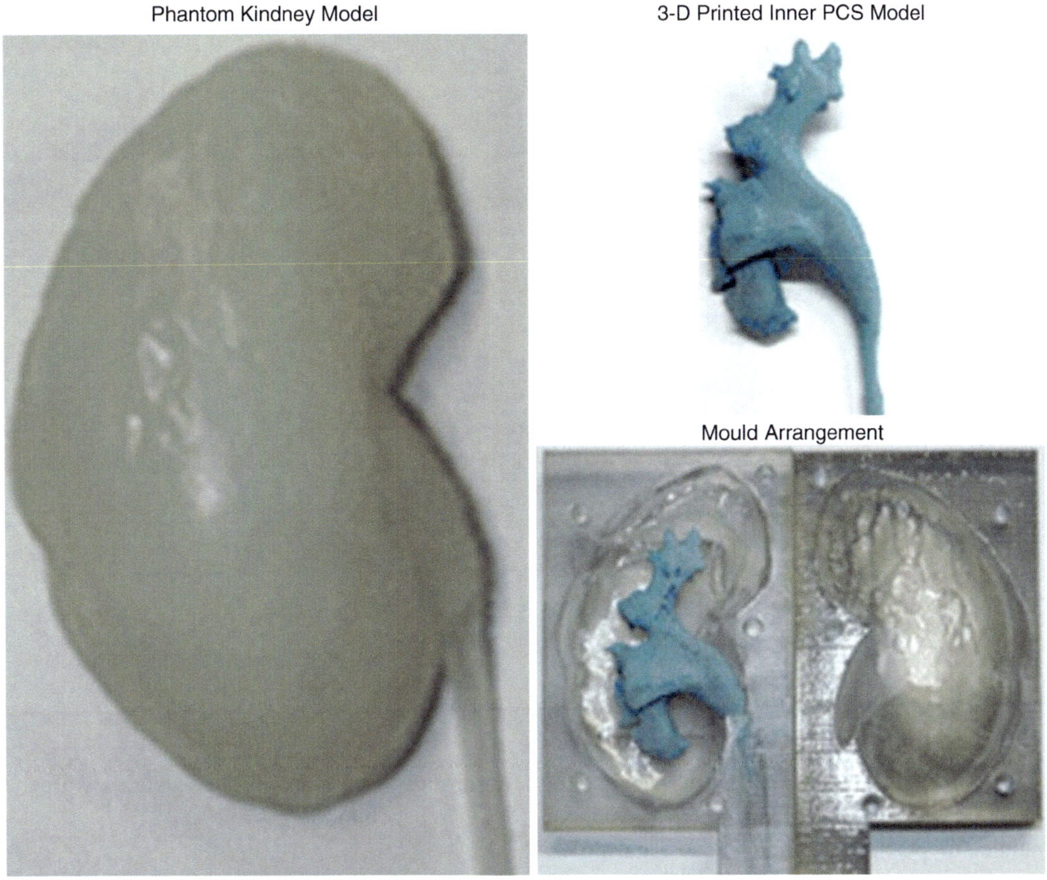


**Fig. 13.11** Three-dimensional kidney model

cutaneous renal access. Computed tomography images of the collecting system are reformatted, a pelvicalyceal system is made and its shape embedded into a silicon replica. Various types of simple to complex collecting systems can be made using the technology. These silicon kidneys are then assembled in a layer of dense foam which replicate tissues between skin and kidney. A limitation of this model includes its incompatibility for ultrasonographic imaging [10, 11]. Fluoroscopic use comes with its radiation hazard. Poor haptics in lieu of the silicon used, and the use of computed tomography, 3-D printing and casting of each model individually add significantly to the cost. These models have a limited usage in terms of various steps of percutaneous renal access and PCNL.

### 13.4.3 Biological Bench Models for Hybrid Labs (Fig. 13.12)

It is difficult to replicate natural tissue haptics with inanimate substrates. Hence various animal tissue-based bench models have been developed. Porcine kidney resembles human pelvicalyceal system but is fragile and less capacious. Hammond and co-workers [18] used porcine kidney prefilled with stones placed in an intact chicken carcass as a model for PCNL. The trainees performed various steps of PCNL under fluoroscopy guidance. No formal assessment of the model was done; but anonymous evaluations submitted by the participants showed high degree of satisfaction with model effectiveness in learning percutaneous renal access and steps of PCNL.

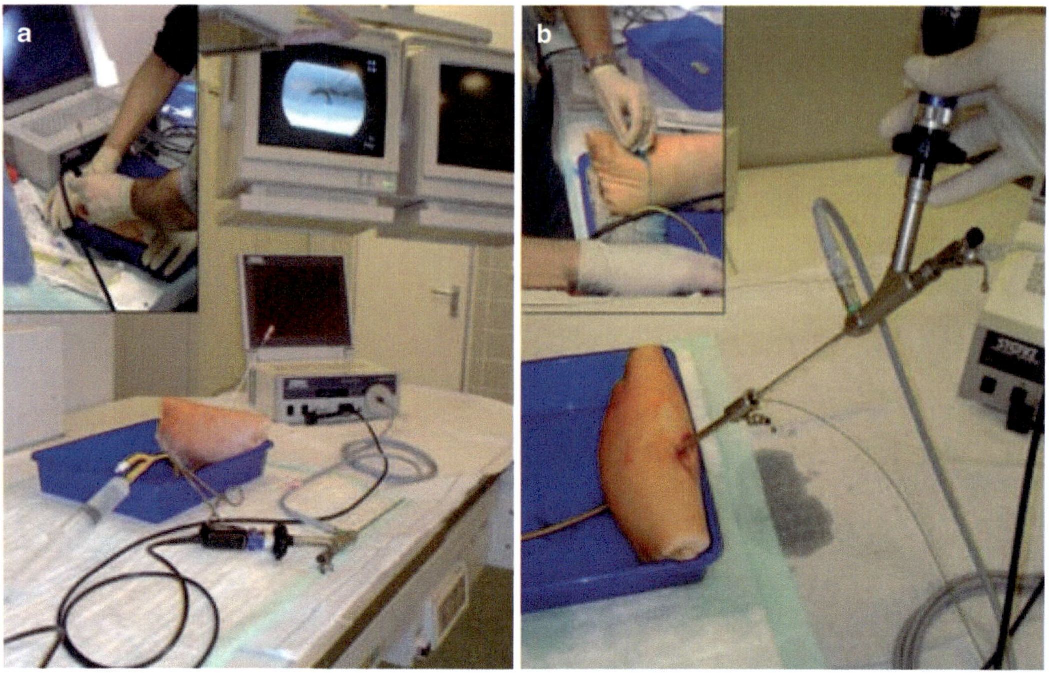


**Fig. 13.12** (**a** & **b**) Biological bench model (porcine kidney wrapped in skin tissue)

Strohmaier and Giese [19] used slaughtered pig kidneys with ureter embedded in a silicon mould for practising percutaneous renal procedures. The ureter was used for saline injection to simulate hydronephrosis and placement of stones. This ex-vivo model was used for training of percutaneous endourological procedures (e.g. percutaneous nephrostomy, percutaneous lithotomy, endopyelotomy). The authors claim good tissue haptics and anatomical resemblance.

An ex-vivo PCNL organ training model was also described by Zhang et al. [20] using a porcine kidney wrapped in a full-thickness skin flap with subcutaneous fascia and muscle and fixed to a wooden board. Various other models [21–23] using the porcine kidney with full-thickness skin cover mounted on various platforms have also been described. All are fluoroscopy and ultrasound compatible and replicate near natural tissue haptics.

Procurement and preservation of porcine kidney along with skin flaps restrict its reusability. There are always issue of cleanliness, specimen preparation, animal borne diseases, tissue disposal and sanitation issues associated with the ex-vivo bench models.

## 13.5 Discussion

PCNL has a steep learning curve. Selection of the correct calyx and initial puncture remains the cornerstone for a successful PCLNL. Mastering PRA requires practice. Primary goal of any teaching programme is to train the residents to acquire the psychomotor skills before they face the real patient. Simulation provides an opportunity to train the novices in a supervised and stress-free environment without harming the patients.

Traditionally animal models were preferred for learning the operative skills till the issues regarding animal rights came into picture. Though live animal models do not represent accurate human anatomy they still provide the best haptics and other intra and postoperative conditions like bleeding, etc., for learning purposes.

Bench models using artificial kidney models were developed to avoid the issues associated with animal models. Various artificial materials like silicone, sponges, foams and other materials are used to simulate the renal and perirenal anatomy. These models show a close resemblance to human renal anatomy. Present-day simulators try to replicate the difference felt between extrarenal tissue and the kidney. There is associated maintenance and recurring cost due to damage of the models following each puncture and tract dilatation. The hybrid models using animal or cadaveric kidney can overcome the difficulties associated with artificial bench models, but the issues of organ procurement, hygiene and animal disease transmission still pose practical problems for these models to be accepted worldwide.

Virtual reality simulators can give the trainee a better visual, auditory feedback, and case scenario variability; but they lack in haptics. Although it has demonstrated its ability to improve the skill of trainees [5, 9]. At present these simulators are expensive and hence are not included in the curriculum at all institutions.

### 13.5.1 Simulation and Teaching Curriculum

Inclusion of simulation-based training in the teaching curriculum is the future of simulation. Paucity of objective parameters, standardisation of simulators, lack of data regarding the validation of simulators are some of the hurdles related. Simulators need to be validated on basis of face, content, construct and predictive validity before they can be incorporated in the curriculum. With the development of instruments such as global rating scale and checklist, it has become possible to assess the acquisition of surgical skills with a higher degree of reliability and validity. Predictive validity which remains the most important end point for any simulator to achieve is not studied much. It measures the ability of the trainee to apply the learned skills to the real operating environment, i.e. the transfer of the skills from simulation room to OR. This validity is practically difficult to establish owing to ethical issues, patient variability and differences in learning capabilities of individual trainee.

In the current situation simulators are being used as an adjunct to formal training in the operating room under supervision of the mentor. Simulators can better be utilised to teach the concept and to make the candidate more oriented to the steps of procedure.

### 13.5.2 Future of Simulation

Simulation in Urology is still in its mid-development and consolidation stages. There is immense potential in this field with regard to training and development of the surgical skills of novice surgeons. There are many unattended arenas in the present-day simulators which need to be looked into. The ideal simulation environment should provide the exact scenario that involves training of all the sensory and motor systems of the trainee. Trainee should be able to learn the planning, decision making, correct techniques, instrument handling, operating room ethics, operating room behaviours, troubleshooting during the procedure, just to mention a few. Simulator should detect the flaws in the trainee and should be able to guide the surgeon to rectify them. This requires algorithms to be developed for each simulation prototype.

Future simulators would be aimed at providing anatomically accurate models which allow various difficulty levels for the trainee, cost effective, non-biologic, hygienic, work with or without radiation exposure depending on the skill level of the surgeon, have near natural haptics and allow for tailored training and practice. They should allow the trainee to practise and master various steps of surgery with real-time experience of various events encountered during the surgery. The future simulators would also have to satisfy the emerging issues of animal rights, trainee and trainer rights, model borne diseases, biocompatibility and easy environment friendly disposability of the model.

The authors have introduced the concept of micro simulation which includes division of the operation of PCNL into smaller steps called microtasks [6]. This is followed by development of micro-simulators and then training the trainee on these micro-simulators which replicate each step of PCNL. The trainees are then oriented to fuse all the micro tasks into a complete procedure in the OR (Fig. 13.13).

The simulation models developed by the authors consists of a wide range of micro-simulators for practising each step of PRA separately. The simulation training module as designed by authors consists of:

(A) Brief overview of calyceal anatomy via didactic lectures, videos and graphical presentations.
(B) Learning the 3-D concept of calyceal orientation on PCNL logic bench.
(C) Concepts of choosing the correct calyx, basics of PRA techniques (Triangulation & Bull's eye) on a fluoroscopy-free simulator.
(D) Practising the same skills on an ultrasound based percutaneous access simulator.
(E) OR training using the fluoroscopy compatible PCNL simulator.
(F) Hands on training in the form of assisting a case of PCNL in OR under supervision.

These simulators help the trainee to get oriented to the three-dimensional anatomy, calyceal orientation, choice of desired calyx, steps of initial puncture, dilatation of tract, stone manipulation separately. This helps the trainee to learn and master every aspect of PCNL at their own pace in a stress-free environment. Post training assessment and transfer of skills from simulation room to operating room need to be focussed while developing new models. Objective assessment tools need to be developed to make it more practical. The lab training will have to be seamlessly fused to the OR training in the near future.

The other facet which would have to be standardised would be the training schedule and algorithms, trainer training, teaching and evaluation algorithms. With further development of these pathways, newer issues would emerge that would need trouble shooting. Till that time the student and the teachers need to adapt to the present simulation avenues and contribute to the existing knowledge of simulation.

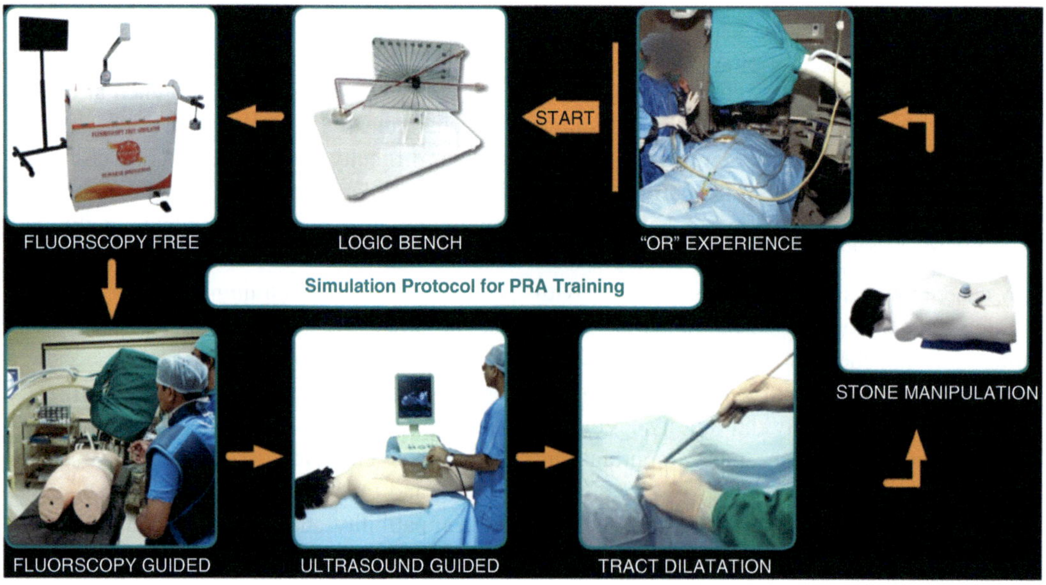


**Fig. 13.13** Simulation protocol

## References


1. De la Rosette JJ, Laguna MP, Rassweiler JJ, et al. Training in percutaneous nephrolithotomy—a critical review. Eur Urol. 2008;54(5):994–1001.
2. Kopta JA. The development of motor skills in orthopaedic education. Clin Orthop. 1971;75:80–5.
3. Fitts PM, Posner MI. Human performance. Belmont: Brooks/Cole; 1967.
4. Mahesh M. Fluoroscopy: patient radiation exposure issues. Radiographics. 2001;21(4):1033–45.
5. Patni L, Rawandale-Patil A, Gade A, S. P. Kaushik construction and assessment of an innovative virtual (radiation free) fluoroscopy PCNL simulator; an indigenous approach to training. Int J Urol. 2019;26(Suppl. 2):216.
6. Patil AR, Patni L, Gulhane P. Training in percutaneous nephrolithotomy. In: Gundeti MS, editor. Surgical techniques in paediatric and adolescent urology. 1st ed. New Delhi: Jaypee Pub; 2019. p. 857–67.
7. Veneziano D, Smith A, Reihsen T, Speich J, Sweet RM. SimPORTAL Fluoro-less C-arm trainer: an innovative device for percutaneous kidney access. J Endourol. 2015;29(2):240–5.
8. Rawandale A, Patni L. Construction and assessment of an innovative indigenious ultrasound guided PERC simulator. J Urol. 2017;197(4S):e693–4.
9. Knudsen BE, Matsumoto ED, Chew BH, et al. A randomized, controlled, prospcctivc study validating the acquisition of percutaneous renal collecting system access skills using a computer based hybrid virtual reality surgical simulator: phase I. J Urol. 2006;176(5):2173–8.
10. Margulis V, Matsumoto ED, Knudsen BE, et al. Percutaneous renal collecting system access: can virtual reality shorten the learning curve? J Urol. 2005;173(Suppl):315.
11. Sainsbury B, Lacki M, Shahait M, Goldenberg M, Baghdadi A, Cavuoto L, et al. Evaluation of a virtual reality percutaneous nephrolithotomy (PCNL) surgical simulator. Front Robot AI Virtual Environ. 2020;6:145. https://doi.org/10.3389/frobt.2019.00145.
12. Sinha M, Krishnamoorthy V. Use of a vegetable model as a training tool for PCNL puncture. Indian J Urol. 2015;31(2):156–9.
13. Tawfik AM, et al. Validity of a sponge trainer as a simple training model for percutaneous renal access. Arab J Urol. 2017;15(3):204–10. https://doi.org/10.1016/j.aju.2017.04.002.
14. Rawandale A, Patni LG, Patil PA. Construction and validation of a novel indigenous PCNL simulator: an innovative approach to training. Euro Urol Supplements. 2013;12(1):e655–6.
15. Park S, Matsumoto ED, Knudsen BE, et al. Face, content and construct validity testing on a percutaneous renal access simulator [abstract]. J Endourol. 2006;20:A4.
16. Benjamin W. Turney: a new model with an anatomically accurate human renal collecting system for training in fluoroscopy-guided percutaneous nephrolithotomy access. J Endourol. 2014;28(3):360–3. https://doi.org/10.1089/end.2013.0616.
17. Adams F, et al. Soft 3D-printed phantom of the human kidney with collecting system. Ann Biomed Eng. 2017;45(4):963–72. https://doi.org/10.1007/s10439-016-1757-5.
18. Hammond L, Ketchum J, Schwartz BF. A new approach to urology training: a laboratory model for percutaneous nephrolithotomy. J Urol. 2004;172(5 Pt 1):1950–2. https://doi.org/10.1097/01.ju.0000140279.15186.20.
19. Strohmaier WL, Giese A. Ex vivo training model for percutaneous renal surgery. Urol Res. 2005;33(3):191–3.
20. Zhang Y, Ou TW, Jia JG, Gao W, Cui X, Wu JT, et al. Novel biologic model for ercutaneous renal surgery learning and training in the laboratory. Urology. 2008;72:513–6.
21. Imkamp F, von Klot C, Nagele U, Herrmann TRW. New ex-vivo organ model for percutaneous renal surgery. Int Braz J Urol. 2011;37(3):388–94.
22. Qiu Z, Yang Y, Zhang Y, Sun YC. Modified biological training model for percutaneous renal surgery with ultrasound and fluroscopy guidance. Chin Med J. 2011;124:1286–9.
23. Jutzi S, Imkamp F, Kuczyk MA, Walcher U, Nagele U, Herrmann TRW. New ex vivo organ model for percutaneous renal surgery using a Laparoendoscopic training box: the Sandwich model. World J Urol. 2014;32(3):783–9. https://doi.org/10.1007/s00345-013-1151-y.

# Part V

# Mini-PCNL Procedure

# 14 Intrarenal Pressure, Fluid Management, and Hydrodynamic Stone Retrieval in Mini-PCNL

Theodoros Tokas and Udo Nagele

## 14.1 Introduction

Mini-PCNL (mPCNL) constitutes an advancing field in active renal stone treatment. Manufacturers have enriched our armamentarium with a variety of instruments. At the same time, different study groups have presented new techniques in patient body positioning, kidney puncture, and stone lithotripsy. Nevertheless, by decreasing instrument caliber to prevent damage caused by instrument access to the kidney, the water inflow–outflow balance is compromised. To achieve better visibility and improve stone clearance, the surgeon must increase irrigation flow (IF). This action results in an increase of inflow/irrigation pressures (IPs). However, subsequent intraoperative intrarenal pressure (IRP) increments can lead to serious complications [1]. This problem becomes more evident when utilizing extra-small instruments. Nonetheless, the majority of endourologists are not aware of normal and pathological IRP ranges during mini-PCNL and their impact on kidney physiology. In this chapter, we will present ways to maintain optimal fluid management to effectively remove stone fragments after lithotripsy and achieve perfect vision during the whole procedure. Furthermore, we are going to discuss the influence of increased IRPs in complication development and prevention measures to control IRPs and, at the same time, maintain optimal irrigation flow.

T. Tokas (✉) · U. Nagele
Department of Urology and Andrology, General Hospital Hall in Tirol, Hall in Tirol, Austria

Training and Research in Urological Surgery and Technology (T.R.U.S.T.)-Group, Hall in Tirol, Austria
e-mail: udo.nagele@tirol-kliniken.at

## 14.2 Adverse Events Due to Increased IRPs

### 14.2.1 Fluid Backflow and Absorption (Fig. 14.1)

Pyelorenal backflow occurs when pelvic or calyceal fluid leaks into the sinus peripelvic tissue (pyelosinous backflow), the collecting ducts and tubules (pyelotubular backflow), the renal interstitium (pyelointerstitial backflow), or the renal vein (pyelointerstitial backflow) (pyelovenous backflow). Animal studies have presented that it occurs at pressures 40.8–47.6 $cmH_2O$ [2]. Backflow to the renal vein may complicate even low pressures (13.6–27.2 $cmH_2O$) [3, 4] and becomes evident at 40.8–68 $cmH_2O$ [5, 6]. At IRPs of 81.6–95.2 $cmH_2O$, different research groups have found a risk of pyelosinous backflow or even fornix rupture in rabbits [7, 8] and at 272 $cmH_2O$ in pigs [9]. Irrigating fluid may reach the retroperitoneum in considerable amounts after renal pelvic perforation [10]. Low urine flow, vesicoureteral reflux, ischemic damage are possible pre-existing conditions that can lower


M. S. Agrawal et al. (eds.), *Minimally Invasive Percutaneous Nephrolithotomy*,
https://doi.org/10.1007/978-981-16-6001-6_14

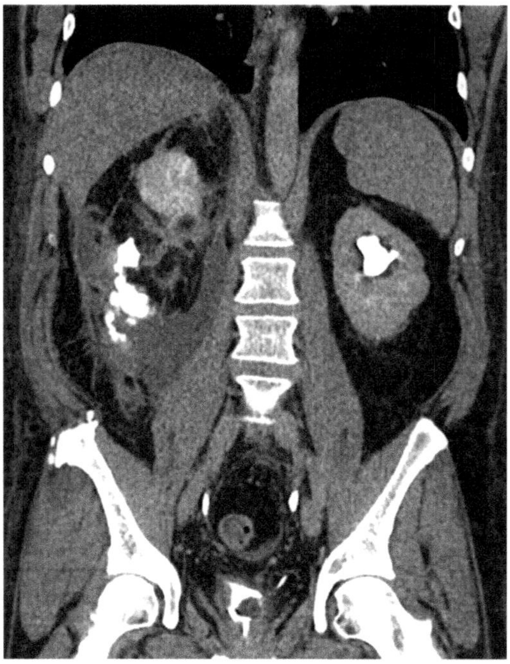

**Fig. 14.1** Backflow and fluid absorption during PCNL demonstrated in a postoperative CT excretory phase

the backflow threshold [7, 11]. The direct intravascular absorption via opened veins, or the intraperitoneal space opening with subsequent peritoneal resorption, lead to the so-called "acute absorption syndrome" [3, 12]. Additional venous hemorrhage and renal pelvis wall lesions are possible contributing factors. Fluid absorption can occur directly into the opened veins or indirectly as a result of a perinephric irrigating fluid accumulation [13]. Reported fluid absorption during conventional PCNL ranges 50–2200 ml [3, 14, 15], but no data exist regarding miniaturized instruments.

### 14.2.2 Infections

Increased IRP, backflow, and urinary tract infections, fever, systemic inflammatory response syndrome (SIRS), and sepsis all have a direct link, demonstrating antibiotics' beneficial effect. The amount of irrigation fluid used is also a potential risk factor for SIRS [16]. In general, postoperative fever after PCNL appears in 10.8% of the cases [17]. Despite its low incidence rates (0.3–1%), septic shock is associated with significant mortality rates (66–80%) [18]. In addition, increments in IRP are a substantial risk factor for postoperative fever and urosepsis [19]. Finally, elevated IPs (272 $cmH_2O$) trigger SIRS more frequently (46%) than low IPs (108.8 $cmH_2O$/11%) [20]. However, information on the occurrence of infections following mini-PCNL is limited.

### 14.2.3 Kidney Damage

Animal studies have proven the direct correlation of increased IRP with irreversible damage [6, 21]. Immensely increased IPs (>200 $cmH_2O$) more probably have a detrimental effect on porcine kidneys in comparison with IPs less than 120 $cmH_2O$. An IRP as high as 250 $cmH_2O$ can lead to a rupture of the collecting system [21]. Furthermore, pyelosinous backflow caused by fornical rupture can be the cause of perirenal pseudocysts, edema and hemorrhage of the retroperitoneum, perinephritic abscess, and fibrolipomatosis [6]. Moreover, increased IRPs might lead to congestion due to calyceal urothelium denudation, and submucosal edema formation [6, 21]. Even 4–6 weeks following a procedure, tubular vacuolization, and degeneration, as well as pericalyceal vasculitis and metaplasia, have been observed [6, 21].

Due to microvessel compression and insufficient venous flow, high IRPs can cause oxidative damage to the kidney and subsequent loss of renal function. Of note, due to ischemia/reperfusion injury, venous outflow obstruction is more harmful than arterial obstruction [22, 23]. Pyelovenous backflow causes venous stagnation to some extent, resulting in perfusion pressure compression of microvessels, reducing the blood supply to the renal parenchyma. The resulting condition may be a renal ischemia, or reperfusion damage [24].

### 14.2.4 Various Complications

Urine leakage is a powerful fibrotic response causative factor [6, 25]. Furthermore, intrarenal backflow may cause papillary damage and consequent pathological stone growth development [26]. Due to fornix or parenchymal rupture, high IRPs can cause subcapsular hematomas [27] and potentially life-threatening perirenal bleedings [28]. The increase of the mean systolic and diastolic blood pressures might be considerable. Moreover, due to large elevations in renin, aldosterone, and ACTH levels, a propensity to hyponatremia and metallic acidosis occurs. These alterations could be attributed to the invasive nature of kidney intervention and continuous irrigation, which has been linked to an increase in IRPs [29, 30].

### 14.2.5 Role of Time

Procedure times independently correlate with postoperative fever and SIRS rates [31, 32]. Additionally, infection risk and postoperative fever rates increase when IRPs remain higher than 40 $cmH_2O$ for more than 10 min [33]. In pig models, renal cellular injury occurs within 1 h at IRPs of 20 $cmH_2O$ or higher [34]. The volume of fluid absorbed during PCNL increases as the IRPs and procedure times increase [3]. After a total irrigation period of 30 min, fluid absorption reaches its peak. The volumes of absorbed irrigant after 30 and 90 min are 154 and 1360 ml, respectively [14]. From the 30th to the 120th irrigation minute, potassium levels drop and do not recover until 24 h after surgery. Researchers discovered an increase in Cl levels at the 120th minute of irrigation, as well as a lowering trend in pH from the beginning to the 120th minute of irrigation, which abates 24 h after surgery [15]. As a result of the prolonged irrigation durations, a trend toward metabolic acidosis can be seen. As a result, based on existing evidence, the total process time should not exceed 2 h [15].

### 14.2.6 Kidney Injury: The Role of Obstruction, Irrigation Pressure, and Irrigation Volume

Renal obstruction is detrimental because IPs starting at 82 $cmH_2O$ are more likely to cause acute kidney damage in rats with substantially obstructed kidneys. Not obstructed kidneys, on the other hand, sustain no renal injuries, whereas partially obstructed kidneys sustain injuries only at pressures of 136 $cmH_2O$ [35]. When rabbits are exposed to renal perfusion pressures of more than 82 $cmH_2O$, severely obstructed kidneys are more sensitive to oxidative damage and mitochondrial injury than slightly obstructed kidneys. Both obstructed and non-obstructed kidneys are damaged by irrigation pressures of 136 $cmH_2O$ [24]. Current research advises keeping perfusion pressure between 70 and 410 $cmH_2O$ during endourological procedures to keep the IRP limit below 30 $cmH_2O$ and avoid kidney injury [36, 37].

## 14.3 IRPs during Mini-PCNL

### 14.3.1 IRP Measurement

Using pressure transducers in animals and people, researchers were able to get precise intraluminal pressure readings in the renal pelvis and ureter [38–40]. The Pressure Flow (PPF)—or Whitaker test—was introduced by Robert H. Whitaker, who created the groundwork by establishing an antegrade pressure measurement of the upper urinary tract [41]. He first used this technique on children, with the goal of identifying obstruction as a cause of urinary tract dilatation [41, 42]. Normal IRPs range from 12 to 15 $cmH_2O$, whereas pressures greater than 20 $cmH_2O$ indicate an obstruction. Intermediate values range from 15 to 20 $cmH_2O$ [43]. Nowadays, surgeons are able to measure intraoperative IRPs by placing a special catheter either antegradely after a kidney punction in a way similar to the Whitaker test, or retrogradely after catheterizing the ureteral orifice [44].

### 14.3.2 IRP Values during Different Conditions

The flow of a fluid through a rigid tube is influenced by the pressure gradient between its ends, the fluid viscosity, the length, and the diameter of the tube, according to the Poiseuille equation (dP = 8VgL/pR4; V = FR through the tube, g = fluid viscosity, L = tube length, and R = tube radius) [45, 46]. Additional parameters, including the difference between internal and exterior pressures, external compression, wall tension, and wall thickness, play an important part in a collapsible tube. The transmural pressure equals the tension per unit length over the radius, according to the Laplace equation. The pressure gradually climbs to a certain capacity during the early filling phase, indicating the upper urinary tract's natural elasticity. The rise of the curve is a proxy for the compliance of the pelvic wall [46].

The IRPs at low urine FRs are not higher than a few $cmH_2O$ in a normal human kidney with no obstruction [47]. During diuresis, however, IRPs may exceed 27.2 $cmH_2O$. They range from 68 to 95 $cmH_2O$ in chronic kidney blockage, and as a result, the values fall until the kidney is no longer functional [2]. In hydronephrosis, mean basal IRPs of 12 $cmH_2O$ have been reported [48], and at flow rates >10 mL/min, the pressure reaches obstructive levels [49, 50]. Of note, there is also direct relevance between changes in intravesical pressure and IRP changes. In hydronephrotic kidneys, bladder pressure at 50% capacity is 8.9 ± 3.1 $cmH_2O$, whereas pelvic pressure is 20.8 ± 2.1 $cmH_2O$, compared to 7.4 ± 1.1 $cmH_2O$ in non-hydronephrotic kidneys [51]. To avoid further increases in IRPs, the urinary bladder should be continually drained during endourological treatments.

### 14.3.3 IRPs during Mini-PCNL

In humans, IRPs have been tested in the following mini-PCNL systems; 9.5 Fr, 12 Fr, 14 Fr, 16 Fr, and 18 Fr with scopes of 7.5–9.8 Fr [32, 52–55]. Additionally, one study group have tested IRPs during micro-PCNL (4.8 Fr) [56]. Irrigation pressures range from 40 to 340 $cmH_2O$, with flow rates ranging from 250 to 580 mL/min. Surgeons usually utilize gravity to achieve adequate irrigation flow. Usually, IRPs are remaining below the critical level of 40 $cmH_2O$, and reach 30 $cmH_2O$ in 14 Fr, 20 $cmH_2O$ in 16 Fr, and 15 $cmH_2O$ in 18 Fr. Maximal IRPs of >40 $cmH_2O$ have been documented with 9.5 F and 14 F sheaths [53, 57].

### 14.3.4 IRPs in Supine Versus Prone Mini-PCNL

Limited data exist comparing the two techniques. However, by taking into account the Poiseuille equation (dP = 8VgL/pR4;) we conclude that the generated IRPs are proportional to the length of the access sheath (L) and reversely proportional to the sheath radius (R). In prone PCNL, the instrument angle ranges from +30° to +90° which means that the sheath adds up 1520 $cmH_2O$ to the estimated IRP. On the other hand, in supine PCNL the instrument angle ranges from 0° to −45°, which sometimes reduces pressures until the collecting system collapses. Therefore, using a slightly longer access sheath during supine position with the absence of a collapsing system may result in increased IRPs. Further research is deemed necessary to support this hypothesis.

## 14.4 Clearance of Fragments and Maintaining Low IRPs by Taking Advantage of Different Hydrodynamic Effects

The big caliber of standard PCNL systems allows maintenance of IRPs below 40 $cmH_2O$ [56, 58–62]. However, irrigation backflow via the access sheath is not achievable with very small-caliber instruments (less than 10 Fr), resulting in a mismatch between in- and outflow. Due to mechanical problems, the open sheath designs of the first-generation miniaturized instruments (15–20 Fr) are sufficient for pressure control [63]. The smaller instrument diameter of miniaturized instruments often results in an increase in the number and decrease in the size of stone fragments to be harvested. With an ever-increasing quantity of microscopic fragments or even dust, stone retrieval is shifting away from mechanical methods and toward hydrodynamic effects. There are numerous essential concepts of hydrodynamic-assisted fragment removal that are independent of access.

### 14.4.1 Passive Washout

It is the secondary natural removal of stones over a period of time, usually specified as one week, one month, or three months. It is commonly accomplished by using a Mono-J stent for a few days, a Double-J stent for a longer period, or even without any stenting postoperatively.

### 14.4.2 Active Washout

It could be used in a variety of ways [64–66]. Transporting fragments within the continuous irrigation backflow through the access sheath alongside the scope is one option. During Chinese mini-PCNL, the surgeon fills the collecting system with high pressure with the nephroscope and then quickly removes it, causing an immediate inversion of irrigation flow and pressure, leading in a spillage-like stone removal throughout the access sheath. The irrigation flow pushes stone particles down the ureter during micro-perc. Finally, during ultra-mini PCNL, the surgeon injects irrigation fluid with a syringe into an extra channel within the access sheath and washes off fragments through the main channel of the access sheath without any pressure peaks.

### 14.4.3 Ureteral Sheaths and Catheters

During conventional PCNL, the concept of a retrograde ureteral catheter or ureteral access sheath (UAS) placement was introduced [36]. When compared to an empty ureter (11–38 $cmH_2O$), a ureteral catheter (15–52 $cmH_2O$), or an occlusion balloon application (16–56 $cmH_2O$), researchers found that using a 10/12 Fr or 12/14 Fr UAS (5–22 $cmH_2O$) resulted in lower IRPs. In the case of mPCNL, the inclusion of a suction device can help with the fluid washing out. In a cadaveric pork model, a combination of pressure irrigation with sensor-controlled suction using a modified transurethral 8-Fr mono-J catheter with expanded drainage holes resulted in enhanced irrigation flow and lower IRP [67].

*Purging effect* [67] is a pressure-controlled irrigation process that transports fragments through a percutaneous entry and outflows through a Mono-J catheter or UAS (Fig. 14.2). It provides a high irrigation fluid turnover as well as effective fragment transportation without causing pressure overload in the collecting system. This approach is particularly appealing for stone clearance in small-caliber percutaneous instruments, where adequate simultaneous in- and outflow irrigation via the same access is not usually possible due to construction and stability issues. IRPs could be reduced by 14% at 100 $cmH_2O$ (19–14.5 $cmH_2O$) and 28% at 150 $cmH_2O$ input pressure (37–26.5 $cmH_2O$) due to the purging action.

### 14.4.4 Vacuum Cleaner Effect (Fig. 14.3) [68]

In a cadaveric pork model, the minimally invasive PCNL (MIP) idea was initially tested using an 18 Fr nephroscope sheath with an open proximal end [63]. In low-pressure settings, the vacuum-cleaner effect is the active and purposeful entrapment of fragments in a hydrodynamic pseudo cavity in front of the scope. The effect resembles mechanical forceps, such as an invisible grasper, and it is not simply a washout phenomenon. It emerges when a slipstream forms in front of the distal end of a round-shaped nephroscope, which is caused by an excursive shift in the width of the fluid flow at the flushing canal's exit. It is determined by the relationship between the diameter of the nephroscope and the diameter of the inner sheath. The greatest benefit is obtained with a 12 Fr nephroscope and a 15 Fr

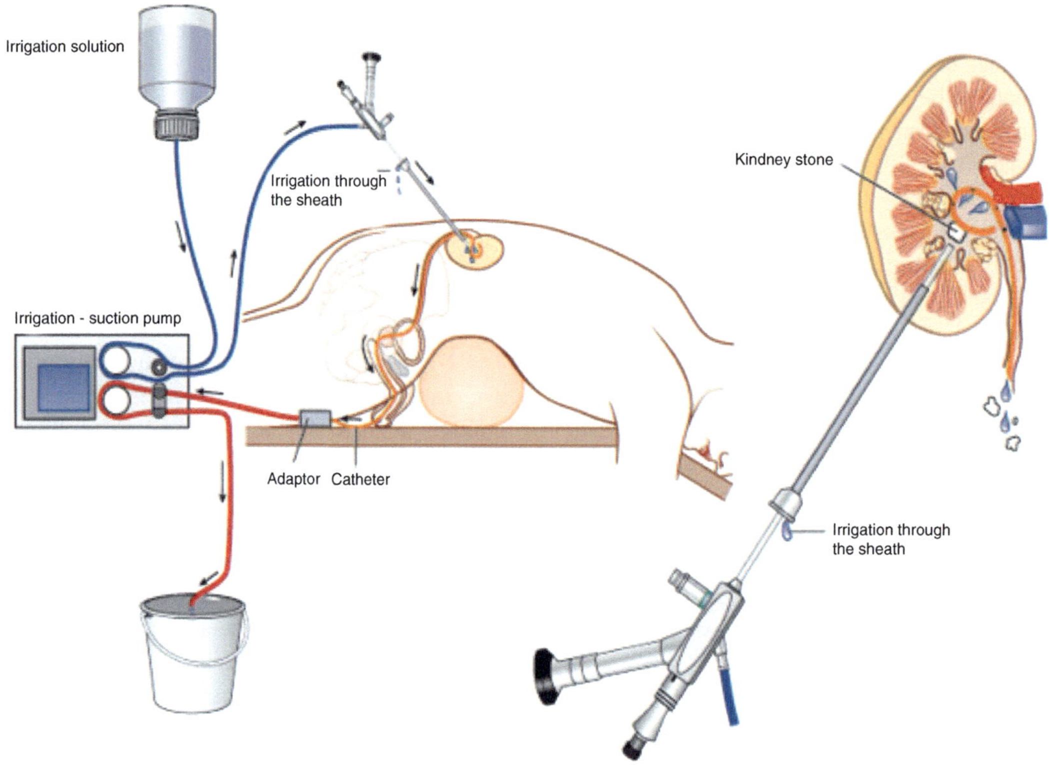


**Fig. 14.2** The *purging effect* is the fragment transportation process by pressure-controlled irrigation using inflow through the percutaneous access and outflow through a Mono-J catheter or UAS

inner sheath diameter; however, utilizing a 16.5 Fr sheath with a 12 Fr scope creates an ideal combination (pressure/stone clearance) at the cost of a high IRP [68].

### 14.4.5 Pressure/Suction Connected with the Nephroscope

During mPCNL, Song et al. introduced a unique irrigation and clearance method (16 Fr). The irrigation volume was 600–800 mL/min, the irrigation pressure was 340–410 $cmH_2O$, and the suction pressure was 140–340 $cmH_2O$. The IRP remained below six $cmH_2O$ on average [69]. Different settings included an irrigation volume of 600–800 mL/min, irrigation pressure of 340–410 $cmH_2O$, and suction pressure of 140–340 $cmH_2O$. IRPs remained below six $cmH_2O$. Yang et al. [70] demonstrated a mini-PCNL (12 Fr) setup with intelligent monitoring and control of IRPs below three $cmH_2O$.

### 14.4.6 Stone Clearance in Small and Extrasmall Instruments (Ultraminiperc, Superperc, Super-Mini Perc, MIP S, MIP XS)

The MIP S system (Karl Storz, Germany) is the smallest instrument with regular backflow via the access sheath in percutaneous surgery, and it was also the smallest percutaneous OR system to create a vacuum cleaner effect in a low-pressure setting [68]. Because irrigation backflow via access sheath was not possible due to the mechanical features of the instruments, all smaller systems, such as the Microperc (Polydiagnost, Germany) and the MIP XS system by Nagele (Karl Storz,

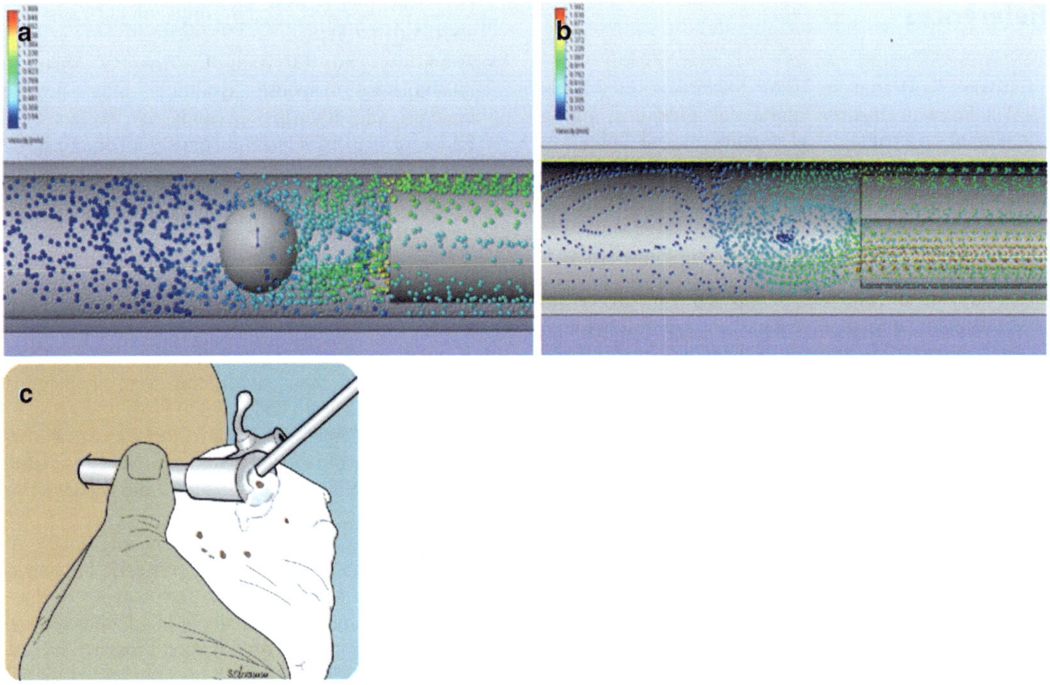


**Fig. 14.3** *Vacuum cleaner effect.* In front of the distal end of the round-shaped nephroscope a slipstream is developing induced by the excursive change of width of the fluid flow on the outlet of the flushing canal (**a**). This allows the adhesion of a stone fragment in the eddy while the fluid flow is circulating around the stone (**b**). By pulling the scope through the sheath the stones are spontaneously evacuated through the proximal end (**c**)

Germany), rely on an outflow utilizing a ureteric catheter. The MIP XS system uses a sensor-controlled dual action pump with purging effect and active pressure control, whereas the Microperc system depends on both active and passive washout without pressure control.

The ultraminiperc uses a 13-Fr access sheath and a 3.5-Fr nephroscope in a 6-Fr inner sheath as a final step in downsizing (Schoelly Fiberoptics GmbH, Denzlingen, Germany) [64]. MIP 2.0, a MIP set expansion by Nagele, is now available in sizes "S" and "X.S." with access sheath diameters of 8.5/9.5 and 11/12 Fr and a nephroscope diameter of 7.5 Fr (Karl Storz GmbH). The isotonic saline can flow beside the inner sheath through the outer sheath due to the unique construction of these instruments [64]. However, this effect can only be achieved with an 11/12 Fr sheath, not an 8.5/9.5 sheath. Following the removal of the inner sheath with the nephroscope during ultraminiperc, the surgeon flushes stone fragments by injecting saline through the integrated channel inside the sheath with a syringe, causing a jet in the calyx and the stones to escape, resulting in the so-called whirlpool effect [64, 71].

The super-miniperc (8 Fr scope, 12 Fr or 14 Fr double-layer metal sheath) [54, 55], superperc (4.5/6 Fr scope, 10/12 Fr sheath, Richard Wolf) [72] and ClearPetra (12 Fr scope, 16 Ch disposable sheath, Well Lead Medical Co., Ltd., China) [73] systems achieve a stone clearance depending on an irrigation-suction mechanism. Stone fragments are removed through an additional tube connected to a negative pressure aspirator.

All currently available small and extra small-caliber instruments offer attractive options in the armamentarium of modern percutaneous stone surgery. Nevertheless, the absence of high-quality data limits their wide distribution and implementation in the everyday clinical praxis. Furthermore, all hydrodynamic benefits are also applicable in conventional modern PCNL instruments, which leads to the term minimally invasive PCNL (MIP) [63, 68].

## References


1. Tokas T, Herrmann TRW, Skolarikos A, Nagele U. Pressure matters: intrarenal pressures during normal and pathological conditions, and impact of increased values to renal physiology. World J Urol. 2018; https://doi.org/10.1007/s00345-018-2378-4.
2. Hinman F, Redewill FH. Pyelovenous back flow. J Am Med Assoc. 1926;87(16):1287–93. https://doi.org/10.1001/jama.1926.02680160035011.
3. Kukreja RA, Desai MR, Sabnis RB, Patel SH. Fluid absorption during percutaneous nephrolithotomy: does it matter? J Endourol. 2002;16(4):221–4. https://doi.org/10.1089/089277902753752160.
4. Stenberg A, Bohman SO, Morsing P, Muller-Suur C, Olsen L, Persson AE. Back-leak of pelvic urine to the bloodstream. Acta Physiol Scand. 1988;134(2):223–34. https://doi.org/10.1111/j.1748-1716.1988.tb08483.x.
5. Boccafoschi C, Lugnani F. Intra-renal reflux. Urol Res. 1985;13(5):253–8.
6. Jung HU, Frimodt-Moller PC, Osther PJ, Mortensen J. Pharmacological effect on pyeloureteric dynamics with a clinical perspective: a review of the literature. Urol Res. 2006;34(6):341–50. https://doi.org/10.1007/s00240-006-0069-x.
7. Thomsen HS, Dorph S, Olsen S. Pyelorenal backflow in normal and ischemic rabbit kidneys. Investig Radiol. 1981;16(3):206–14.
8. Thomsen HS, Dorph S, Olsen S. Pyelorenal backflow in rabbits following clamping of the renal vein and artery: radiologic and microscopic investigation. Acta Radiol Diagn. 1982;23(2):143–8.
9. Thomsen HS, Larsen S, Talner LB. Pyelorenal backflow during retrograde pyelography in normal and ischemic porcine kidneys. A radiologic and pathoanatomic study. Eur Urol. 1982;8(5):291–7.
10. Carson CC, Nesbitt JA. Peritoneal extravasation during percutaneous lithotripsy. J Urol. 1985;134(4):725–7.
11. Hodson CJ. The effects of disturbance of flow on the kidney. J Infect Dis. 1969;120(1):54–60.
12. Sinclair JF, Hutchison A, Baraza R, Telfer AB. Absorption of 1.5% glycine after percutaneous ultrasonic lithotripsy for renal stone disease. Br Med J (Clin Res Ed). 1985;291(6497):691–2.
13. Dimberg M, Norlen H, Hoglund N, Allgen LG. Absorption of irrigating fluid during percutaneous transrenal lithotripsy. Scand J Urol Nephrol. 1993;27(4):463–7.
14. Malhotra SK, Khaitan A, Goswami AK, Gill KD, Dutta A. Monitoring of irrigation fluid absorption during percutaneous nephrolithotripsy: the use of 1% ethanol as a marker. Anaesthesia. 2001;56(11):1103–6.
15. Xu S, Shi H, Zhu J, Wang Y, Cao Y, Li K, Wang Y, Sun Z, Xia S. A prospective comparative study of haemodynamic, electrolyte, and metabolic changes during percutaneous nephrolithotomy and minimally invasive percutaneous nephrolithotomy. World J Urol. 2014;32(5):1275–80. https://doi.org/10.1007/s00345-013-1204-2.
16. Zhong W, Leto G, Wang L, Zeng G. Systemic inflammatory response syndrome after flexible ureteroscopic lithotripsy: a study of risk factors. J Endourol. 2015;29(1):25–8. https://doi.org/10.1089/end.2014.0409.
17. Seitz C, Desai M, Hacker A, Hakenberg OW, Liatsikos E, Nagele U, Tolley D. Incidence, prevention, and management of complications following percutaneous nephrolitholapaxy. Eur Urol. 2012;61(1):146–58. https://doi.org/10.1016/j.eururo.2011.09.016.
18. Michel MS, Trojan L, Rassweiler JJ. Complications in percutaneous nephrolithotomy. Eur Urol. 2007;51(4):899–906. discussion 906. https://doi.org/10.1016/j.eururo.2006.10.020.
19. Kreydin EI, Eisner BH. Risk factors for sepsis after percutaneous renal stone surgery. Nat Rev Urol. 2013;10(10):598–605. https://doi.org/10.1038/nrurol.2013.183.
20. Omar M, Noble M, Sivalingam S, El Mahdy A, Gamal A, Farag M, Monga M. Systemic inflammatory response syndrome after percutaneous nephrolithotomy: a randomized single-blind clinical trial evaluating the impact of irrigation pressure. J Urol. 2016;196(1):109–14. https://doi.org/10.1016/j.juro.2016.01.104.
21. Schwalb DM, Eshghi M, Davidian M, Franco I. Morphological and physiological changes in the urinary tract associated with ureteral dilation and ureteropyeloscopy: an experimental study. J Urol. 1993;149(6):1576–85.
22. Li X, Liu M, Bedja D, Thoburn C, Gabrielson K, Racusen L, Rabb H. Acute renal venous obstruction is more detrimental to the kidney than arterial occlusion: implication for murine models of acute kidney injury. Am J Physiol Renal Physiol. 2012;302(5):F519–25. https://doi.org/10.1152/ajprenal.00011.2011.
23. Park Y, Hirose R, Dang K, Xu F, Behrends M, Tan V, Roberts JP, Niemann CU. Increased severity of renal ischemia-reperfusion injury with venous clamping compared to arterial clamping in a rat model. Surgery. 2008;143(2):243–51. https://doi.org/10.1016/j.surg.2007.07.041.
24. Cao Z, Yu W, Li W, Cheng F, Rao T, Yao X, Zhang X, Larre S. Oxidative damage and mitochondrial injuries are induced by various irrigation pressures in rabbit models of mild and severe hydronephrosis. PLoS One. 2015;10(6):e0127143. https://doi.org/10.1371/journal.pone.0127143.
25. Hodson CJ. Neuhauser lecture. Reflux nephropathy: a personal historical review. AJR Am J Roentgenol. 1981;137(3):451–62. https://doi.org/10.2214/ajr.137.3.451.
26. Thomsen HS. Pyelorenal backflow. Clinical and experimental investigations. Radiologic, nuclear, medical and pathoanatomic studies. Dan Med Bull. 1984;31(6):438–57.
27. Meng H, Chen S, Chen G, Tan F, Wang C, Shen B. Renal subcapsular hemorrhage complicating

ureterolithotripsy: an unknown complication of a known day-to-day procedure. Urol Int. 2013;91(3):335–9. https://doi.org/10.1159/000350891.
28. Xu L, Li G. Life-threatening subcapsular renal hematoma after flexible ureteroscopic laser lithotripsy: treatment with superselective renal arterial embolization. Urolithiasis. 2013;41(5):449–51. https://doi.org/10.1007/s00240-013-0585-4.
29. Atici S, Zeren S, Aribogan A. Hormonal and hemodynamic changes during percutaneous nephrolithotomy. Int Urol Nephrol. 2001;32(3):311–4.
30. Mohta M, Bhagchandani T, Tyagi A, Pendse M, Sethi AK. Haemodynamic, electrolyte and metabolic changes during percutaneous nephrolithotomy. Int Urol Nephrol. 2008;40(2):477–82. https://doi.org/10.1007/s11255-006-9093-6.
31. Dogan HS, Sahin A, Cetinkaya Y, Akdogan B, Ozden E, Kendi S. Antibiotic prophylaxis in percutaneous nephrolithotomy: prospective study in 81 patients. J Endourol. 2002;16(9):649–53. https://doi.org/10.1089/089277902761402989.
32. Zhong W, Zeng G, Wu K, Li X, Chen W, Yang H. Does a smaller tract in percutaneous nephrolithotomy contribute to high renal pelvic pressure and postoperative fever? J Endourol. 2008;22(9):2147–51. https://doi.org/10.1089/end.2008.0001.
33. Guo HQ, Shi HL, Li XG, Gan WD, Zeng LQ, Liu GX, Yang Y, Liu TS. [Relationship between the intrapelvic perfusion pressure in minimally invasive percutaneous nephrolithotomy and postoperative recovery]. Zhonghua wai ke za zhi [Chinese J Surgery]. 2008;46(1):52–4.
34. Fung LC, Atala A. Constant elevation in renal pelvic pressure induces an increase in urinary N-acetyl-beta-D-glucosaminidase in a nonobstructive porcine model. J Urol. 1998;159(1):212–6.
35. Cao Z, Yu W, Li W, Cheng F, Xia Y, Rao T, Yao X, Zhang X, Larre S. Acute kidney injuries induced by various irrigation pressures in rat models of mild and severe hydronephrosis. Urology. 2013;82(6):1453.e9–16. https://doi.org/10.1016/j.urology.2013.08.024.
36. Landman J, Venkatesh R, Ragab M, Rehman J, Lee DI, Morrissey KG, Monga M, Sundaram CP. Comparison of intrarenal pressure and irrigant flow during percutaneous nephroscopy with an indwelling ureteral catheter, ureteral occlusion balloon, and ureteral access sheath. Urology. 2002;60(4):584–7.
37. Shao Y, Shen ZJ, Zhu YY, Sun XW, Lu J, Xia SJ. Fluid-electrolyte and renal pelvic pressure changes during ureteroscopic lithotripsy. Minim Invasive Ther Allied Technol. 2012;21(4):302–6. https://doi.org/10.3109/13645706.2011.595419.
38. Rattner WH, Fink S, Murphy JJ. Pressure studies in the human ureter and renal pelvis. J Urol. 1957;78(4):359–62.
39. Struthers NW. The role of manometry in the investigation of pelvi-ureteral function. Br J Urol. 1969;41(2):129–62.
40. Weaver RG, Yelderman JJ. The positive pressure catheter for measurement of intracavital pressures and pressure patterns. J Urol. 1967;98(6):718–20.
41. Whitaker RH. Methods of assessing obstruction in dilated ureters. Br J Urol. 1973;45(1):15–22.
42. Whitaker RH. An evaluation of 170 diagnostic pressure flow studies of the upper urinary tract. J Urol. 1979;121(5):602–4.
43. Veenboer PW, de Jong TP. Antegrade pressure measurement as a diagnostic tool in modern pediatric urology. World J Urol. 2011;29(6):737–41. https://doi.org/10.1007/s00345-011-0717-9.
44. Doizi S, Letendre J, Cloutier J, Ploumidis A, Traxer O. Continuous monitoring of intrapelvic pressure during flexible ureteroscopy using a sensor wire: a pilot study. World J Urol. 2020; https://doi.org/10.1007/s00345-020-03216-w.
45. Pfitzner J. Poiseuille and his law. Anaesthesia. 1976;31(2):273–5.
46. Bullock KN. The biomechanical principles of upper urinary tract pressure-flow studies. Br J Urol. 1983;55(2):136–9.
47. Kiil F. Pressure recordings in the upper urinary tract. Scand J Clin Lab Invest. 1953;5(4):383–4. https://doi.org/10.3109/00365515309094217.
48. Kinn AC. Pressure flow studies in hydronephrosis. Scand J Urol Nephrol. 1981;15(3):249–55.
49. Lupton EW, Holden D, George NJ, Barnard RJ, Rickards D. Pressure changes in the dilated upper urinary tract on perfusion at varying flow rates. Br J Urol. 1985;57(6):622–4.
50. Pfister RC, Newhouse JH, Hendren WH. Percutaneous pyeloureteral urodynamics. Urol Clin North Am. 1982;9(1):41–9.
51. Fichtner J, Boineau FG, Lewy JE, Sibley RK, Vari RC, Shortliffe LM. Congenital unilateral hydronephrosis in a rat model: continuous renal pelvic and bladder pressures. J Urol. 1994;152(2 Pt 2):652–7.
52. Guohua Z, Wen Z, Xun L, Wenzhong C, Yongzhong H, Zhaohui H, Ming L, Kaijun W. The influence of minimally invasive percutaneous nephrolithotomy on renal pelvic pressure in vivo. Surg Laparosc Endosc Percutan Tech. 2007;17(4):307–10. https://doi.org/10.1097/SLE.0b013e31806e61f4.
53. Huusmann S, Wolters M, Schilling D, Kruck S, Bader M, Tokas T, Herrmann TR, Nagele U. [Pressure study of two miniaturised amplatz sheaths of 9.5 F and 12 F outer diameter for minimal invasive percutaneous nephrolithotomy (MIP): an ex vivo organ model measurement]. Aktuelle Urol. 2018. https://doi.org/10.1055/a-0759-0140.
54. Zeng G, Zhu W, Liu Y, Fan J, Lam W, Lan Y, Cai C, Deng T, Li X, Zhao Z. Prospective comparative study of the efficacy and safety of new-generation versus first-generation system for super-mini-percutaneous nephrolithotomy: a revolutionary approach to improve endoscopic vision and stone removal. J Endourol. 2017;31(11):1157–63. https://doi.org/10.1089/end.2017.0558.

55. Zeng G, Zhu W, Liu Y, Fan J, Zhao Z, Cai C. The new generation super-mini percutaneous nephrolithotomy (SMP) system: a step-by-step guide. BJU Int. 2017;120(5):735–8. https://doi.org/10.1111/bju.13955.
56. Tepeler A, Akman T, Silay MS, Akcay M, Ersoz C, Kalkan S, Armagan A, Sarica K. Comparison of intrarenal pelvic pressure during micro-percutaneous nephrolithotomy and conventional percutaneous nephrolithotomy. Urolithiasis. 2014;42(3):275–9. https://doi.org/10.1007/s00240-014-0646-3.
57. Tokas T, Skolarikos A, Herrmann TRW, Nagele U. Pressure matters 2: intrarenal pressure ranges during upper-tract endourological procedures. World J Urol. 2018; https://doi.org/10.1007/s00345-018-2379-3.
58. Saltzman B, Khasidy LR, Smith AD. Measurement of renal pelvis pressures during endourologic procedures. Urology. 1987;30(5):472–4.
59. Goble NM, Hammonds JC. An in vitro study of intracavitary pressures during percutaneous nephrolithotomy. Br J Urol. 1987;60(4):307–11.
60. Low RK. Nephroscopy sheath characteristics and intrarenal pelvic pressure: human kidney model. J Endourol. 1999;13(3):205–8. https://doi.org/10.1089/end.1999.13.205.
61. Troxel SA, Low RK. Renal intrapelvic pressure during percutaneous nephrolithotomy and its correlation with the development of postoperative fever. J Urol. 2002;168(4 Pt 1):1348–51. https://doi.org/10.1097/01.ju.0000030996.64339.f1.
62. Mager R, Balzereit C, Reiter M, Gust K, Borgmann H, Husch T, Nagele U, Haferkamp A, Schilling D. Introducing a novel in vitro model to characterize hydrodynamic effects of percutaneous nephrolithotomy systems. J Endourol. 2015;29(8):929–32. https://doi.org/10.1089/end.2014.0854.
63. Nagele U, Horstmann M, Sievert KD, Kuczyk MA, Walcher U, Hennenlotter J, Stenzl A, Anastasiadis AG. A newly designed amplatz sheath decreases intrapelvic irrigation pressure during mini-percutaneous nephrolitholapaxy: an in-vitro pressure-measurement and microscopic study. J Endourol. 2007;21(9):1113–6. https://doi.org/10.1089/end.2006.0230.
64. Desai J, Solanki R. Ultra-mini percutaneous nephrolithotomy (UMP): one more armamentarium. BJU Int. 2013;112(7):1046–9. https://doi.org/10.1111/bju.12193.
65. Desai MR, Sharma R, Mishra S, Sabnis RB, Stief C, Bader M. Single-step percutaneous nephrolithotomy (microperc): the initial clinical report. J Urol. 2011;186(1):140–5. https://doi.org/10.1016/j.juro.2011.03.029.
66. Li X, He Z, Wu K, Li SK, Zeng G, Yuan J, He Y, Lei M. Chinese minimally invasive percutaneous nephrolithotomy: the Guangzhou experience. J Endourol. 2009;23(10):1693–7. https://doi.org/10.1089/end.2009.1537.
67. Nagele U, Walcher U, Bader M, Herrmann T, Kruck S, Schilling D. Flow matters 2: how to improve irrigation flow in small-calibre percutaneous procedures-the purging effect. World J Urol. 2015; https://doi.org/10.1007/s00345-015-1486-7.
68. Nicklas AP, Schilling D, Bader MJ, Herrmann TR, Nagele U. The vacuum cleaner effect in minimally invasive percutaneous nephrolitholapaxy. World J Urol. 2015; https://doi.org/10.1007/s00345-015-1541-4.
69. Song L, Chen Z, Liu T, Zhong J, Qin W, Guo S, Peng Z, Hu M, Du C, Zhu L, Yao L, Yang Z, Huang J, Xie D. The application of a patented system to minimally invasive percutaneous nephrolithotomy. J Endourol. 2011;25(8):1281–6. https://doi.org/10.1089/end.2011.0032.
70. Yang Z, Song L, Xie D, Deng X, Zhu L, Fan D, Peng Z, Guo S, Ye Z. The new generation mini-PCNL system—monitoring and controlling of renal pelvic pressure by suctioning device for efficient and safe PCNL in managing renal staghorn calculi. Urol Int. 2016;97(1):61–6. https://doi.org/10.1159/000442002.
71. Nagele U, Nicklas A. Vacuum cleaner effect, purging effect, active and passive wash out: a new terminology in hydrodynamic stone retrival is arising-does it affect our endourologic routine? World J Urol. 2016;34(1):143–4. https://doi.org/10.1007/s00345-015-1575-7.
72. Shah K, Agrawal MS, Mishra DK. Superperc: a new technique in minimally-invasive percutaneous nephrolithotomy. Indian J Urol. 2017;33(1):48–52. https://doi.org/10.4103/0970-1591.194784.
73. Zanetti SP, Lievore E, Fontana M, Turetti M, Gallioli A, Longo F, Albo G, De Lorenzis E, Montanari E. Vacuum-assisted mini-percutaneous nephrolithotomy: a new perspective in fragments clearance and intrarenal pressure control. World J Urol. 2020; https://doi.org/10.1007/s00345-020-03318-5.

# Tract Dilatation, Nephroscopy, Stone Fragmentation, and Retrieval

15

Dilip K. Mishra and Madhu S. Agrawal

## 15.1 Introduction

It has now been well established that PCNL (Percutaneous nephrolithotripsy) can achieve a high stone-free rate over a short treatment period in most patients. At the present time, when a post-operative CT scan is considered the standard method of confirming stone clearance, no other procedure can match the primary stone-free rates of PCNL for upper tract urolithiasis.

The procedure of PCNL is based on the creation of a direct percutaneous renal access to the pelvicalyceal system, followed by fragmentation and removal of the stone. Recent efforts to decrease the complications of PCNL have focused on reducing access size, leading to the development of Mini-PCNL. There is now enough evidence to suggest that decreasing the tract size for PCNL could decrease bleeding and reduce morbidity [1]. The most important aspect of the performance of a PCNL procedure revolves around a correct and accurate puncture. Once the puncture is achieved, tract dilatation, nephroscopy, and stone removal comprise the bulk of the PCNL procedure. We shall discuss these important aspects of PCNL in this chapter.

## 15.2 Tract Dilatation

Tract dilatation refers to increasing the percutaneous tract to the required size for placement of Amplatz sheath to allow the introduction of nephroscope and retrieval of stone. The various techniques of dilatation include metal telescopic dilatation (MTD), single-step dilatation (SSD), balloon dilatation (BD), and fascial Amplatz dilatation (AD) [2, 3]. In the case of standard PCNL, tract dilatation goes up to 24–30 Fr, whereas in Mini-PCNL, the tract dilatation is mostly done up to 15–18 Fr.

### 15.2.1 Puncture Prerequisites

"Mini-PCNL" essentially signifies the use of nephroscope and Amplatz sheaths of smaller caliber as compared to the conventional PCNL. It utilizes a nephroscope of 12 F size with an Amplatz sheath size of 15–18 F. However, the technique of initial puncture remains the same *(discussed in Sect. 4, Chaps. 9–13 of this book).*

D. K. Mishra (✉)
Kasturba Medical College, Manipal, Karnataka, India

Head, Department of Urology, Pushpanjali Hospital and Research Center, Agra, Uttar Pradesh, India

Department of Urology, Center for Minimally-Invasive Endourology, Global Rainbow Healthcare, Agra, Uttar Pradesh, India

M. S. Agrawal
Professor and Head, Department of Urology, Global Rainbow Healthcare, Agra, Uttar Pradesh, India

SN Medical College, Agra, Uttar Pradesh, India


M. S. Agrawal et al. (eds.), *Minimally Invasive Percutaneous Nephrolithotomy*,
https://doi.org/10.1007/978-981-16-6001-6_15

Access is obtained to the desired calyx with either USG or fluoroscopic guidance and a Terumo or extra-stiff guidewire is inserted in the pelvicalyceal system. It is important to place a good length of the wire in the pelvicalyceal system, preferably in the upper ureter, to avoid slippage of the wire. The puncture should be in line with the infundibulum through which access is intended, to minimize the torque effect on the parenchyma. If multiple tracts are needed in a given case, it is advisable to obtain all accesses at the beginning itself, with separate guidewires for each access. These tracts can be dilated later on a preferential basis as needed.

### 15.2.2 Metal Telescopic Dilatation (MTD)

This was the first described method for percutaneous tract dilatation, proposed by Alken et al. [4] An Alken's cannula is introduced over the guidewire under fluoroscopic control which is followed by a guide rod. This is followed by an introduction of serial telescopic metal dilators which slide one over the other till the required diameter of Amplatz sheath to be placed is reached. The advantage of this system is that a central rod is always there to guide the dilator, and if the initial angle and depth are maintained, there is minimal chance of under- or over-dilatation. The equipment, being metallic, is reusable and thus cost-effective, and remains a popular approach in conventional PCNL. However, it has largely been replaced by the simpler single-step dilatation (SSD) in mini-PCNL.

### 15.2.3 Single-step Dilatation (SSD)

This system was proposed by Frattini et al. [5] in 2001. Herein the desired tract size is created in a single step with the dilator of appropriate size without resorting to multiple steps. After initial puncture and guidewire placement, the desired sized dilator is passed over the Alken rod followed by the access sheath. This takes considerably less time and the amount of radiation exposure is also less with this technique. In mini-PCNL, this is the preferred form of dilatations; the tract size is also small (Fig. 15.1).

An alternative, which is our preferred choice, is to use a single-step screw dilator. The dilator is made of PTFE and is flexible to allow easy passage through the muscles and fascia. This has a considerable advantage over conventional dila-

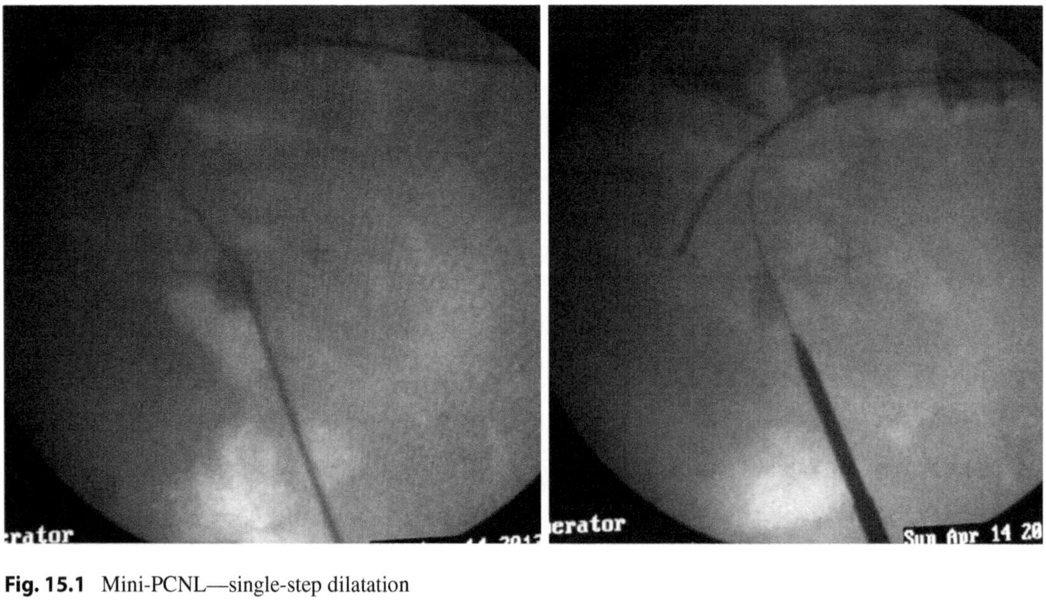

**Fig. 15.1** Mini-PCNL—single-step dilatation

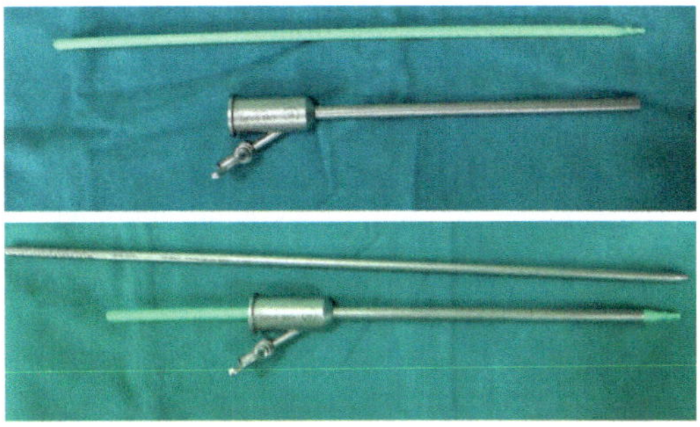

**Fig. 15.2** Screw dilator

tors, as this screw dilator can be passed straight over the initial guidewire. The dilator is advanced in a screwing motion till it reaches the desired position. The access sheath can be back-loaded over the dilator and can be slid in all the way once the dilator is in place. The entire process is over quickly, saving on time as well as radiation exposure. Figure 15.2 (screw dilator with sheath).

### 15.2.4 Balloon Dilatation (BD)

The use of a balloon dilator for tract dilatation was proposed by Clayman et al. [6] in 1983. This involved passing a balloon over the guidewire into the pelvicalyceal system over which the desired access sheath can be passed. This has been a popular approach in conventional PCNL where a tract size of 30 Fr was used. The balloon dilates the tract in one shot; however, the procedure must be done under complete fluoroscopic control, resulting in greater radiation exposure. The balloon dilator (Nephromax; Boston Scientific, MA) is available in size of 30 F which is suitable for standard PCNL.

The procedure involves the passing of a 0.035- or 0.038-inch guidewire into the pelvicalyceal system through the puncture needle once an appropriate puncture is made. A 10-F fascial dilator is advanced over the guidewire. After these steps, tract dilatation is performed with a balloon dilator which is inflated with a LeVeen inflator (Boston Scientific) until all "waisting" in the balloon disappears. The Amplatz sheath is passed over the balloon to create the final tract [7].

### 15.2.5 Fascial Amplatz Dilatation (FAD)

This method of tract dilatation is like telescopic metal dilatation. In standard PCNL, serial passage of Amplatz dilators is done, progressing from 8 to 30 F followed by placement of the Amplatz sheath over the last dilator [8]. The disadvantage is that when one dilator is withdrawn, it allows bleeding in the tract until the next dilator comes in. In mini-PCNL, the number of steps is less as the dilatation needs to proceed only up to 15–18 Fr, which also provides an opportunity to use one-step dilatation in these cases.

### 15.2.6 Trouble Shooting

Tract dilatation in PCNL holds as much importance as an initial puncture. If this step goes wrong, it may cause severe hemorrhage and may lead to loss of tract, and may result in abandoning the procedure. In cases of under-dilatation wherein the Amplatz sheath is still in the parenchyma or outside the PCS, the dilator needs to be passed yet again over the guidewire till it is inside the PCS and the full process of dilatation is repeated and the Amplatz sheath advanced and secured before a relook. In such cases, it is not unusual to encounter bleeding and collection of clots inside the PCS.

The guidewire should always be retained in place without letting it slip out until the tract is fully secured. The initial angle of the tract must be maintained throughout the dilatation procedure, failing which the guidewire may kink at the fascial interfaces during dilatation. The tip of the guide rod should be kept at the point in a calyx and care should be taken not to advance the dilator beyond that point. The final dilator and sheath should be passed to the pre-desired point only and any further advancement of the Amplatz sheath is to be done under nephroscopic vision.

Sometimes, over-dilatation may lead to shearing of the infundibulum and hemorrhage. In cases of over-dilatation, we need to assess the damage done during nephroscopy. If there is bleeding from the infundibulum, it may be controlled by advancing the Amplatz beyond the traumatized area, to create a tamponade effect. In severe cases, the procedure may be curtailed with the placement of a Nephrostomy.

If the dilator is advanced more, it may sometimes lead to a counter-puncture of the opposite wall of pelvicalyceal system, leading to extravasation of fluid and extrusion of stone fragments. In counter-puncture cases, if the injury is minor, one may proceed to finish quickly under low-pressure irrigation, while avoiding extrusion of stone fragments. However, if there is major perforation, it is wise to abandon the procedure and place a JJ Stent and a nephrostomy to allow drainage and healing of the system.

## 15.3 Nephroscopy

Nephroscopy refers to the introduction of a nephroscope through the access sheath placed in the tract created, to inspect the PCS and remove the stone. In the case of mini-PCNL, the tract size is <20Fr, so only mini-nephroscopes are used in these settings. Mini-nephroscopes are supplied by several manufacturers, and the most popular size is 12 Fr (Fig. 15.3). Smaller sizes including 7.5 Fr, called by several names including "ultra-mini" PCNL and "MIP XS" are also available (Fig. 15.4). The various nephroscopes have been discussed in Chap. 5.

With the initial introduction of nephroscope, we must assess the adequacy of dilatation and any trauma to the PCS. The Amplatz sheath must be advanced or retracted as required under vision to get a clear view of the PCS and the stone. It should be our endeavor to have a direct access to the stone without much torque on the renal parenchyma. Any clot if present should be either washed out or removed with appropriate grasping forceps. Once the PCS is clear of clots and debris, stone fragmentation should be started.

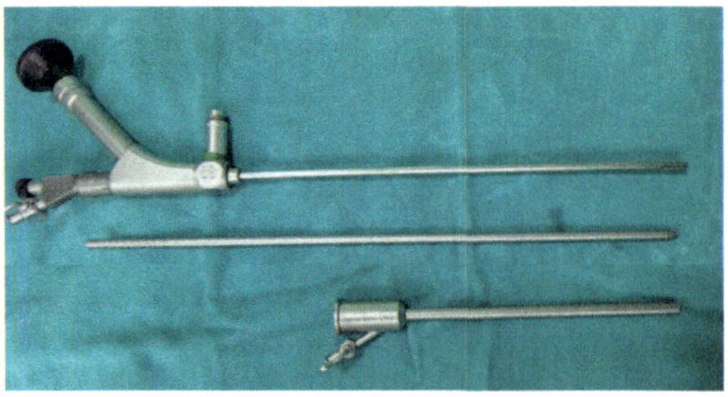

**Fig. 15.3** Mini-PCNL Equipment (12 Fr Nephroscope and 15 Fr Amplatz sheath)

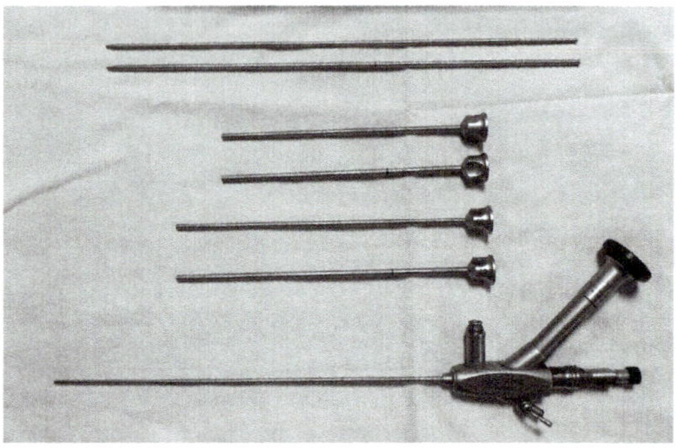

**Fig. 15.4** MIP XS Equipment (7.5Fr Nephroscope and 8.5 and 11 Fr Amplatz sheaths)

Working with an Amplatz sheath of 15–18 Fr and a 12 Fr nephroscope leaves adequate space between the telescope and sheath for the outflow of irrigation fluid during nephroscopy. This helps in keeping the intra-renal pressures low and also allows egress of any stone dust and fragments, clots, and infected urine and debris.

Nephroscope is also useful to pass a guidewire across the Pelvi-Ureteric Junction (PUJ) for placement of a DJ stent at completion. Stenting is optional in mini-PCNL (discussed elsewhere in this book) but is often required in the case of upper ureteric stones, edematous pelvi-ureteric junction, or in presence of bleeding or significant trauma to the mucosa.

## 15.4 Stone Fragmentation and Retrieval

Various lithotripsy devices are available for stone fragmentation, ranging from pneumatic lithotripters which work very well for larger stone bulk, to Lasers that can do effortless lithotripsy for any stone type. All these have been discussed in Chap. 6 of this book. The type of lithotripter chosen is decided by the stone bulk and type of stone.

In cases of small and medium stone burden (<2 cm size), Lasers work very well. The major advantages offered by Lasers are smooth operation, smaller fragments and limited retropulsion. Holmium is the most popular laser for stone fragmentation, as being a pulsed laser, it is highly efficient in stone fragmentation. There are various settings available for stone fragmentation or dusting during Laser lithotripsy. In mini-PCNL, fragmentation may be chosen as the primary modality to clear the stone completely and rapidly. The usual laser settings are frequency ranging from 10 to 30 Hz with the energy of 1.5–3 Joules with power outputs ranging from 15 to 50 Watts. One can work with 550 μm fiber, which passes easily through the working channel of nephroscope [9]. High-power settings in Holmium YAG laser, beyond 50 watts, can be very useful for large and hard stones but should be used with caution.

A new addition to the laser armamentarium is the Thulium Fiber Laser (TFL). TFL has been found to be effective for soft tissue application as well as lithotripsy. Due to its continuous-wave form and high-frequency format, it has been found to have a special benefit for stone dusting and is believed to produce less retropulsion as compared to conventional holmium laser [10].

A remarkable feature of mini-PCNL is the "vacuum-cleaner effect" which allows stone fragments to get washed out with the in-and-out movement of the telescope without the use of any graspers [11]. The hydrodynamics of the outflow of irrigation fluid through the Amplatz sheath creates a "Venturi effect," producing a low-pressure bubble in front of the telescope which entraps the freshly produced fragments and allows them to be retrieved as the telescope is withdrawn through the Amplatz sheath (Fig. 15.5).

In addition, various bi-pronged and tri-pronged graspers of 3–5 Fr size are also available, which can be passed through the working channel of nephroscope. These devices help to remove clots or stone fragments that may be stuck to the mucosa and fail to get washed out with irrigation flow. A stone basket of appropriate size can also be used to grasp and remove any fragments.

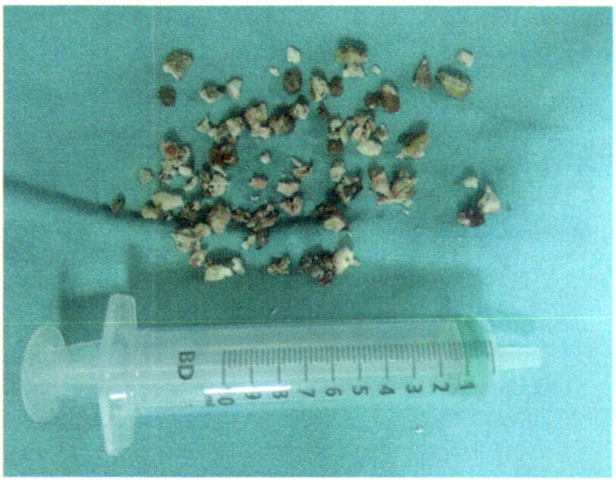


**Fig. 15.5** Stone fragments after Spontaneous expulsion (Extracted fragments)

Another new addition to the mini-PCNL armamentarium is suction, either in the sheath or in the lithotripsy probe. In mini-PCNL, sheaths with suction have begun to play a major role in getting quick and good clearance. The Super Mini Perc (SMP), and the Super perc (Shah Sheath), both work on a similar principle, explained in Chaps. 19 and 20 of this book, with suction as an integral part of the sheath. The stone fragments are sucked inside the sheath as the stone is fragmented and delivered to a stone collection bottle.

For large volume stones, as in multiple or staghorn stones, we now have dual-energy lithotripters like Trilogy (EMS) or Shock-pulse (Olympus), which use a combination of Ballistic and Ultrasonic lithotripsy. The third component in these advanced combined lithotripters is the availability of suction through the channel of the lithotripsy probe, which allows rapid clearance of the stone fragments, and thus is extremely helpful in large stone bulk. The details about these new gadgets are available in a separate chapter in this book.

## References


1. Monga M, Oglevie S. Minipercutaneous nephrolithotomy. J Endourol. 2000;14(5):419–21. https://doi.org/10.1089/end.2000.14.419.
2. Wu Y, Xun Y, Lu Y, Hu H, Qin B, Wang S. Effectiveness and safety of four tract dilatation methods of percutaneous nephrolithotomy: a meta-analysis. Exp Ther Med. 2020;19(4):2661–71. https://doi.org/10.3892/etm.2020.8486. Epub 2020 Feb 4
3. Yamaguchi A, Skolarikos A, Buchholz NP, Chomón GB, Grasso M, Saba P, Nakada S, de la Rosette J, Clinical Research Office of The Endourological Society Percutaneous Nephrolithotomy Study Group. Operating times and bleeding complications in percutaneous nephrolithotomy: a comparison of tract dilatation methods in 5,537 patients in the Clinical Research Office of the Endourological Society Percutaneous Nephrolithotomy Global Study. J Endourol. 2011;25(6):933–9. https://doi.org/10.1089/end.2010.0606. Epub 2011 May 13
4. Alken P, Hutschenreiter G, Günther R. Percutaneous kidney stone removal. Eur Urol. 1982;8(5):304–11. https://doi.org/10.1159/000473540.
5. Frattini A, Barbieri A, Salsi P, Sebastio N, Ferretti S, Bergamaschi E, Cortellini P. One shot: a novel method to dilate the nephrostomy access for percutaneous lithotripsy. J Endourol. 2001;15(9):919–23. https://doi.org/10.1089/089277901753284143.
6. Clayman RV, Castañeda-Zuñiga WR, Hunter DW, et al. Rapid balloon dilatation of the nephrostomy track for nephrostolithotomy. Radiology. 1983;147:884–5.
7. Gönen M, Istanbulluoglu OM, Cicek T, Ozturk B, Ozkardes H. Balloon dilatation versus Amplatz dilatation for nephrostomy tract dilatation. J Endourol. 2008;22(5):901–4. https://doi.org/10.1089/end.2007.0167.
8. Al-Kandari AM, Jabbour M, Anderson A, Shokeir AA, Smith AD. Comparative study of degree of renal trauma between Amplatz sequential fascial dilation and balloon dilation during percutaneous renal surgery in an animal model. Urology. 2007;69(3):586–9. https://doi.org/10.1016/j.urology.2007.01.025.
9. Bujons A, Millán F, Centeno C, Emiliani E, Sánchez Martín F, Angerri O, Caffaratti J, Villavicencio H. Mini-percutaneous nephrolithotomy with high-power holmium YAG laser in pediatric patients with staghorn and complex calculi. J Pediatr Urol. 2016;12(4):253.e1–5. https://doi.org/10.1016/j.jpurol.2016.04.027. Epub 2016 May 26
10. Korolev D, Akopyan G, Tsarichenko D, Shpikina A, Ali S, Chinenov D, Corrales M, Taratkin M, Traxer O, Enikeev D. Minimally invasive percutaneous nephrolithotomy with SuperPulsed thulium-fiber laser. Urolithiasis. 2021;49(5):485–91. https://doi.org/10.1007/s00240-021-01258-2. Epub ahead of print
11. Nicklas AP, Schilling D, Bader MJ, Herrmann TR, Nagele U, Training and Research in Urological Surgery and Technology (T.R.U.S.T.)-Group. The vacuum cleaner effect in minimally invasive percutaneous nephrolitholapaxy. World J Urol. 2015;33(11):1847–53. https://doi.org/10.1007/s00345-015-1541-4. Epub 2015 Apr 2

# 16 Exit Strategy After PCNL

Palaniappan Sundaram, Mukhilesh Ramesh,
Dilip K. Mishra, and Madhu S. Agrawal

## 16.1 Introduction

Let us look at a case scenario: the PCNL has been done successfully, complete clearance of all stone fragments has been achieved. Now a decision needs to be made, what next? Placement of a nephrostomy tube has been the traditional approach, regardless of the complexity of the PCNL. Nephrostomy tube can be a Nelaton catheter, Malecot tube, pigtail catheter, Foley catheter, or a nephro-ureteral stent.

However, over the years, our understanding of the procedure of PCNL has evolved greatly. It is now understood that a tubeless or totally tubeless procedure can be performed safely, avoiding nephrostomy altogether. "Tubeless" refers to a procedure where an indwelling double-J (DJ) stent or a ureteric catheter alone (with no nephrostomy) is placed. "Totally tubeless" refers to a case where there is no internal or external drainage. In such situations, the normal ureter will be the only drainage for the kidney.

The initial purpose of the nephrostomy was to allow good drainage of the pelvicalyceal system, and additionally, aid in the healing of the percutaneous tract. Small stone fragments and clots may pass via the nephrostomy without causing significant obstruction to the urinary tract. Hence, the nephrostomy would prevent renal colic, urinary extravasation, and possible urinoma formation. This is crucial particularly in procedures where there is ureteral or pelvi-ureteric junction edema or obstruction. Moreover, nephrostomy provides access for future procedures through the same tract. This may be a planned re-look procedure, antegrade nephrostogram, or percutaneous chemolysis. Importantly, it was often thought to reduce bleeding by allowing tamponade of the tract. However, there is sufficient evidence to support this assumption, as seen in studies where bleeding complications were found to be no worse when tubeless procedures are performed [1].

P. Sundaram (✉)
Department of Urology, Sengkang General Hospital, Singapore, Singapore
e-mail: palaniappan.sundaram@singhealth.com.sg

M. Ramesh
KKS Hospital and Kidney Care Center, Gobichettipalayam, Tamil Nadu, India

D. K. Mishra
Kasturba Medical College, Manipal, Karnataka, India

Head, Department of Urology, Pushpanjali Hospital and Research Center, Agra, Uttar Pradesh, India

Department of Urology, Center for Minimally-Invasive Endourology, Global Rainbow Healthcare, Agra, Uttar Pradesh, India

M. S. Agrawal
Professor and Head, Department of Urology, Global Rainbow Healthcare, Agra, Uttar Pradesh, India

SN Medical College, Agra, Uttar Pradesh, India


M. S. Agrawal et al. (eds.), *Minimally Invasive Percutaneous Nephrolithotomy*,
https://doi.org/10.1007/978-981-16-6001-6_16

## 16.2 Large Tube Versus Small Tube

Several authors have investigated whether the smaller size of the nephrostomy tube had any benefits. Liatsikos et al. studied the benefit of an 18-F nephrostomy over the 24-F nephrostomy using a randomized trial [2] while Pietrow and colleagues compared 22-F nephrostomy with a 10-F pigtail catheter in a randomized fashion [3]. Another randomized study by Desai et al. assessed the differences between 20-F nephrostomy, 9-F pigtail catheter, and a tubeless approach with an indwelling stent [4]. All three studies found that smaller nephrostomy induced less pain and hence reduced the analgesic requirements. It also resulted in less urine leakage [2, 4, 5]. The tract contracts around the smaller tube and hence seals earlier without much urine leaking after the tube removal. No increase in bleeding rates was seen in these studies. In addition, postoperatively patients with smaller tubes were found to have a short hospitalization period. It was found that patients with larger percutaneous nephrostomy had an increased risk of urine leakage after tube removal. This was most likely related to the tract not collapsing as the large tube kept it splinted open, leaving a fistula that may take longer to close off.

However, CROES PCNL database presented contradictory results, with the smaller bore (<18F) nephrostomy group having significantly greater bleeding, higher fever, and higher complications than the larger bore nephrostomy group (>18F). The rates of urine leakage, duration of hospital stay, and stone-free rates were no different between the two groups. The conclusion of this study was if there was a need to place a nephrostomy, especially in complicated cases, the larger tube was preferable. These results may be attributed to the heterogeneous population and unmatched groups included in this study [6].

## 16.3 Tubeless PCNL

Although tubeless PCNL was proposed as early as 1984 by Wickham [7], within the next 2 years Winfield reported poor outcomes of severe discomfort and prolonged hospital stay in two patients, putting the progress of tubeless PCNL on a long hold [8]. Eventually, Bellman and colleagues revived this technique in 1997 with an internal stent in place of an external nephrostomy [9]. This tubeless technique refers to the absence of a nephrostomy, but often a stent is left in place for a period of 1–2 weeks (Fig. 16.1). However, any ureteral drainage is acceptable, which could be in the form of a DJ stent on an external string or even a retrograde ureteral catheter.

The supposed hemostatic advantage of leaving the nephrostomy that was equal to the size of the initial access sheath was found to be less plausible as the use of small caliber nephrostomy did not result in an increased risk of bleeding from the tract. On the other hand, early tract closure due to the absence of the nephrostomy may actually result in better tamponade of the tract.

The tubeless approach has significant advantages, which have been demonstrated practically. Firstly, there is decreased pain leading to lower

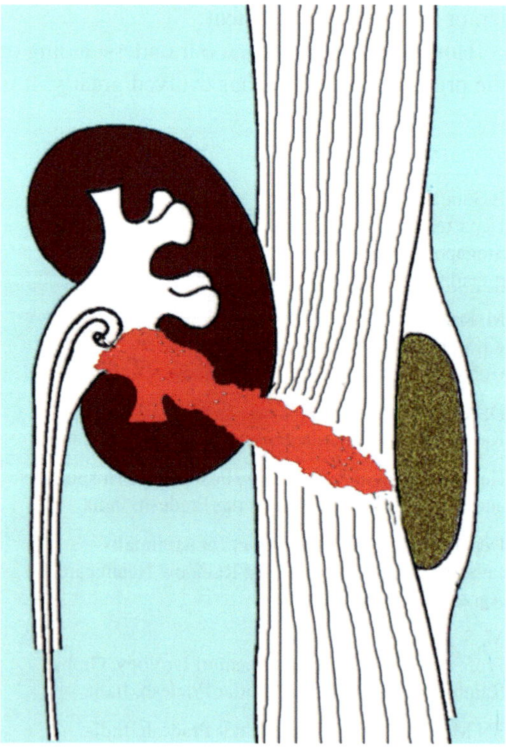

**Fig. 16.1** Tubeless PCNL with DJ stent

analgesic usage and greater patient comfort. Secondly, there is avoidance of external drainage of the kidney. Thirdly, tract contracts completely after removal of the Amplatz sheath reducing the likelihood of protracted urine leakage which is more commonly associated with nephrostomy placement. The presence of the nephrostomy would lead to the maturation of the tract which may lead to prolonged urinary leakage. Lastly, with all the above benefits, the hospital stay is reduced to a minimum, and healthcare costs are kept low.

### 16.3.1 Tubeless PCNL with Ureteric Catheter for Drainage

As these tubeless procedures usually had double-J stents placed, this created a new set of issues for the patients. They reported more discomfort related to the indwelling stent and required medications to cope with the symptoms [10]. Moreover, they required an additional procedure, cystoscopy, to remove the stent at a later date. Hence a ureteral catheter [11] or a DJ stent on a string [12] could be an alternative. Meta-analysis comparing drainage of tubeless procedures by ureteric catheter and DJ stent showed no differences in complication rate, change in hemoglobin, postoperative pain, need for analgesia, operative time, and hospital stay [13]. When an external ureteric catheter was used for 1 or 2 days, stent-related symptoms could be avoided, thus improving the quality of life for the patients. In minimally invasive PCNL, the use of an external ureteric catheter for 24 hours or even less, with a correspondingly short hospital stay, is feasible as demonstrated in a study conducted at our center using Ultra-Mini-PCNL (UMP) [14].

### 16.3.2 Tubeless PCNL with DJ Stent on an External String

An alternative option is the placement of a double-J stent on completion of the procedure in an antegrade fashion leaving an external string

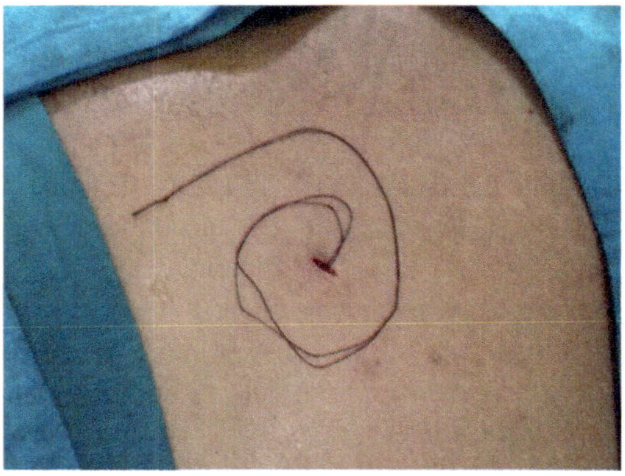

**Fig. 16.2** Tubeless PCNL with tether exiting through external tract

[15], which exits through the nephrostomy tract (Fig. 16.2). This allows the stent to be removed from the flank as an office procedure without the need for cystoscopy. The tether exiting from the flank also provides access to pelvicalyceal system for a re-look procedure. The tether can be used to pull the proximal end of the stent to the skin level, to allow passing a guidewire down the ureter to gain access to the pelvicalyceal system.

## 16.4 Early Nephrostomy Tube Removal

Early nephrostomy tube removal was also considered as an alternative to address the issue of stent-related symptoms in tubeless procedures. This involves removal of the nephrostomy after the first postoperative day instead of later in the postoperative period. Mishra et al. performed a randomized study and found analgesic requirement, drop in hemoglobin and hospital stay in early nephrostomy removal patients to be equivalent to the tubeless group. However, the stone clearance was better in the early tube removal group while urine leak was of shorter duration in the tubeless group. The presence of the tube gives the option of the second-look nephroscopy to improve stone clearance if at all required [16, 17].

## 16.5 Impact of Mini and Ultra-mini-PCNL on the Exit Strategy

Bleeding is an inherent part of PCNL. This starts as soon as the puncture and dilatation is performed which causes blunt trauma to the kidney. In recent years, it has been understood that reducing the caliber of the percutaneous access reduces bleeding complications significantly [18]. Mini-PCNL was first described by Jackman and colleagues [19]. Its advantages were reproducible and together with the use of holmium laser, advances in optics, smaller accessories, and fragmentation devices, mini-PCNL established itself as an important armamentarium for the treatment of urolithiasis. With mini-PCNL, the differences between small-bore nephrostomy and tubeless procedure became less apparent. Mini-PCNL has opened up the possibilities of doing away with drainage altogether, allowing urologists to perform more frequently "totally tubeless PCNL."

## 16.6 Totally Tubeless PCNL

Since the presence of a stent adds further morbidity to the patient in the form of bothersome stent symptoms, "totally tubeless" procedure came about in order to reduce the patient morbidity [20, 21]. This proved to be a safe and feasible option in a selected population. The length of stay as well as the need for analgesia were significantly lower in the totally tubeless group as compared to the standard PCNL group.

A meta-analysis showed totally tubeless procedure resulted in shorter operative time, shorter hospital stay, and reduced postoperative analgesia requirements. No significant difference existed in terms of drop in hemoglobin, postoperative fever, and stone-free rates [22]. Another network meta-analysis of 16 trials reported a comparison of large tube, small tube, tubeless, and totally tubeless [23]. Totally tubeless and small tube PCNL groups were superior to tubeless procedure in terms of the drop in hemoglobin while the length of hospital stay was shorter in totally tubeless and tubeless groups. It was postulated by the authors that the presence of the stent in the tubeless group may have caused more hematuria compared to the other groups. This reinforces the fact that leaving any tube in the patient adds to the morbidity, and the earliest removal results in best outcomes. However, we must remain mindful that these studies are conducted in selected populations by experienced surgeons in high-volume centers.

## 16.7 Adjuncts for Hemostasis and Sealants

Innovative techniques have been described to aid in the hemostasis of the tract created for PCNL. Specifically for mini-PCNL, mechanical compression for some minutes after the procedure usually stops the small amount of bleeding from the tract. Placing stitches in the deep fascia may help sometimes. Other adjuncts have also been described to aid tubeless procedures, such as direct diathermy of the bleeding points and cryotherapy to the tract prior to the removal of the tube.

Instillation of various hemostatic agents has been used as quicker alternatives to achieve hemostasis [24]. These include oxidized cellulose, gelatin, and fibrin sealants. Examples of gelatin matrix products are Floseal, Surgiflo, and Spongostan. These do not contain fibrinogen so thrombin present in the product would activate the patient's own fibrinogen to form the fibrin clot. In addition, they expand to many times greater than their original volume to produce a compressive effect. Examples of fibrin sealants include Tisseel, Evicel, and Tachosil. Tachosil may produce the clot regardless of patient factors as they contain both thrombin and fibrinogen. The clinical utility of these agents is still unclear as experimental studies show some adverse effects. Gelatin matrix products become a fine suspension of particles when it is in contact with urine whereas fibrin sealants form a thicker semi-solid material, which may remain even after 5 days of contact in urine and hence may predispose to stone formation [25]. Though the use of sealants remains controversial with respect to earlier hemostasis, the quick closure of the tract will aid recovery and encourage more tubeless procedures.

## 16.8 Specific Situations

### 16.8.1 Bleeding

Bleeding is commonly from two sources. It can occur if the opposite wall is injured during dilatation when the dilators overshoot past the renal parenchyma. The other area of bleeding is from the tract itself. In both these situations, the best immediate treatment is to place a nephrostomy across the bleeding site and leave it clamped. A clot that forms will tamponade further bleeding. If the bleeding from the tract is very severe, a Foley catheter with traction or a Kaye nephrostomy catheter may be used.

### 16.8.2 Perforation of Pelvicalyceal System

Perforation of the pelvicalyceal system may lead to fluid extravasation and lead to perinephric collection or even fluid overload if absorbed into the intravascular space. In addition, when there is large perforation, stone fragments may extrude outside the kidney. The irrigation fluid does not remain in the pelvicalyceal system in the event of a large perforation. Hence, there will be no distension and the pelvicalyceal system will collapse. This makes it difficult to progress with stone fragmentation and retrieval. In these large perforations, it would be prudent to stage the procedure by placing a DJ stent and a nephrostomy away from the perforation site. This would allow healing of the perforation as urine is drained away from the perforation via the stent and the nephrostomy. Whereas with a small perforation, no specific treatment is needed.

### 16.8.3 Complex and Staghorn Stones

In PCNL for complex stone or staghorn stone, multiple tracts may be used. In such instances, following the same tubeless principle, placing multiple tubes is not necessary, a single nephrostomy tube drainage is adequate [26]. It should be placed in the largest tract to provide adequate drainage and to allow re-entry if there is a need for a re-look.

### 16.8.4 PCNL in Children

The exit strategy after PCNL in children needs to be individualized. The age of the patent is not the deciding criterion. Saleem et al. [27] assessed the outcome of tubeless PCNL in children (mean age 7.5 years) and found out that tubeless PCNL was less painful, less troublesome, and shortens the hospital stay of the child. In this study, the procedure was a standard PCNL with 24 Fr sheath and drainage was through an externalized ureteric catheter, removed 24–48 hours postoperatively. The miniaturization of PCNL has also made the tubeless PCNL feasible and safe. Bilen et al. [28] showed a tubeless mini-PCNL safe option for children with stone disease. The mean age in this study was 3 years and the tubeless procedure was found to have a short hospitalization course.

### 16.8.5 PCNL in Patients with Previous Open Surgery

PCNL in patients with a history of previous open surgery can be done tubeless. Shah et al. [29] in their study showed 25 patients who underwent tubeless PCNL with a history of open surgery for calculus in the ipsilateral renal unit had a short hospital stay and low analgesia requirement. They did not have any compromise in stone-free rate or increased complication. Lojanapiwat [30] performed tubeless PCNL in similar patients and found out that there was no increased complication rate.

### 16.8.6 Bilateral Tubeless PCNL

Simultaneous bilateral tubeless PCNL is a safe and effective exit strategy [31–34]. Shah et al. [31] studied the outcome of bilateral tubeless PCNL in 10 patients with those who underwent bilateral PCNL with a nephrostomy tube. They showed that bilateral tubeless PCNL is safe and effective without increasing the complication rate. The outcome of bilateral tubeless PCNL in staghorn calculus was compared with staged PCNL by Wang et al. [32]. They reported that there was no increase in complication rate as well as blood loss. The stone-free rate was similar to staged PCNL with nephrostomy tube while pain, analgesic requirement, hospital stay, and cost were low.

### 16.8.7 Ambulatory Tubeless PCNL

Tubeless PCNL as an ambulatory procedure is feasible [35, 36]. Singh et al. [35] performed tubeless PCNL under spinal anesthesia (bupivacaine with fentanyl) in 10 consecutive patients. The patients were discharged the next day with no complications. The advantage of tubeless PCNL, combined with spinal anesthesia, makes ambulatory tubeless PCNL effective and feasible.

### 16.8.8 PCNL in Renal Anomalies

The ectopic position of kidneys does not make the tubeless PCNL impossible. Matlaga and associates [37] showed lap-assisted PCNL in 6 patients with pelvic kidney to be successful. Aghamir et al. [38] published their randomized study comparing totally tubeless PCNL with standard PCNL in renal anomalies. Their results showed that even for moderate to large stone burden the tubeless PCNL had decreased pain, hospitalization days, and early return to activity.

### 16.8.9 PCNL in Obese Patients

The outcome of tubeless PCNL in obese patients was analyzed by Yang et al. [39] in their study; they analyzed the data of 45 patients who had normal BMI (18.5–25), 55 overweight (BMI 25–30), 28 obese (BMI 30–40), and 5 morbid obese (BMI greater than 40). A stone-free rate of 94.5% was achieved. BMI does not affect the stone-free rate or complication rate of tubeless PCNL [40]. Kazem Aghamir et al. [41] in their study compared standard PCNL with totally tubeless PCNL in obese patients (BMI >35). They showed that early return of activity in totally tubeless PCNL and recommended it for the obese.

## 16.9 Summary

Recent meta-analyses have shown that tubeless procedures resulted in a shorter operative duration, shorter hospital stay, earlier convalescence, lesser postoperative pain, and lower analgesia requirements [16]. In terms of complications, urine leakage rates were markedly lower. No significant difference in rates of fever, bleeding and other complications were seen. Moreover, the stone-free rates were not significantly different between patients who underwent tubeless procedures and those who had nephrostomy placement [1, 4, 42, 43]. A comparison of the advantages and disadvantages of tubeless procedure vs conventional PCNL is provided in Table 16.1.

Regardless, we need to remain mindful of the need for a nephrostomy in certain situations such as prolonged multi-tract procedures, bilateral procedures, pyonephrosis or infection, significant bleeding, large pelvicalyceal system perforation, pleural injury, patient on antiplatelets, patients with renal impairment, or when re-look nephroscopy is needed.

**Table 16.1** Comparison of tube and tubeless procedures

| | PCNL with Nephrostomy Tube | Tubeless PCNL |
|---|---|---|
| Advantages | Able to drain kidney even if ureter is obstructed<br>Possible re-look procedure can be performed if residual stones are present | Less pain<br>Shorter hospitalization<br>Shorter duration of urine leak from puncture site |
| Disadvantages | More pain<br>Longer hospitalization<br>Longer duration of urine leak from puncture site | Clot colic<br>Unable to perform re-look nephroscopy for residual stones |

## References


1. Agrawal MS, Agrawal M, Gupta A, Bansal S, Yadav A, Goyal J. A randomized comparison of tubeless and standard percutaneous nephrolithotomy. J Endourol. 2008;22(3):439–42. https://doi.org/10.1089/end.2007.0118.
2. Liatsikos EN, Hom D, Dinlenc CZ, et al. Tail stent versus re-entry tube: a randomized comparison after percutaneous stone extraction. Urology. 2002;59:15–9.
3. Pietrow PK, Auge BK, Lallas CD, et al. Pain after percutaneous nephrolithotomy: impact of nephrostomy tube size. J Endourol. 2003;17:411–4.
4. Desai MR, Kukreja RA, Desai MM, et al. A prospective randomized comparison of type of nephrostomy drainage following percutaneous nephrostolithotomy: large bore versus small bore versus tubeless. J Urol. 2004;172:565–7.
5. Marcovich R, Jacobson AI, Singh J, Shah D, El-Hakim A, Lee BR, Smith AD. No panacea for drainage after percutaneous nephrolithotomy. J Endourol. 2004;18(8):743–7. https://doi.org/10.1089/end.2004.18.743.
6. Cormio L, Preminger G, Saussine C, Buchholz NP, Zhang X, Walfridsson H, Gross AJ, de la Rosette J. Nephrostomy in percutaneous nephrolithotomy (PCNL): does nephrostomy tube size matter? Results from the Global PCNL Study from the Clinical Research Office Endourology Society. World J Urol. 2013;31(6):1563–8.
7. Wickham JE, Miller RA, Kellett MJ, Payne SR. Percutaneous nephrolithotomy: one stage or two? Br J Urol. 1984;56(6):582–5.
8. Winfield HN, Weyman P, Clayman RV. Percutaneous nephrostolithotomy: complications of premature nephrostomy tube removal. J Urol. 1986;136(1):77–9. https://doi.org/10.1016/s0022-5347(17)44733-1.
9. Bellman GC, Davidoff R, Candela J, Gerspach J, Kurtz S, Stout L. Tubeless percutaneous renal surgery. J Urol. 1997;157(5):1578–82.
10. Shah HN, Kausik VB, Hegde SS, Shah JN, Bansal MB. Tubeless percutaneous nephrolithotomy: a prospective feasibility study and review of previous reports. BJU Int. 2005;96(6):879–83.
11. Goh M, Wolf JS Jr. Almost totally tubeless percutaneous nephrolithotomy: further evolution of the technique. J Endourol. 1999;13:177–80.
12. Choi M, Brusky J, Weaver J, et al. Randomized trial comparing modified tubeless percutaneous nephrolithotomy with tailed stent with percutaneous nephrostomy with smallbore tube. J Endourol. 2006;20:766–70.
13. Chen Y, Feng J, Yue Y, Zhao Z, Deng T, Wu W, Zeng G. Externalized ureteral catheter versus double-J stent in tubeless percutaneous nephrolithotomy for upper urinary stones: a systematic review and meta-analysis. J Endourol. 2018 Jul;32(7):581–8.
14. Agrawal MS, Agarwal K, Jindal T, Sharma M. Ultra-mini-percutaneous nephrolithotomy: a minimally-invasive option for percutaneous stone removal. Indian J Urol. 2016;32:132–6.
15. Agrawal MS, Sharma M, Agarwal K. Tubeless percutaneous nephrolithotomy using antegrade tether: a randomized study. J Endourol. 2014;28(6):644–8.
16. Mishra S, Sabnis RB, Kurien A, Ganpule A, Muthu V, Desai M. Questioning the wisdom of tubeless percutaneous nephrolithotomy (PCNL): a prospective randomized controlled study of early tube removal vs tubeless PCNL. BJU Int. 2010;106(7):1045–8.
17. Xun Y, Wang Q, Hu H, Lu Y, Zhang J, Qin B, Geng Y, Wang S. Tubeless versus standard percutaneous nephrolithotomy: an update meta-analysis. BMC Urol. 2017;17(1):102. https://doi.org/10.1186/s12894-017-0295-2.
18. Yamaguchi A, Skolarikos A, Buchholz NP, Chomón GB, Grasso M, Saba P, Nakada S, de la Rosette J, Clinical Research Office of The Endourological Society Percutaneous Nephrolithotomy Study Group. Operating times and bleeding complications in percutaneous nephrolithotomy: a comparison of tract dilation methods in 5,537 patients in the Clinical Research Office of the Endourological Society Percutaneous Nephrolithotomy Global Study. J Endourol. 2011;25(6):933–9.
19. Jackman SV, Docimo SG, Cadeddu JA, Bishoff JT, Kavoussi LR, Jarrett TW. The "mini-perc" technique: a less invasive alternative to percutaneous nephrolithotomy. World J Urol. 1998;16(6):371–4.
20. Karami H, Gholamrezaie HR. Totally tubeless percutaneous nephrolithotomy in selected patients. J Endourol. 2004;18:475–6.
21. Istanbulluoglu MO, Ozturk B, Gonen M, et al. Effectiveness of totally tubeless percutaneous nephrolithotomy in selected patients: a prospective randomized study. Int Urol Nephrol. 2009;41:541–5.
22. Li Q, Gao L, Li J, Zhang Y, Jiang Q. Total tubeless versus standard percutaneous nephrolithotomy: a meta-analysis. Minim Invasive Ther Allied Technol. 2020;29(2):61–9.
23. Lee JY, Jeh SU, Kim MD, Kang DH, Kwon JK, Ham WS, Choi YD, Cho KS. Intraoperative and postoperative feasibility and safety of total tubeless, tubeless, small-bore tube, and standard percutaneous nephrolithotomy: a systematic review and network meta-analysis of 16 randomized controlled trials. BMC Urol. 2017;17(1):48.
24. Nagele U, Schilling D, Anastasiadis AG, et al. Closing the tract of mini-percutaneous nephrolithotomy with gelatine matrix hemostatic sealant can replace nephrostomy tube placement. Urology. 2006;68(3):489–94. https://doi.org/10.1016/j.urology.2006.03.081.
25. Uribe CA, Eichel L, Khonsari S, Finley DS, Basillote J, Park HK, Li CC, Abdelshehid C, Lee DI, McDougall EM, Clayman RV. What happens to hemostatic agents in contact with urine? An in vitro study. J Endourol. 2005;19(3):312–7. https://doi.org/10.1089/end.2005.19.312.

26. Agrawal MS, Agrawal M. Are multiple nephrostomy tubes necessary after multi-tract percutaneous nephrolithotomy? A randomized comparison of single versus multiple nephrostomy tubes. J Endourol. 2009;23(11):1831–4.
27. Salem HK, Morsi HA, Omran A, Daw MA. Tubeless percutaneous nephrolithotomy in children. J Pediatr Urol. 2007;3:235–8.
28. Bilen C, Gunay M, Ozden E, Inci K, Sarikaya S, Tekgul S. Tubeless mini percutaneous nephrolithotomy in infants and preschool children: a preliminary report. J Urol. 2010;184:2498–502. https://doi.org/10.1016/j.juro.2010.08.039.
29. Shah HN, Mahajan AP, Hegde SS, Bansal M. Tubeless percutaneous nephrolithotomy in patients with previous ipsilateral open renal surgery: a feasibility study with review of literature. J Endourol. 2008;22:19–24.
30. Lojanpiwat B. Previous open nephrolithotomy: does it affect the percutaneous nephrolithotomy techniques and outcomes? J Endourol. 2006;20:17–20.
31. Shah HN, Kausik VB, Hegde SS, Shah JN, Bansal MB. Safety and efficacy of bilateral simultaneous tubeless percutaneous nephrolithotomy. Urology. 2005;66:500–4.
32. Wang CJ, Chang CH, Huang SW. Simultaneous bilateral tubeless percutaneous nephrolithotomy of staghorn stones: a prospective randomized controlled study. Urol Res. 2011;39(4):289–94. https://doi.org/10.1007/s00240-010-0342-x. Epub 2010 Dec 16
33. Weld KJ, Wake RW. Simultaneous bilateral tubeless percutaneous nephrolithotomy. Urology. 2000;56:1057.
34. Gupta NP, Kumar P, Aron M, Goel R. Bilateral simultaneous tubeless percutaneous nephrolithotomy. Int Urol Nephrol. 2003;35:313–4.
35. Singh I, Kumar A, Kumar P. "Ambulatory PCNL" (tubeless PCNL under regional anesthesia): a preliminary report of 10 cases. Int Urol Nephrol. 2005;37:35–7.
36. Beiko D, Lee L. Outpatient tubeless percutaneous nephrolithotomy: the initial case series. Can Urol Assoc J. 2010;4(4):E86–90. https://doi.org/10.5489/cuaj.886.
37. Matlaga BR, Kim SC, Watkins SL, Kuo RL, Munch LC, Lingeman JE. Percutaneous nephrolithotomy for ectopic kidneys: over, around, or through. Urology. 2006;67:513–7.
38. Aghamir SM, Mohammadi A, Mosavibahar SH, Meysamie AP. Totally tubeless percutaneous nephrolithotomy in renal anomalies. J Endourol. 2008;22(9):2131–4. https://doi.org/10.1089/end.2008.0015.
39. Yang RM, Bellman GC. Tubeless percutaneous renal surgery in obese patients. Urology. 2004;63:1036–41.
40. Kuntz NJ, Neisius A, Astroza GM. Does body mass index impact the outcomes of tubeless percutaneous nephrolithotomy? BJU Int. 2014;114:404–11.
41. Aghamir SMK, Mohseni MG, Hosseini SR, Salavati A, Ganjali H, Fallah MA, Rezaei H, Modaresi SS. Totally tubeless percutaneous nephrolithotomy is feasible in morbidly obese patients. Turk J Urol. 2017;43(2):162–4. https://doi.org/10.5152/tud.2017.03185. Epub 2017 Jun 1.
42. Feng MI, Tamaddon K, Mikhail A, Kaptein JS, Bellman GC. Prospective randomized study of various techniques of percutaneous nephrolithotomy. Urology. 2001;58(3):345–50. https://doi.org/10.1016/s0090-4295(01)01225-0.
43. Shah HN, Sodha HS, Khandkar AA, et al. A randomized trial evaluating type of nephrostomy drainage after percutaneous nephrolithotomy: small bore v tubeless. J Endourol. 2008;22:1433–9.

# Part VI

# Newer Advances in Mini PCNL

# 17 Ultra-mini PCNL

Ramandeep S. Chalokia and Janak Desai

## 17.1 Introduction

Percutaneous nephrolithotomy (PCNL) remains the treatment of choice for large and complex renal stones leading to a higher rate of stone clearance as compared to Shockwave lithotripsy (SWL) and retrograde intrarenal surgery (RIRS) [1, 2]. It all began in 1941 when Rupel and Brown from Indianapolis removed a stone through an already formed nephrostomy track [3]. Fernstrom and Johansson further pioneered the concept of stone removal with percutaneous access using radiologic control in the late 1970s [4]. Further progress in the optics and imaging techniques, three-dimensional computed tomography reconstruction, improved telescopes, novel, and efficient energy devices contributed to the rapid development of this technique to a well-recognized method of minimally invasive method of renal stone treatment [5, 6].

Although PCNL is considered safe, it can, however, be associated with significant morbidity with complications which include postoperative sepsis (2%), fever (10–16%), blood transfusion (3–6%), and significant bleeding (8%) [7]. Sheath size is the key parameter associated with blood loss. The incidence of transfusion was about 1.1% for smaller sheaths (less than 18Fr) as compared to 5.9% for the standard large sheaths (27 Fr, 28 Fr, 30 Fr) and 12% in the largest sheaths (32 Fr, 33 Fr, and 34 Fr) in the analysis found by the Clinical Research Office of the Endourological Society (CROES) PCNL global study [8]. An ongoing global effort to reduce the rate of bleeding complication, potential damage to the renal parenchyma, and postoperative pain resulted in the creation of smaller cross-sectional endoscopes and sheaths for use in smaller size tracks to remove renal stones. These innovations resulted in various minimally invasive percutaneous methods to treat renal stones.

## 17.2 Ultra-mini PCNL

One of the above many methods was the development of ultra-mini PCNL (UMP) by Desai et al. from Ahmedabad, India [9]. This technique limits the dilatation to either 11 Fr or 13 Fr. This concept was borne out of the observation while performing standard PCNL, renal parenchyma was generally resilient up to a dilatation of 14–15 Fr. However, dilatation beyond 15 Fr resulted in lateral tears leading to increase in bleeding complication and renal parenchymal damage. A set of particularly designed instruments include a telescope of 1 mm with a resolution of 17,000 pixels; an inner sheath of 6.0 Fr, which has two ports

R. S. Chalokia
Warrington and Halton Teaching Hospitals, NHS Foundation Trust, Warrington, UK

J. Desai (✉)
Samved Hospital, Ahmedabad, Gujarat, India



M. S. Agrawal et al. (eds.), *Minimally Invasive Percutaneous Nephrolithotomy*,
https://doi.org/10.1007/978-981-16-6001-6_17

(one for the irrigation and the other for a laser fiber); and an outer sheath of 11 Fr or 13 Fr with a side-port that connects to a very thin tube running parallel to its lumen. The access is performed with the aid of ultrasound and dilatation done under fluoroscopy after the initial placement of a 6-Fr ureteric catheter cystoscopically under general anesthesia.

The stone fragmentation is done with a holmium laser of 200 or 365 μm with an aim to produce small fragments of 1.5–2.0 mm. The laser settings are set at high energy (12 W) and low frequency (8 Hz). The stone fragments are removed by creating a whirlpool effect by injecting saline through the side port of the outer sheath (see video).

Alternatively, a vortex can be created by injecting saline through the ureteric catheter. The fluid moves from a high-pressure zone of the renal pelvis and calyces into a low-pressure zone which is the lumen of the outer sheath. Frequently the fragments will be evacuated automatically by the vortex. On certain occasions, a low suction can be placed on the end of the outer sheath to remove the fragments. The mini whirlpool effect can be viewed in the small video (see video).

The results from the initial study were quite promising with SFR at 1 month of 86.66% on a cohort of 62 patients. Two patients required conversion into mini-PCNL due to bleeding and the average hemoglobin decrease was 1.4 gm/dl. The mean stone size was 16.8 mm.

The UMP can be used as a primary modality of renal stone treatment up to 20 mm or as a complement to the standard PCNL for removal of a stone in a difficult calyx while treating staghorn stone. The deemed advantage of the UMP over RIRS is the relative speed of the procedure and the use of minimal disposables which may result in UMP being more cost-effective. UMP and RIRS are compared in Table 17.1 [10].

Our results have been compared to other high stone volume centers using this modality of minimally invasive PCNL. Agrawal et al. used this method of renal stone treatment for stones measuring between 8 and 20 mm on a cohort of 120 patients. Complete stone fragmentation was seen in 114 out of 120 patients (95%). A 2-week follow-up revealed a stone-free rate of more than 99% (119/120) and there were no significant postoperative complications [11].

**Table 17.1** Comparison between ultra-mini-percutaneous nephrolithotomy and retrograde intrarenal surgery [10]

| | RIRS | UMP |
|---|---|---|
| Total cases | 20 | 32 |
| Operation time (min) | 98 | 46 |
| Hospitalization (h) | 32 | 24 |
| Cost of disposables (euros) | 484 | 80 |
| Complication rate | 8% | 6% |
| Stone-free rate | 80% | 88% |
| Auxiliary procedure | 100% | 1% |
| Fever (percentage of patients) | 20% | 12.5% |

*UMP* ultra-mini percutaneous nephrolithotomy, *RIRS* retrograde intrarenal surgery

## 17.3 Synopsis

UMP is a minimally invasive option of PCNL and demands a high level of experience before undertaking it. The availability of this technique along with the others such as Mini-PCNL, Micro-perc, Mini-micro PCNL, and Super-mini-PCNL provide a range of available treatment options along with standard PCNL for renal stones. The common driving factor for the introduction of these techniques is to minimize the risk of bleeding encountered during standard PCNL. Kukreja et al. analyzed potential factors leading to blood loss during PCNL. They found that using smaller tracts in pediatrics, non-hydronephrotic systems, and those with narrow infundibulum and secondary tracts in a multiple-tract procedure where the main bulk of the stone has been cleared with a wider tract may reduce the blood loss [12].

The need for a routine nephrostomy placement can be avoided in this technique which would have an important factor in minimizing the postoperative pain and hence quicker discharge [13].

For large renal stone burden, the standard PCNL would still be considered the gold standard. For renal stones of 1–2 cm size, either UMP or RIRS can be an option and the choice would also depend on the surgeon and familiarity with the technique and the stone location. UMP may

**Table 17.2** Observational comparison among minimally invasive treatment modalities for kidney stones [14]

| | Mini-PCNL | UMP | RIRS | Micro-perc |
|---|---|---|---|---|
| Cost of equipment | Moderate | Moderate | High | Moderate |
| Learning curve | High | High | Moderate | High |
| Stone-free rate | Good; even for large | Good, up to 1.8 cm size stone | Good, up to 1.8 cm size stone | Good, up to 1.0 cm size stone |
| Auxiliary procedure | Almost nil | Almost nil | Stent removal; pre-procedure stenting sometimes | Stein Strasse removal sometimes |
| Hospitalization | Two days | One day | One day | One day |

**Table 17.3** Comparison between miniaturized percutaneous nephrolithotomy instruments [14]

| | Mini-PCNL | UMP | Micro-perc |
|---|---|---|---|
| Smallest size of sheath | 17.5 Fr | 11.0 Fr | 4.85 FR |
| Stone removal | Forceps and fluid dynamics | Creating a fluid vortex | Leave for natural expulsion |
| Telescope size | 3 mm | 1 mm | 0.9 mm |
| Resolution of telescope | 30,000 pixels | 17,000 pixels | 10,000 pixels |

be preferred in lower pole stone. UMP can also be used as an auxiliary procedure to standard PCNL; the main bulk of the stone being dealt with standard PCNL and the UMP used for a small stone in an inaccessible calyx.

It is important to recognize the familiarity with the available surgical options and with the necessary skills one could facilitate a minimally invasive treatment of the renal stone without compromising the safety. Of course, these many options would create a dilemma of the choice of the treatment one could offer to a patient. This again may be reflected in the availability of instruments and experience of a particular technique familiar to the urologist (Tables 17.2 and 17.3) [14].

It is not surprising to note that there will be more advances in these modalities in the future and possibly more high-quality evidence to shed more light on the recommendations for their use. A lot would depend on the skill of the surgeon, availability of resources, patient factors and the financial implications to decide the best treatment for renal stones. The least invasive option of SWL, however, must be kept in mind before offering these modalities to the patient. One must remember that size of the tract does matter but more vital is the correct indication and the skill of the surgeon [15].

## References


1. EAU Guidelines Office, Arnhem, The Netherlands. http://uroweb.org/guidelines/compilations-of-all-guidelines/
2. Ganpule AP, Vijayakumar M, Malpani A, Desai MR. Percutaneous nephrolithotomy (PCNL) a critical review. Int J Surg. 2016;36(Pt D):660–4. https://doi.org/10.1016/j.ijsu.2016.11.028. Epub 2016 Nov 14
3. Rupel E, Brown R. Nephroscopy with removal of stone following nephrostomy for obstructive calculous anuria. J Urol. 1941;46:177.
4. Fernström I, Johansson B. Percutaneous pyelolithotomy. A new extraction technique. Scand JUrol Nephrol. 1976;10(3):257–9. https://doi.org/10.1080/21681805.1976.11882084.
5. Patel U, Walkden RM, Ghani KR, et al. Three-dimensional CT pyelography for planning of percutaneous nephrostolithotomy: accuracy of stone measurement, stone depiction and pelvicalyceal reconstruction. Eur Radiol. 2009;19:1280. https://doi.org/10.1007/s00330-008-1.
6. Lowe G, Knudsen BE. Ultrasonic, pneumatic and combination intracorporeal lithotripsy for percutaneous nephrolithotomy. J Endourol. 2009;23(10):1663–8. https://doi.org/10.1089/end.2009.1533.
7. Armitage JN, Irving SO, Burgess NA, For the British Association of Urological Surgeons Section of Endourology. Percutaneous nephrolithotomy in the United Kingdom: results of a prospective data registry. Eur Urol. 2012;61:1188–93.
8. Yamaguchi A, Skolarikos A, Buchholz N-PN, et al. Operating times and bleeding complications in percutaneous nephrolithotomy: a comparison of tract

dilatation methods in 5537 patients in the clinical research Office of the Endourological Society Percutaneous Nephrolithotomy Global Study. J Endourol. 2011;25:933.
9. Desai J, Solanki R. Ultra-mini percutaneous nephrolithotomy (UMP): one more armamentarium. BJUI Int. 2013;112:1046.
10. Desai J, Solanki R. E93 comparison of UMP v/s RIRS for lower calyx stone. Eur Urol Suppl. 2013;3:62.
11. Agrawal MS, Agarwal K, Jindal T, Sharma M. Ultra-mini-percutaneous nephrolithotomy: a minimally-invasive option for percutaneous stone removal. Indian Journal of Urology. 2016;32(2):132–6. https://doi.org/10.4103/0970-1591.174778.
12. Kukreja R, Desai M, Patel S, et al. Factors affecting blood loss during percutaneous nephrolithotomy: prospective study. J Endourol. 2004;18:715.
13. Akman T, Binbay M, Yuruk E, et al. Tubeless procedure is most important factor in reducing length of hospitalization after percutaneous nephrolithotomy: results of univariable and multivariable models. Urology. 2011;77:299–304.
14. Desai J, Miernik A. Chapter 24: Small-caliber percutaneous nephrolithotomy: mini, UMP and micro-perc. In: Smith AD, Preminger GM, Kavoussi LR, Badlani GH, Rastinehad AR, editors. Smith's textbook of endourology. 4th ed. Wiley; 2018. p. 301–9.
15. Knoll T. Is mini-percutaneous nephrolithotomy the way to go for renal stones? No! Curr Opin Urol. 2019;29(3):312–3. https://doi.org/10.1097/MOU.0000000000000614.

# 18 Micro-PCNL

Ravindra B. Sabnis and Abhijit P. Patil

## 18.1 Introduction

PCNL since its invention in the 1980s has undergone a lot of modifications. From open surgery to PCNL was a conceptual change & because of its minimally invasive nature, it became standard of care for treating renal stones. However, over a period of years, it was realized that PCNL is not without many complications and some can be disastrous. It became evident that the large tract was associated with many complications. In the year 2000, Miniperc was introduced with a tract size of 16–18 F, which had many advantages. Impressed with the success of Miniperc, several innovations were introduced like Ultra-Miniperc, super-miniperc, MIP-XS, Microperc, reducing the tract size to as low as 4.85 F. Microperc is the lowest tract size instrument used for the removal of kidney stones as of today.

## 18.2 How Microperc Came into Existence

Laparoscopy has a small needloscope which is used to see if the tract is proper or not especially if adhesions are expected in the abdomen, and with this 2 mm scope, the tract is created under vision to avoid any injury. Markus Badar thought to use the same technique for PCNL—to ensure that the PCS access was proper [1]. He called it "All-seeing needle"—purpose of which was to establish the tract under vision—so that tract can be made through papilla and complications of a wrong puncture could be avoided. His objective of using this method was only to get access to the kidney and once proper access is established, then proceed to regular PCNL. However, Desai et al. thought—why cannot this tract be utilized to complete the treatment of stone fragmentation [2]. This is how "Microperc" came into existence.

## 18.3 Concept of Microperc

All forms of PCNL have a similar concept, which involves multiple steps—(access to pelvicalyceal system (PCS), putting guide wire, dilating tract to whatever size, and nephroscopy) before stone disintegration. Microperc is different from other formats, as it is a one-step procedure. Once you get access, you can start doing nephroscopy and stone dusting. The steps of inserting guidewire and dilatation are avoided. Hence, many complications and problems arising out of wire insertion and tract dilatation are avoided. There are two ways in which PCS access can be obtained. The first method is by inserting a needle under vision. The optical needle avoids the risk of traversing through

R. B. Sabnis (✉) · A. P. Patil
Department of Urology, Muljibhai Patel Urological Hospital (MPUH), Nadiad, Gujarat, India


M. S. Agrawal et al. (eds.), *Minimally Invasive Percutaneous Nephrolithotomy*,
https://doi.org/10.1007/978-981-16-6001-6_18

the viscera and confirms the selection of the correct papilla [3]. Another method is getting access like any PCNL—fluro guided or USG guided.

## 18.4 Instruments (Fig. 18.1)

1. 3 part −16 G (4.85 F) needle (also called as all-seeing needle)
2. 0.9 mm Telescope which is flexible and has 10,000-pixel resolution—whose distal end has light cable and camera attachment provision
3. 3 part plastic adaptor
4. 200-micron laser fiber
5. Irrigation tubing which goes to irrigation pump.

## 18.5 Technique

It is performed under general or spinal anesthesia. The procedure can be performed in prone as well as supine position. In lithotomy position, ureteric catheter (preferably 6 or 7 F open-ended, multi-hole) is passed. Then, the patient is positioned in a prone or modified Valdivia position. The puncture of the desired calyx is done under fluoroscopic or ultrasonic guidance or using the direct visual guidance of the "all-seeing needle." Confirmation of PCS access can be done by fluid coming out of needle or by direct vision. Then a three-way adapter is connected to the hub. The latter serves as the inlet for—laser fiber (200/272 μ) via "Touhy Borst" adapter, saline irrigation, and 0.9 mm flexible telescope. Saline irrigation is under pressure irrigation enough for proper vision. Multi-hole ureteric catheter continuously drains the PC system to maintain the intrarenal pressures in physiological limit. A laser fiber is passed and stone is dusted. Once the stone is powdered completely and clearance is confirmed on fluoroscopy, then the needle is withdrawn. Ureteric catheter and foley are kept for 24 hrs. In case DJ stenting is desired, a ureteric catheter can be changed to DJ at the end of the procedure.

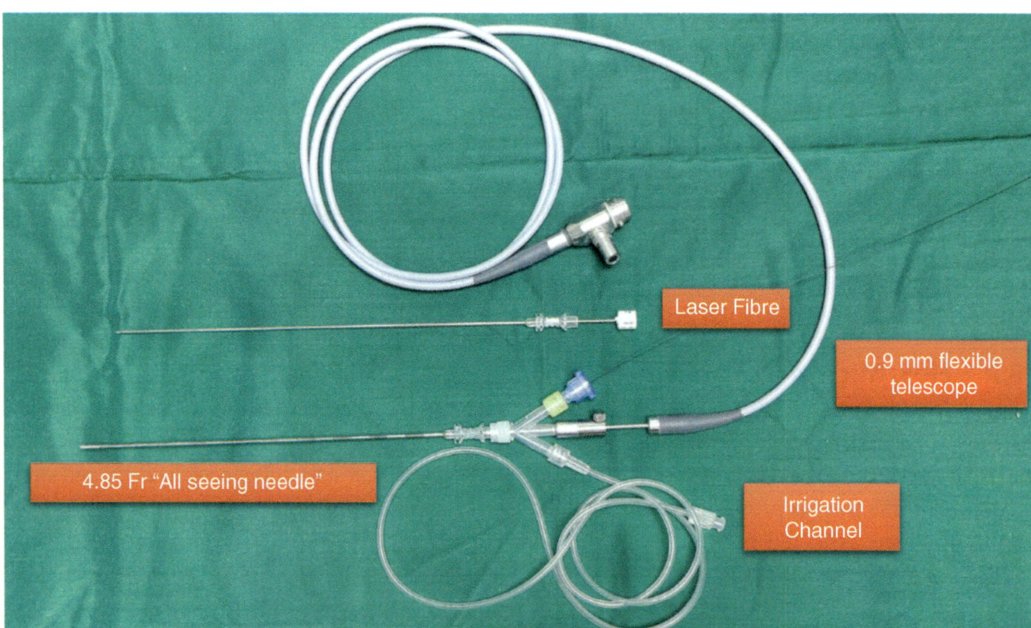


**Fig. 18.1** Microperc assembly consisting of—0.9 mm flexible telescope, 4.85 Fr "All-seeing needle" with three-way adaptor for laser fiber, scope, and irrigation channel

**Important Points**

1. Space inside the 16 G needle is limited—which has to accommodate a 0.9 mm telescope, laser fiber, and fluid irrigation. Hence, only 240 or less size laser fiber can be passed, irrigation will have to be used under pressure.
2. Telescope carries light as well as captures images. The camera or light cable is not attached near the needle as the needle will not take the weight of the camera as well as the light cable. Hence, light cable and camera attachments are at the other end of the cable. Camera and light cable are mounted away by an articulating arm (Fig. 18.2).
3. Better to use a large diameter multi-hole ureteric catheter—if a single-hole ureteric catheter is used, it can get blocked by stone fragments. If it gets blocked, free drainage from the ureteric catheter will not happen and thereby intrarenal pressures will increase.
4. It is a closed system; hence, irrigation pressure should be adjusted in such a way that it is just sufficient to keep vision good. Too much pressure and flow will distend the system and increase pressure. Flow should keep vision good and amount should match outflow coming out from the ureteric catheter.
5. Laser setting should be of dusting as there is no way to remove the fragments. Once the powder is formed, it will clear over a period of time.

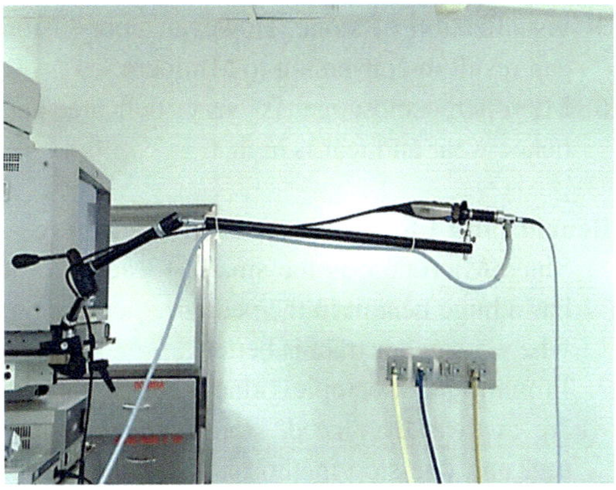

**Fig. 18.2** An articulating arm to mount the camera and light cable for Microperc

6. Since it is a needle puncture—it is always tubeless procedure.
7. In case DJ stenting is required (if any problem, for example—fragments are slightly bigger, injury to PCS), then this will have to be done at the end of the procedure—retrogradely.
8. In Microperc, usually, the desired calyx is calyx containing stone. Hence, generally, it is stone-guided puncture. Since the sheath is just a needle, there is no way to move from one calyx to other calyces. If you try to do that, the needle gets bent at abdominal wall level, as the needle has no strength. Hence, whether calyx is anterior or posterior is immaterial.
9. Since this is a one-step procedure, even if the puncture is not perfect or maybe a little oblique, it may not matter how much provided vision is good. Sub-optimal punctures pose problems and complications once such tract is dilated.
10. If stones migrate to some other calyx, it may be difficult to approach other calyces with Microperc and may require conversion to Miniperc. Hence, laser settings are very important—to dust the stone and prevent migration.
11. Fragment retrieval is not possible in Microperc—so in that way, it may be similar to RIRS or ESWL, where stones are blasted and stone fragments are expected to pass out.
12. Mostly, Microperc is used for a therapeutic purpose—stone removal. There are hardly any reports for only puncture purposes as originally was thought of.

## 18.6 Modifications of Microperc

Mini-Microperc (Fig. 18.3) is a modification of using 8/10 Fr outer sheath for better intrarenal manipulation and stability. The additional benefit is the admission of a 1.6-mm Ultrasonic Lithotripter (which helps with faster fragmentation and extracting of fragments) and basket or fine forceps (3 Fr) [4, 5].

Penbegul et al. used a double angiocath technique. Earlier, the author used a 14-gauge

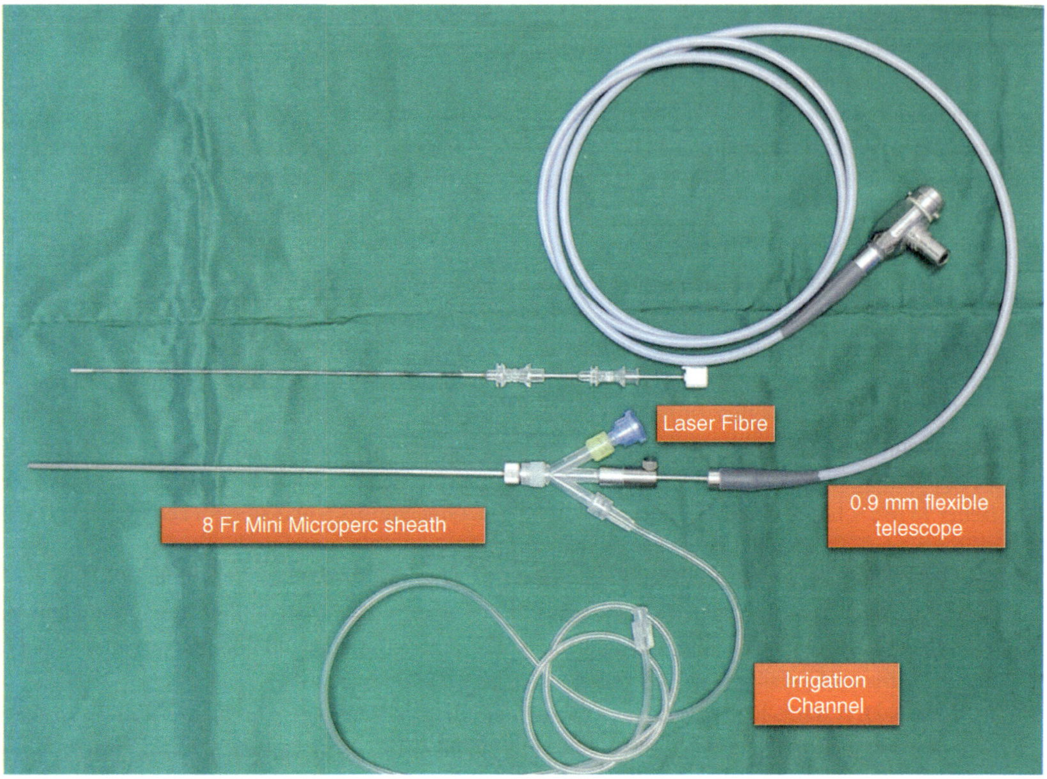


**Fig. 18.3** Mini-Microperc assembly: it is the same as conventional Microperc assembly except the 4.85 Fr needle is replaced with an 8 Fr Mini-Microperc sheath

angiocath needle and sheath (micro sheath) during microperc surgery for pediatric patients to reduce the IPP [6]. Now, a second angiocath is used to drain fluid during surgery [7].

Ibrahim Buddu et al. combined microperc with standard PCNL for complex renal stones to improve stone clearance rates without increasing the morbidity of the procedure [8].

**Drawbacks**

1. Thicker puncture needle (16 G–1.65 mm versus 20 G—0.9 mm or 18 G—1.27 mm)
2. Though it is an all-seeing needle, vision through the scope is red till calyx is reached.
3. Intrarenal pressure may rise. Even though a large multi-hole ureteric catheter is used, as it may not be sufficient to drain the same amount of fluid that is coming through irrigation.
4. There is no active stone retrieval mechanism. It depends on the natural passage of stone. Hence, clearance of stone from a calyx with a very thin infundibulum may be difficult.
5. Even if there is a small amount of blood/clot in the system, then vision will be hampered. There is no way to remove clots. Sometimes, clots cover stone. Laser disintegration of stone can be started to disperse clots and proper visualization of stone. However, poor vision can result in conversion to Miniperc.
6. Microperc telescope is very delicate and hence wear and tear is high.

**Benefits and Ideal Indications of Microperc**

1. Since Microperc is the smallest tract size, it has a huge benefit in the pediatric population, where a smaller tract is better.
2. In malrotated, ectopic kidneys, often calyces are awkwardly placed, stone targeted puncture and one-step method is most beneficial. In ectopic kidneys, USG-guided, puncture

and finishing procedure in one step can prevent a lot of complications. Just puncture usually does not have morbidity, even if it has hit surrounding structures. No requirement of dilatation makes it the most suitable method in anomalous kidneys provided stones are small.

3. Compact calyceal stone—where there is no space for wire placement, tract dilatation may not be complete, in that situation, stone-guided puncture and immediate laser disintegration makes it an ideal indication.
4. As additional tract in association with standard or miniperc has the benefit of achieving one more access without additional morbidity.
5. Stones for Microperc preferably should be less than 1.5 cm. Larger stones will take time and will need the necessity of fragment retrieval—which is not possible in microperc.

## 18.7 Outcomes and Need for Conversion [2, 4, 9–18]

The stone-free rates in various studies on microperc have been 82–97%, with a mean hospital stay of around 1–2 days. The hemoglobin drop in various studies ranged from 0.1 to 1.4 gm%. The majority of the complications of microperc are of low Clavien grade like fever, urinary tract infection, renal colic, intra–/extravasation, and need for DJ stenting. Many studies have reported steinstrasse and renal colic after microperc requiring medical management or DJ stenting. This could be attributed to the procedural technicality of clearance of stone using laser and depending upon spontaneous passage of stone fragments. The stone fragments cannot be actively retrieved. Some studies (Armagan et al. [16], Desai et al. [2], Tepeler et al. [10], and Piskin et al. [11]) have mentioned about conversion of microperc to mini-microperc or Miniperc. The 4.85 Fr sheath has limited ability to irrigate the system. Thus, there was a need to convert due to the inability to maneuverer the scope from one calyx to another and poor visibility due to intraoperative bleeding.

## 18.8 Comparison with Other Techniques

Microperc after its introduction in 2011 is widely practiced across the globe. Various authors have published their results. Obviously, when there are several modalities available to treat stones up to 1.5 cm, Microperc will have to be compared with all other modalities.

### 18.8.1 Microperc Versus EWSL

Hatipoglu et al. retrospectively compared microperc with ESWL and found lower treatment rates in microperc [15].

### 18.8.2 Microperc Versus RIRS

Sabnis et al. (2013) performed a randomized controlled trial of Microperc versus RIRS for renal calculi <1.5 cm. They concluded that Microperc is safe and has similar stone clearance and complication rates as RIRS for small renal calculi. Microperc is associated with higher hemoglobin loss, increased pain, and higher analgesic requirements, while RIRS is associated with a higher requirement for JJ stenting [13].

Fata et al. (2014) compared the efficacy of microperc with RIRS for intermediate renal calculi (1–3 cm). They concluded that both these techniques have comparable stone clearance and compilation rates [14].

Armagan et al. (2015) retrospectively compared microperc with RIRS for moderate (<2 cm) lower pole stones and concluded that microperc is safe and efficacious with significantly higher stone-free rates [17].

Bagcioglu M et al. (2016) performed a cost-effectiveness analysis of 111 procedures of microperc and RIRS. They concluded that microperc is less expensive than RIRS due to additional required treatments and ancillary equipment in RIRS. RIRS is more effective than microperc in terms of operation time and more effective use of operation rooms [19].

Baş O et al. (2016) retrospectively compared microperc and RIRS for 10–20 mm calculi in pediatric patients. Both the techniques were equally efficacious and had similar complication rates. Hospital stay and radiation exposure were significantly lower in the RIRS group [20].

Cepeda M et al. (2017) prospectively compared microperc and RIRS for <2 cm renal calculi. Stone-free and complication rates, hospital stay, and JJ stenting were similar for both groups. The hemoglobin drop was more in the microperc group [32].

Kandemir A et al. (2017) prospectively randomized 60 patients with <15 mm lower pole renal stones into microperc and RIRS groups. Both techniques have comparable stone-free and complication rates. Microperc had the disadvantage of prolonged hospital and scopy times [21].

Li X et al. (2018) performed a meta-analysis of nine studies (842 patients) comparing microperc with RIRS. Microperc was associated with higher stone-free rate (SFR) (OR: 1.6; 95% CI, 1.03 to 2.48), significantly longer hospital stays (MD: 0.66 day; 95% CI, 0.17 to 1.15), longer fluoroscopy time (MD: 78.12 s; 95% CI, 66.08 to 90.15), and larger decreases in hemoglobin (MD: 0.59 g/dl; 95% CI, 0.16 to 1.02) than was RIRS. No significant differences were observed with respect to operative time, stone-free rate, complication rate, or auxiliary procedures [22].

Zhang B et al. (2020) in a systematic review and meta-analysis of three RCTs and four non-RCTs of Microperc versus RIRS concluded that Microperc is associated with fewer DJ stent insertions and higher SFR at the expense of a greater drop in hemoglobin and longer hospital stay. On subset analysis of lower pole and non-lower pole stones, the SFR, auxiliary procedure and complication rates were comparable. The hemoglobin drop was greater for Microperc in both lower or non-lower pole stones group, while the operative time was comparable for RIRS and Microperc for lower pole stones [23].

### 18.8.3 Microperc Versus Miniperc

Karatag T et al. (2015) compared Microperc and Miniperc for treatment of pediatric renal stones of sizes 10–20 mm in retrospective multicentric analysis. An analysis of 119 patients concluded that Microperc has similar stone clearance and complications rates with lower hemoglobin drop, shorter hospitalization stay, and fluoroscopy time. The stone-free rate at 1 month was 92.8% for Microperc versus 93.6% for Miniperc [24].

Tok A et al. (2016) compared clinical outcomes of 98 patients of Miniperc with Microperc for treatment of lower calyx stones of 10–20 mm. The stone-free and complications rates in both the arms were comparable. They concluded that Microperc is a treatment option for medium-sized lower calyx stone, being associated with lower blood loss, reduced fluoroscopy, procedure time, hospitalization time, and a higher tubeless rate [25].

Dundar G et al. (2016) compared Miniperc with Microperc in 43 pediatric patients for stones less than 2 cm. These patients had undergone unsuccessful SWL procedures. The mean operative duration and hospitalization duration was less in Microperc as compared to Miniperc. The stone clearance rate for Microperc (93.8%) and Miniperc (92.6%) was comparable. The hemoglobin drop was less in Microperc but was statistically comparable with that of Miniperc [26].

## 18.9 Microperc in Pediatric Population

Sen H et al. (2017) compared Microperc and RIRS in 48 pediatric patients. They had comparable operative duration and stone-free rate in both arms. They concluded Microperc and RIRS are safe first-line minimal-invasive treatment in pediatric patients [27].

Caione P et al. (2015) evaluated the feasibility of Microperc in Valdivia-modified position in five pediatric patients. They concluded that Microperc is a new cost-effective and time-saving technique that demonstrated as safe and effective in the minimally invasive procedure for lower pole and pelvic renal stones of small size [28].

The feasibility and safety of Microperc in the pediatric population have been well described in literature. Microperc has been performed in a 7-month-old kid (Sancaktutar AA et al. [29]), 2-year-old kid (Kaynar M [30]), and Laparoscopic-assisted microperc of a stone in a pelvic kidney of a 3-year-old girl (Tepeler A et al. [31]).

## 18.10 Where Microperc Stands Today

Microperc should not be considered as an alternative but as complementary to other modalities like Miniperc, ESWL, or RIRS. As mentioned above, there are specific benefits and ideal indications for Microperc. In carefully selected cases, Microperc is very useful.

## References


1. Bader M, Gratzke C, Schlenker B, Tilki D, Reich O, Gozzi C, et al. 1890 The "all-seeing needle"–an optical puncture system confirming percutaneous access in Pcnl. J Urol. 2010;183(4s):E734–5.
2. Desai MR, Sharma R, Mishra S, Sabnis RB, Stief C, Bader M. Single-step percutaneous nephrolithotomy (microperc): the initial clinical report. J Urol. 2011;186(1):140–5.
3. Desai M, Mishra S. 'Microperc'micro percutaneous nephrolithotomy: evidence to practice. Curr Opin Urol. 2012;22(2):134–8.
4. Sabnis RB, Ganesamoni R, Ganpule AP, Mishra S, Vyas J, Jagtap J, et al. Current role of microperc in the management of small renal calculi. Indian J Urol. 2013;29(3):214.
5. Sabnis RB, Chhabra JS, Ganpule AP, Abrol S, Desai MR. Current role of PCNL in pediatric urolithiasis. Curr Urol Rep. 2014;15(7):423.
6. Penbegul N, Bodakci MN, Hatipoglu NK, Sancaktutar AA, Atar M, Cakmakci S, et al. Microsheath for microperc: 14-gauge angiocath. J Endourol. 2013;27(7):835–9.
7. Penbegul N, Utangac MM, Daggulli M, Dede O, Bozkurt Y, Bodakci MN, et al. A novel drainage technique during micropercutaneous nephrolithotomy in pediatric patients: double angiocath. J Pediatr Surg. 2016;51(6):1051–3.
8. Buldu İ, Tepeler A, Karatağ T, İnan R, Armağan A, İstanbulluoğlu O. Combined micro-and standard percutaneous nephrolithotomy for complex renal calculi. Turk J Urol. 2016;42(3):150.
9. Silay MS, Tepeler A, Atis G, Sancaktutar AA, Piskin M, Gurbuz C, et al. Initial report of microperc in the treatment of pediatric nephrolithiasis. J Pediatr Surg. 2013;48(7):1578–83.
10. Tepeler A, Armagan A, Sancaktutar AA, Silay MS, Penbegul N, Akman T, et al. The role of microperc in the treatment of symptomatic lower pole renal calculi. J Endourol. 2013;27(1):13–8.
11. Piskin MM, Guven S, Kilinc M, Arslan M, Goger E, Ozturk A. Preliminary, favorable experience with microperc in kidney and bladder stones. J Endourol. 2012;26(11):1443–7.
12. Hatipoglu NK, Tepeler A, Buldu I, Atis G, Bodakci MN, Sancaktutar AA, et al. Initial experience of micro-percutaneous nephrolithotomy in the treatment of renal calculi in 140 renal units. Urolithiasis. 2014;42(2):159–64.
13. Sabnis RB, Ganesamoni R, Doshi A, Ganpule AP, Jagtap J, Desai MR. Micropercutaneous nephrolithotomy (microperc) vs retrograde intrarenal surgery for the management of small renal calculi: a randomized controlled trial. BJU Int. 2013;112(3):355–61.
14. de Fata FR, García-Tello A, Andrés G, Redondo C, Meilán E, Gimbernat H, et al. Comparative study of retrograde intrarenal surgery and micropercutaneous nephrolithotomy in the treatment of intermediate-sized kidney stones. Actas Urol Esp Engl Ed. 2014;38(9):576–83.
15. Hatipoglu NK, Sancaktutar AA, Tepeler A, Bodakci MN, Penbegul N, Atar M, et al. Comparison of shockwave lithotripsy and microperc for treatment of kidney stones in children. J Endourol. 2013;27(9):1141–6.
16. Armagan A, Tepeler A, Silay MS, Ersoz C, Akcay M, Akman T, et al. Micropercutaneous nephrolithotomy in the treatment of moderate-size renal calculi. J Endourol. 2013;27(2):177–81.
17. Armagan A, Karatag T, Buldu I, Tosun M, Basibuyuk I, Istanbulluoglu MO, et al. Comparison of flexible ureterorenoscopy and micropercutaneous nephrolithotomy in the treatment for moderately size lower-pole stones. World J Urol. 2015;33(11):1827–31.
18. Karatag T, Buldu I, Inan R, Istanbulluoglu MO. Is micropercutaneous nephrolithotomy technique really efficacicous for the treatment of moderate size renal calculi? Yes Urol Int. 2015;95(1):9–14.
19. Bagcioglu M, Demir A, Sulhan H, Karadag MA, Uslu M, Tekdogan UY. Comparison of flexible ureteroscopy and micropercutaneous nephrolithotomy in terms of cost-effectiveness: analysis of 111 procedures. Urolithiasis. 2016;44(4):339–44.
20. Baş O, Dede O, Aydogmus Y, Utangaç M, Yikilmaz TN, Damar E, et al. Comparison of retrograde intrarenal surgery and micro-percutaneous nephrolithotomy in moderately sized pediatric kidney stones. J Endourol. 2016;30(7):765–70.

21. Kandemir A, Guven S, Balasar M, Sonmez MG, Taskapu H, Gurbuz R. A prospective randomized comparison of micropercutaneous nephrolithotomy (microperc) and retrograde intrarenal surgery (RIRS) for the management of lower pole kidney stones. World J Urol. 2017;35(11):1771–6.
22. Li M-M, Yang H-M, Liu X-M, Qi H-G, Weng G-B. Retrograde intrarenal surgery vs miniaturized percutaneous nephrolithotomy to treat lower pole renal stones 1.5-2.5 cm in diameter. World J Clin Cases. 2018;6(15):931.
23. Zhang B, Hu Y, Gao J, Zhuo D. Micropercutaneous versus retrograde intrarenal surgery for the management of moderately sized kidney stones: a systematic review and meta-analysis. Urol Int. 2020;104(1–2):94–105.
24. Karatag T, Tepeler A, Silay MS, Bodakci MN, Buldu I, Daggulli M, et al. A comparison of 2 percutaneous nephrolithotomy techniques for the treatment of Pediatric kidney stones of sizes 10-20 mm: microperc vs Miniperc. Urology. 2015;85(5):1015–8.
25. Tok A, Akbulut F, Buldu I, Karatag T, Kucuktopcu O, Gurbuz G, et al. Comparison of microperc and mini-percutaneous nephrolithotomy for medium-sized lower calyx stones. Urolithiasis. 2016;44(2):155–9.
26. Dundar G, Gokce G, Gokcen K, Korgali E, Asdemir A, Kaygusuz K. Microperc versus miniperc for treatment of renal stones smaller than 2 cm in pediatric patients. Urol J. 2016;13(5):2829–32.
27. Sen H, Seckiner I, Bayrak O, Dogan K, Erturhan S. A comparison of micro-PERC and retrograde intrarenal surgery results in pediatric patients with renal stones. J Pediatr Urol. 2017;13(6):619.e1–5.
28. Caione P, De Dominicis M, Collura G, Matarazzo E, Nappo SG, Capozza N. Microperc for pediatric nephrolithiasis: technique in Valdivia-modified position. Eur J Pediatr Surg Off J Austrian Assoc Pediatr Surg Al Z Kinderchir. 2015;25(1):94–9.
29. Sancaktutar AA, Adanur S, Ziypak T, Hatipoglu NK, Bodakcı MN, Soylemez H, et al. Micropercutaneous nephrolithotomy in the Management of Bilateral Renal Stones in a 7-month-old infant: the youngest case in the literature. Urol Int. 2016;96(2):238–40.
30. Kaynar M, Sümer A, Şalvarcı A, Tekinarslan E, Cenker A, Istanbulluoğlu MO. Micropercutaneous nephrolithotomy (microperc) in a two-year-old with the 'all-seeing needle'. Urol Int. 2013;91(2):239–41.
31. Tepeler A, Silay MS, Armagan A, Basibuyuk I, Akman T, Akcay M, et al. Laparoscopic-assisted "microperc" of a stone in a pelvic kidney of a 3-year-old girl. J Laparoendosc Adv Surg Tech A. 2013;23(2):174–6.
32. Cepeda M, Amón JH, Mainez JA, de la Cruz B, Rodríguez V, Alonso D, Martínez-Sagarra JM. Retrograde intrarenal surgery and micro-percutaneous nephrolithotomy for renal lithiasis smaller than 2 CM. Actas Urol Esp. 2017;41(8):516–521. English, Spanish. https://doi.org/10.1016/j.acuro.2017.02.003. Epub 2017 Apr 25. PMID: 28389028.

# 19 Superperc

Kaushikkumar V. Shah, Ulhas Sathaye, and Arabind Panda

## 19.1 Introduction

Percutaneous nephrolithotomy (PCNL), since its introduction by Fernstrom and Johansson in 1976, has been the modality of choice for treating complex upper tract urolithiasis [1]. It has several advantages over shock wave lithotripsy (SWL) and retrograde intra renal surgery (RIRS). The ease of treating a larger stone burden, stones with distal obstruction, infection stones, a higher stone free rate, one-stage procedure, and cost-effectiveness in developing countries, with wide applicability in most cases, are some of the advantages.

Appropriate access to the pelvicalyceal system is critical to remove all stone burdens effectively. Access has two components—correct puncture and an appropriate tract size. Tract size is related to significant morbidity like bleeding, need for transfusion and duration of hospital stay [1]. Major advances in PCNL were possible due to improvement in areas like optics, lithotripsy devices and stone fragment evacuation systems. Advances in optics allowed reduced size of nephroscope without losing the quality of vision.

Another major advance is related to reducing tract size without losing efficacy, safety, and cost-effectiveness of the procedure. Now we have a mini perc nephroscope from a number of manufacturers, an ultra mini PCNL (UMP) telescope and even a Microperc telescope [2]. Lithotripsy devices include pneumatic, holmium laser and thulium fiber laser. Thinner probes of pneumatic lithotripsy allowed the nephroscope size to be reduced from 24–26 F size to 12–18 F size with high efficacy with almost no maintenance cost. Holmium laser lithotripsy allowed the nephroscope size to go down further. It paved the way for small tract size PCNL, especially for small volume stone burden with excellent efficacy, reduced morbidity and increased tubeless procedures. However, Holmium laser lithotripsy may be relatively slow in the treatment of large-sized stones due to prolonged operative time, increased intrarenal pressure with delayed or reduced stone clearance.

In minimally-invasive PCNL techniques, there is difficulty in the removal of the fragments using conventional methods. Alternative systems to remove stone fragments emerged like flushing fragments down the ureter (Microperc), whirlpool effect (UMP) or vacuum cleaner effect (miniperc from Karl Storz). Efforts to increase the speed of fragmentation with simultaneous fragment retrieval have resulted in the development of advanced lithotripters using suction—Lithovac, Shock Pulse lithotripsy and Trilogy. However, the addition of suction channel inside

K. V. Shah (✉)
Varun Hospital, Surat, Gujarat, India

U. Sathaye
Sahayog Speciality Hospital, Jamnagar, Gujarat, India

A. Panda
Department of Urology, Krishna Institute of Medical Sciences (KIMS) Hospital, Secunderabad, India


M. S. Agrawal et al. (eds.), *Minimally Invasive Percutaneous Nephrolithotomy*,
https://doi.org/10.1007/978-981-16-6001-6_19

the probe increases the size of the lithotripsy probe needing a bigger nephroscope and thereby a bigger tract size. These offer a definite advantage in large stone volumes.

An alternative approach is the addition of suction to the sheath rather than the lithotripsy probe. Superperc and Super Mini PCNL have added suction in the sheath itself. This breakthrough allowed the nephroscope and lithotripsy device to be smaller. The addition of suction in the renal sheath along with retrograde irrigation in Superperc has resulted in a number of advantages while offering a wide range of sheath and nephroscope sizes to choose for PCNL depending upon the size of stone.

## 19.2 Armamentarium

Superperc uses the same principle of minimally-invasive PCNL, with added suction to the sheath, which would create negative pressure and augment the vacuum cleaner effect to help egress of the fragments. The sheath has been finalized as Shah sheath, and it has now been patented in China and subsequently in US.

**Set up for Superperc** is almost the same as in any PCNL (Fig. 19.1). Few of the instruments we use are modified to meet the need. It includes (1) multihole ureteral catheter in place of the conventional open-end ureteral catheter, (2) a set of Shah sheath as renal sheath, (3) stone catcher bottle (4) low-power suction machine along with a suction bottle with a tap.

### 19.2.1 Multihole Ureteral Catheter

Multihole ureteral catheter is an open-ended ureteral catheter with a few holes in the sidewalls for a few centimeters at the distal end that is placed in the renal pelvis and upper ureter. It has to be placed on a guidewire under C arm guidance so that the tip of the ureteral catheter is in the upper calyx. This will ensure that some of the holes are in the renal pelvis and a few are in the upper ure-

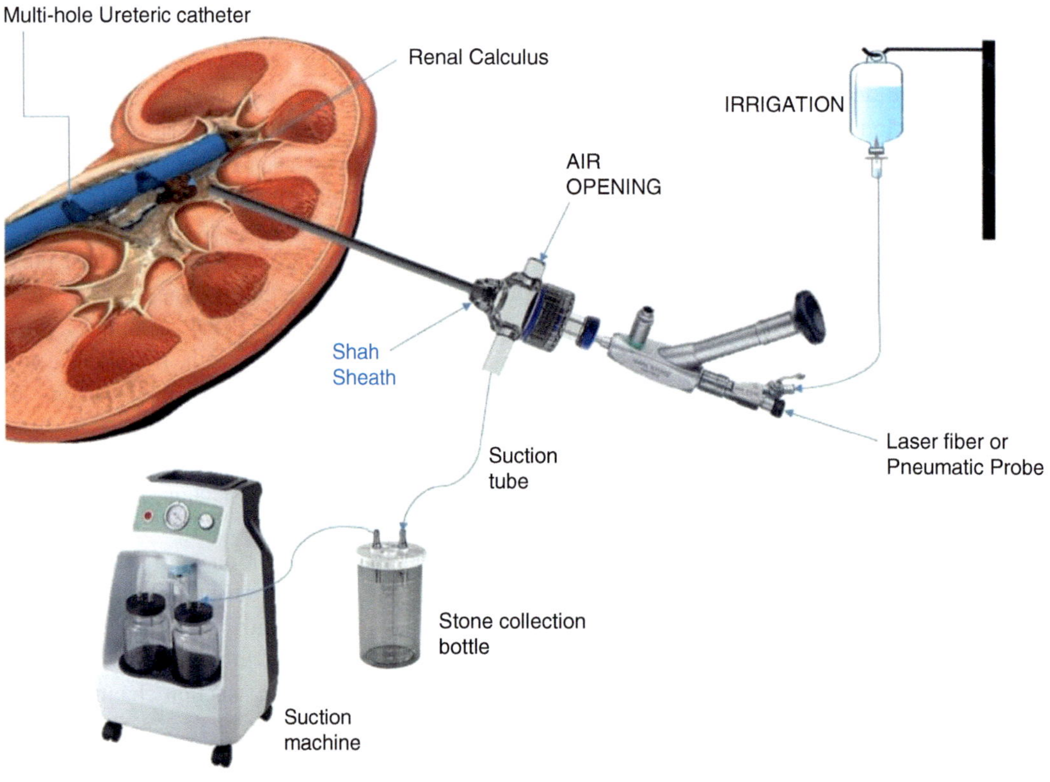


**Fig. 19.1** Set up for Superperc

ter. It is to fill/empty the whole pelvicalyceal system and upper ureter simultaneously and effectively. It is aimed at (1) effective, simultaneous visualization of the pelvicalyceal system while doing renal calyceal puncture, (2) good retrograde irrigation during lithotripsy in the renal pelvis and upper ureter, (3) as an exit strategy at the end of procedure leaving only ureteral catheter for drainage.

### 19.2.2 Shah Superperc Sheath

Shah Superperc sheath (Fig. 19.2) has two components: (1) tubular metal sheath along with dedicated metal dilator (2) connector. It has evolved over the years from being a pure metal design with detachable parts to having a clear suction master and dilator integrated into the sheath. It is available as reusable, both autoclavable and non-autoclavable version. This allows for reducing one step in placing sheath, visualization of the fragments, significant reduction in the weight of the sheath with improved ergonomics.

The tubular metal sheath is available in different working lengths −10 cm, 12 cm, and 14 cm, the default being 14 cm. It is also available in different sizes—12 F, 15 F, 18 F, 21 F, and 24 F. This is to suit different tract lengths and widths needed for a particular patient. For a shorter tract, as in children, one can use a shorter length sheath-like 10 cm sheath for better ergonomics. For a smaller tract size as in UMP, one can use 12 F, and for miniperc size tract, one can use 15 F, 18 F, and 21 F size sheath. For a bigger tract size, as in large stone volume, one can use 21 F or 24 F sheath. Thus, the system provides a lot of flexibility in choosing the most appropriate sheath length and width (Fig. 19.3).

A dedicated metal dilator is provided for each size of the sheath. For 12 F,15 F, and 18 F sheath, a dilator is designed to be introduced over a guide wire as a one-step dilatation. For 21 F and 24 F, a dilator is designed to be used over a guide rod as a one-step dilatation.

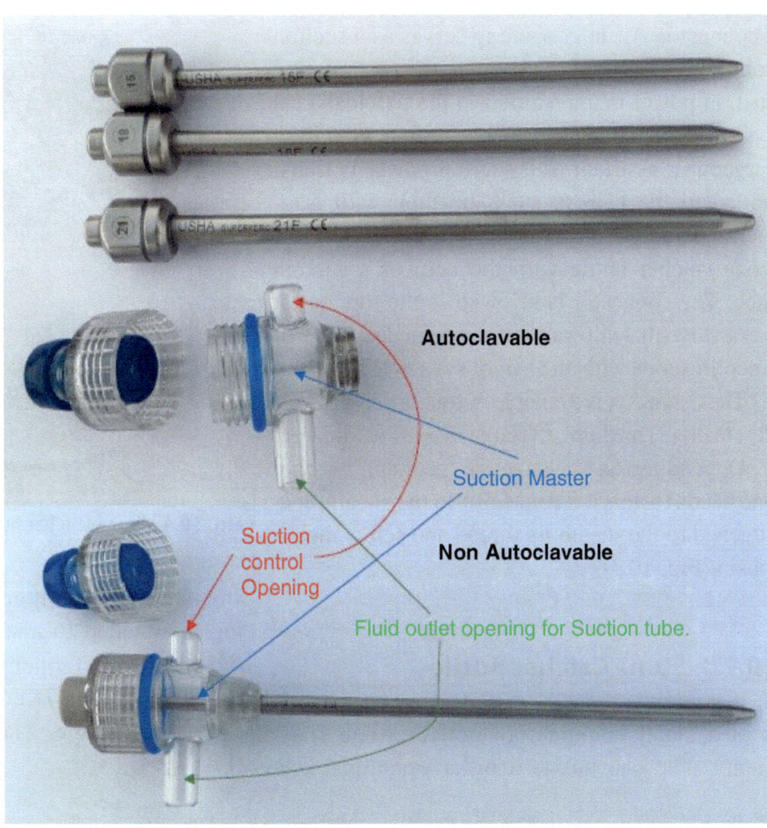


**Fig. 19.2** The Shah Superperc Sheath

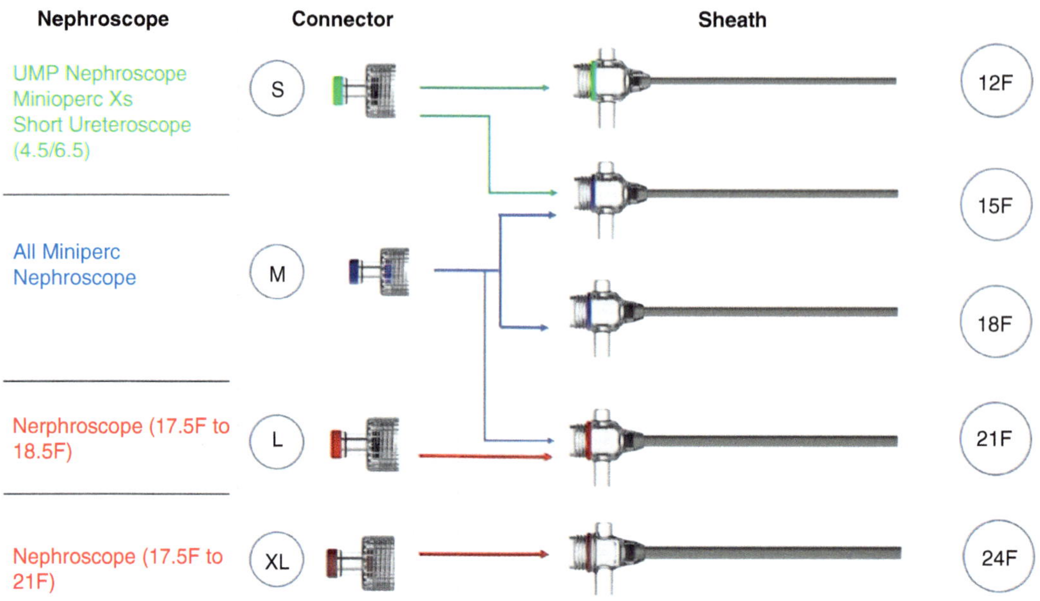


**Fig. 19.3** The appropriate nephroscope for each sheath

The suction master attached to the tubular sheath has two pillar openings (1) air inlet opening (2) fluid outlet opening with an area to attach a connector. Air inlet opening serves as a suction control opening. If it is open to air, minimal suction power is transmitted to the pelvicalyceal system (PCS). If it is closed by the finger of either surgeon or assistant, full suction power is transmitted to the PCS to suck the fluid with fragments. The fluid outlet opening is connected to a stone catcher bottle with the help of a suction tube. The connector is screwed to the top, and it has a valve that allows for the repeated passage of a nephroscope with an airtight system (Fig. 19.2).

The connector is available in four different sizes: (1) small, (2) medium, (3) large and (4) extra-large.

Depending on the size of the nephroscope, one needs to attach a connector to the sheath. It is attached to the sheath by thread and screw mechanism (Fig. 19.3).

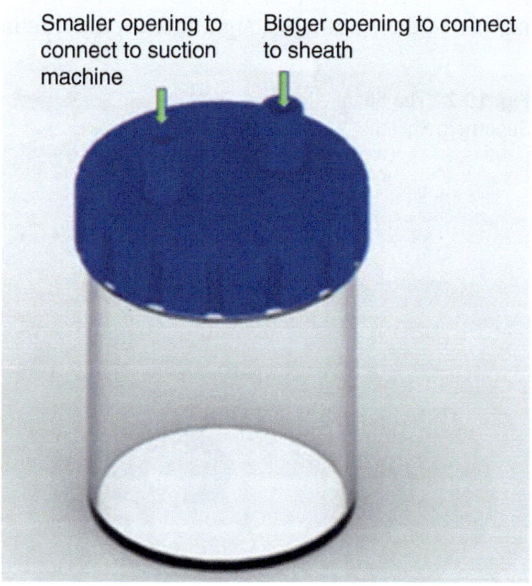


**Fig. 19.4** Stone catcher bottle

### 19.2.3 Stone Catcher Bottle

It is a small container to collect stone fragments. The cap has two pillar openings, one smaller and one bigger in diameter. Big opening is attached to a suction tube coming from the fluid outlet opening of the Shah sheath. Smaller opening is connected to a low-power suction machine via another suction tube (Fig. 19.4).

### 19.2.4 Low-Power Suction Machine and a Suction Bottle with a Tap

Low power suction machine is designed to provide low-power suction with a control knob to vary the suction power. Set the power of the suction machine to 0.020 to 0.026 megapascal or 0.2 to 0.26 Bar or 150 to 200 mm of Hg. Start with the lowest setting and increase if necessary. It has a tap attached by T connection. The suction bottle has a tap at the bottom part of it. When the suction bottle is filled with returning fluid, tap on suction bottle and tap on T tube connection of suction machine are opened. This will allow the bottle to be emptied easily, quickly, and safely. When the bottle is empty, both taps are again closed (Fig. 19.5).

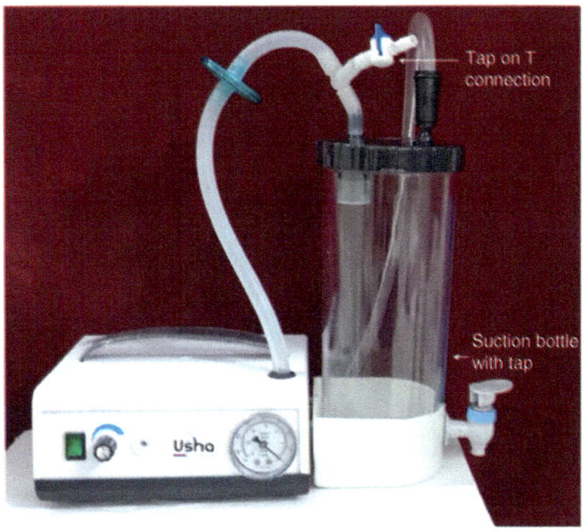


**Fig. 19.5** Low power suction machine and a suction bottle with a tap

## 19.3 Technique

Technique for Superperc is almost the same as in any form of PCNL (Fig. 19.6). There are four minor differences from conventional technique.1. Insertion of a multihole ureteral catheter instead of the simple ureteral catheter. 2. Placement of Shah sheath instead of other renal sheath. 3. Attaching a low-power suction machine with a stone catcher bottle to the fluid outlet port of the sheath. 4. Adding a retrograde irrigation via ureteric catheter [3, 4].

Once we decide to offer PCNL to a particular patient, one has to plan the technique like prone, supine, or ECIRS. First step is to put a multihole ureteral catheter over a straight tip guide wire, under C arm guidance to keep the tip of the ureteral catheter in the upper calyx. Insert A foley catheter and fix the ureteral catheter well so that it does not slip down.

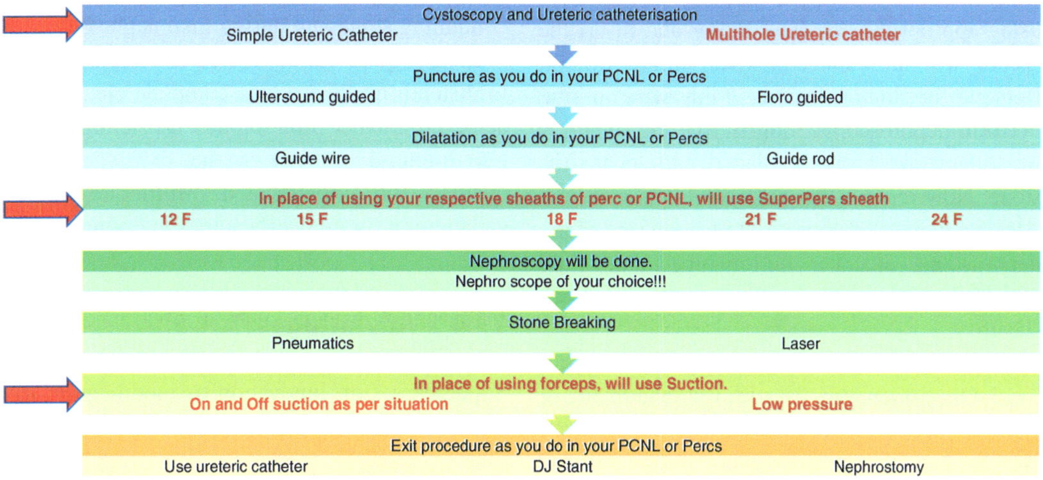


**Fig. 19.6** Adapting conventional PCNL to Superperc

### 19.3.1 Preparing for Suction

After draping the patient, keep the stone catcher bottle at an appropriate place. Attach a suction tube of 8 mm inner diameter to the bigger opening of the bottle and keep it ready so that it can be easily attached to the fluid outlet opening of the Shah Sheath. Attach another suction tube from the stone catcher bottle to the low-power suction machine. Set the suction power to 150 to 250 mm of Hg/0.02 to 0.025 mega pascal. Adjust the suction power of the machine to minimum and increase as and when needed.

During retrograde pyelography, multihole ureteral catheter fills all the calyces simultaneously due to multiple holes in the ureteral catheter. That will help to delineate all the calyces and upper ureter well. Due to multihole ureteral catheter, the system empties fast and one needs to refill the system if repeated attempts to puncture are required. Air does not drain out easily as compared to saline. Decide the position of calyx and size of infundibulum to puncture. Depending on the nephroscope/s available, characteristics of stone/s and surgeon's preference, tract size, along expected tract length are decided. Select the appropriate size and length of the Shah sheath.

Create a tract under sonography or fluoro guidance or combined, as per personal preference. Dilate tract as per individual choice or using appropriate one-step dilator and insert the sheath without connector over/with a dilator. Remove the dilator, leaving guide wire in situ. Perform nephroscopy, confirm that the sheath is in system and properly placed and locate the stone. Now remove the guide wire under vision. Attach a connector appropriate for the size of the nephroscope, attach a suction tube to the fluid outlet opening of the suction master of Shah sheath.

Nephroscopy is started as per individual protocol. Once orientation is achieved, pneumatic or laser lithotripsy is started. Retrograde irrigation is started. Suction machine is always kept on. When air inlet opening is open to the air, only minimal suction is transmitted to renal pelvis and fluid is coming by overflowing from PCS, augmented by minimal suction. When extra suction is required, air inlet opening is closed either by a surgeon or assistant's finger. Suction is activated with a nephroscope in situ or during withdrawal of the nephroscope to remove fragments of varying sizes. Suction is activated in the following situations. (1) during lithotripsy to remove small fragments by the side of the nephroscope so that vision is maintained. (2) if you feel that stone/fragment is migrating into distant calyx or ureter due to irrigation from nephroscope. It will reduce the chances of migration. (3) when enough fragments of size smaller than sheath size are present, suction is activated while withdrawing the nephroscope. It will allow multiple bigger fragments to come out due to space created by the gradual removal of the nephroscope. Few repeated passages of the nephroscope will remove all small fragments. Now the stone fragments are bigger than sheath size. They are again fragmented and the cycle is repeated. Advancing the tip of the sheath near the stone fragments and retrograde irrigation will augment the stone clearance. Suction is very useful in the severely hydronephrotic system, obese patient, infected system and if you want low pressure in PCS while doing Superperc. The use of forceps is reduced significantly.

At the end, all calyces are inspected for stone clearance. One can distend the system by detaching the suction tube and closing both air inlet opening and fluid outlet opening. This is very useful to find out narrow calyceal neck openings containing stone and during final nephroscopy. It is extremely useful in ECIRS and supine PCNL to distend the PCS. Once complete clearance is achieved, the decision to put a DJ stent/nephrostomy/ureteral catheter as an exit strategy is decided and implemented. Multihole ureteral catheter is extremely efficacious in draining PCS.

## 19.4 Advantages [3, 4, 5]:

Superperc as an innovation or modification has established itself as another method of stone management.

Some of the advantages of this method are:

1. Ease of use.
2. Ergonomically optimal. Lightweight, length of the sheath as per need, in and out movements of the nephroscope is very easy.

3. Quicker because of continuous circulation of fluid and washing of the dust results in clearer vision.
4. When using the smaller sheaths, tubeless surgery is possible.
5. For larger stone bulk, a bigger sheath with the same suction capabilities is available.
6. Continuous suction can potentially prevent the migration of stone fragments into inaccessible calyces after the fragmentation of the stone.
7. Convenience of using stone forceps or graspers if required.
8. Convenience of placing a stent under direct vision.

## 19.5 Disadvantages and Troubleshooting

1. The ureteric catheter is always placed under C Arm guidance.
2. Because of the multiple holes in the ureteric catheter, the initial puncture may take time when performed under C Arm guidance because contrast leaks off in the upper ureter and does not allow the PCS to fill optimally.

   Solution: The assistant needs to inject diluted contrast in small pulsatile increments to keep the system full, till the puncture is completed or few cc of air can be injected to delineate the desired calyx. Air will not drain out spontaneously.
3. The procedure is compromised if the catheter tip slips out of the upper calyx during the procedure. Displaced tip of the catheter will not allow the pelvicalyceal system to fill optimally, and renal puncture will be difficult.

   Solution: The ureteric catheter has to be fixed to the urethral catheter. Ensure that the urethral catheter is draining and the bladder does not fill up. Ureteral catheter can get displaced with a full bladder.
4. If the suction is more than the inflow, the PCS wall collapses on the sheath and can be traumatized.

   Solution: Ask the assistant to increase the force and speed of retrograde irrigation. With a little bit of practice, one gets to know when to stop using the suction by optimal use of air inlet opening. Reduce suction power if possible.
5. Suction settings and functioning may be a distraction in case of an operative challenge during the procedure and preclude concentrating fully on the procedure.

   Solution: Before starting the procedure, delegate the suction functioning to a dedicated person with instructions for all eventualities. Use a dedicated low-pressure suction machine rather than using existing suction machines or central suction.
6. Though the procedure can be performed for impacted pelvic and upper ureteric stones, the advantages of the ureteric catheter cannot be utilized fully because of the inability to place the ureteric catheter tip proximal to the stone.

   Solution: Try to negotiate a glide wire proximal to the stone. Once that is done, the ureteric catheter can be negotiated, and the procedure started. Occasionally pushing 2% lidocaine jelly diluted in water with enough pressure can push up the stone, and the procedure can commence. As a last resort, use a simple open-ended ureteral catheter rather than the multihole ureteral catheter. Place tip just distal to the stone. Make the puncture and commence the fragmentation. If the stone gets dislodged, the ureteric catheter tip can be seen, pull it up and place optimally if needed. Then Superperc can continue.
7. In case there is a small bleed, the blood flow keeps on coming in line of vision and may compromise the ease of the procedure.

   Solution: Stop the procedure for a couple of minutes. The small bleed usually stops. Once it stops, restart the procedure but avoid rushing into using the suction.

## 19.6 Discussion

The basic technique of PCNL has remained unchanged for decades. Superperc with its novel Shah sheath that incorporates suction has modified the way the ureteric catheter, renal sheath, and lithotripsy devices are used.

As urologists became aware of the reduced morbidity in a smaller tract size, there has been widespread adoption of mini PCNL techniques. With a smaller tract size, the technical challenge was to achieve complete clearance within a reasonable time.

In the quest towards achieving a smaller tract for access, each mini PCNL technique had to evolve their own system of managing the stone fragments. In Microperc, the calculi are dusted by a laser, and the fragments are washed away by the irrigating fluid down the ureter with its own consequences. UMP redesigned the renal sheath and used forceful irrigation through the side channel of UMP sheath to cause a whirlpool effect for fragment removal [2]. In the Miniperc, there is a "vacuum cleaner effect" by repeated in and out movements of the nephroscope to remove fragments through the sheath. The ultimate aim is to try to remove the fragments completely and relatively easily.

Intermittent suction has always been an important part of standard PCNL. It reduced the intrarenal pressure, removed small fragments, improved vision during lithotripsy and helped to achieve complete clearance with ease, safety, efficacy, and speed. The traditional way in standard PCNL is to use intermittent suction with a suction cannula through a nephroscope. Later multiple manufacturers introduced inbuilt suction in the ultrasonic lithotripter. Both these techniques meant that a minimum size of the nephroscope and working channel was necessary as these instruments were of a larger caliber. Miniaturization was not possible.

Superperc and Super miniperc use a renal sheath with the capability of continuous suction and the ability to change the force of suction by occluding the air vent without interrupting the procedure. During withdrawal of the scope with suction, it is possible to suck the renal pelvic mucosa with subsequent injury. To prevent mucosal injury during blind suction during withdrawal of the nephroscope and to flush the stone fragments into the sheath, retrograde irrigation is done with the ureteric catheter. To provide flow of saline from multiple areas rather than from the tip of the ureteric catheter, with even fluid pressure distribution, Dr. Shah designed the multihole ureteral catheter. It irrigated the pelvicalyceal junction and all the calyces simultaneously to flush out fragments towards the renal sheath to be sucked out.

In the initial series of 20 patients with stone sizes ranging in size from 10 to 29 mm in varying locations (renal pelvic stone, upper ureteric stone, low volume partial stag horn stone and 10 cases of multiple stones), 95% complete clearance was achieved with tract size of 10 F/12 F. The drop in Hemoglobin was 0.8 gm% without need for any blood transfusion. A nephrostomy was not placed in any patient. Eleven patients were totally tubeless procedures without even a D J stent. (4) Compared to Microperc and UMP, the straight working channel allowed the use of biprong and tri prong forceps when it was occasionally needed. Tract size was almost the same as UMP and slightly more than microperc.

A year later Shah and Agarwal reported a series of 43 cases of Superperc in upper tract urolithiasis (upper ureteric stones, multiple renal stones, stones in horseshoe and anomalous kidney and pediatric renal calculus) and renal stone >1.5 cm. A tract size of 10 F/12 F was used. In 2 cases, conversion to a 15 F tract and to 22 F in another case was done. A single patient needed a 2nd stage procedure to achieve 100 percent clearance. Average length of hospital stay was 2 days. There was no transfusion requirement. Only one patient had a nephrostomy, 20 had only DJ stents, and the rest were totally tubeless. These results were comparable or better than any form of PCNL [5].

In another prospective observational study of 52 cases of Superperc, stone size ranged from 10 to 37 mm, mean operative time was 40.9 minutes. 32 patients were totally tubeless with a hospital stay of 31.5 hours with 96.15% stone clearance. Only 3 patients had mild fever with a drop in hemoglobin of 0.32 gm%. These results clearly showed high clearance with minimal infective and bleeding complications with tubeless procedures with reduced hospital stay [3].

Superperc sheath is now available in sizes ranging from 12 F to 24 F. The sizes are compatible with pneumatic lithotripsy and nephroscope of 12 F to 22 F size. Trial comparing Superpec with a pneumatic lithotripsy probe using suction and standard PCNL with Shock pulse lithotripsy and/or Trilogy will be interesting.

## 19.7 Future

PCNL is an important technique in the armamentarium in the management of upper tract urolithiasis. The addition of suction to the nephoscope sheath makes the Shah sheath a very attractive option. It is hoped that the obvious advantages may result in the Shah sheath completely replacing the conventional renal sheath over a period of time. Multiple studies from different centers by urologists from across the world will evaluate its true position in the coming decade.

## References


1. Yamaguchi A, Skolarikos A, Buchholz NP, Chomón GB, Grasso M, Saba P, Nakada S, de la Rosette J. Clinical Research Office Of The Endourological Society Percutaneous Nephrolithotomy Study Group. Operating times and bleeding complications in percutaneous nephrolithotomy: a comparison of tract dilation methods in 5,537 patients in the Clinical Research Office of the Endourological Society Percutaneous Nephrolithotomy Global Study. J Endourol. 2011 Jun;25(6):933–9.
2. Desai JD, Ultra-mini PNL. (UMP): material, indications, technique, advantages and results. Arch Esp Urol. 2017 Jan;70(1):196–201.
3. Shah K, Agrawal MS, Mishra DK. Superperc: a new technique in minimally-invasive percutaneous nephrolithotomy. Indian. J Urol. 2017 Jan–Mar;33(1):48–52.
4. Shah K. AIO (All in one) Shah sheath 10/12F for superperc in upper tract urolithiasis. In: abstracts—USICON 2015. Indian J Urol. 2015;31(Suppl S1):39–152.
5. Shah K, Agrawal M. Superperc in varieties of upper tract urolithiasis and for renal stone >1.5 cm. Abstracts—USICON 2016. Indian J Urol. 2016;32(Suppl S1):38–165.

# 20 Super-Mini-PCNL (SMP)

Guohua Zeng and Wei Zhu

## 20.1 Introduction

According to the European Association of Urology, the latest guidelines suggest PCNL as the therapy of choice for renal calculus greater than 20 mm and also for smaller stones from 10 to 20 mm of the lower calyceal when SWL is unfavorable [1]. Comparing to traditional open surgery, PCNL offers significantly higher stone-free rates. However, the significant complication risks associated with PCNL may compromise its efficacy [1]. Potential significant associated morbidities include bleeding, injury to the kidney and its adjacent visceral or vascular organs, etc. PCNL complications are usually associated with inaccurate sizing and placement of the nephrostomy tracts. To reduce morbidity associated with conventional-sized PCNL, miniaturized PCNL such as minimally invasive PCNL, mini-PCNL, and miniperc were developed. These procedures include the use of miniaturized endoscopes via smaller percutaneous tracts (14–20 F), and are generally termed into multiple sessions. In addition to miniperc, Desai et al. [2] first reported the ultra-mini PCNL (UMP), and later micro-PCNL was introduced for clinical use [3]. In order to reduce nephrostomy tract size, research and development of miniaturized nephroscopes and access sheaths are necessary. However, using smaller nephrostomy tracts may result in compromised visual quality, therefore, increases stone extraction difficulties. Utilizing a pressure pump helps increase irrigation pressure while improving visual fields and passive extractions of stone fragments but may meanwhile increase intra-luminal pressure.

The super-mini-PCNL (SMP) treatment was created to alleviate further the critical limitations of conventional miniaturized PCNLs [4, 5]. SMP technique is a recent addition to the armamentarium of miniaturized PCNL, with the use of a recently engineered access sheath of 10–14 F. The unique design of the access sheath has been shown to be able to prevent excessive intrarenal pressure while providing excellent endoscopic visual quality for stone fragmentation and extraction at the same time.

## 20.2 Armamentarium

The key components of the SMP system consist of an 8 F miniaturized nephroscope with a working channel of 3.3 F and an irrigation-suction sheath [6].

### 20.2.1 Miniaturized Nephroscope

The SMP nephroscope is a miniaturized nephroscope with a dismountable sheath. The sheath has

G. Zeng (✉) · W. Zhu
Department of Urology and Guangdong Key Laboratory of Urology, The First Affiliated Hospital of Guangzhou Medical University, Guangzhou, China



M. S. Agrawal et al. (eds.), *Minimally Invasive Percutaneous Nephrolithotomy*,
https://doi.org/10.1007/978-981-16-6001-6_20

an outer diameter of 8 F and an inner diameter of 7.5 F. The telescope consists of a 4.2 F fiber-optic bundle, delivering 120° angle of view and up to 40,000 pixels. During the procedure, after insertion of the telescope into the sheath, a 3.3 F space remains in the bottom half of the dismountable sheath, which serves as the working channel (Fig. 20.1). This working channel can accommodate a laser fiber up to 550 $\mu$m in size for stone fragmentation. Alternatively, a 2.4 F (0.8 mm) pneumatic lithotripter probe, or a 3 F stone basket or forceps, could also pass through the working channel. The nephroscope has a working length of up to 25.2 cm.

### 20.2.2 Irrigation-Suction Sheath

The irrigation-suction sheath is the key element of the SMP technique, as its design essentially allows efficient irrigation and stone clearance within a miniaturized mechanism which consists of a straight sheath as well as a handle.

The straight sheath component consists of a double-layered metallic, tubular structure with measures between 12 F and 14 F and provides a working length of 8 or 14 cm. The gap between the two sheath layers works as the irrigation channel, while the central lumen of the sheath acts as a conduit for continuous suction. Side holes are located at the distal tip, which allows irrigation fluid to outflow to the target area.

The handle component includes a straight tube, an irrigation port with an integrated stopcock, as well as an oblique bifurcated suction tube at 45° placed around the mid-shaft. The straight tube is connected to the central lumen of the straight sheath. Lithotripsy instruments or endoscopic baskets could be inserted through the rubber cap end of the straight tube. During the SMP procedure, the irrigation port is mounted to a pump for irrigation inflow, while the bifurcated suction port is connected to a negative pressure aspirator. Suction pressure could be modified by pressing or releasing the pressure vent located in the axis of the suction tube (Fig. 20.2). A specimen collection bottle is connected to the suction port and the aspirator to facilitate the efficient collection of stone fragments.

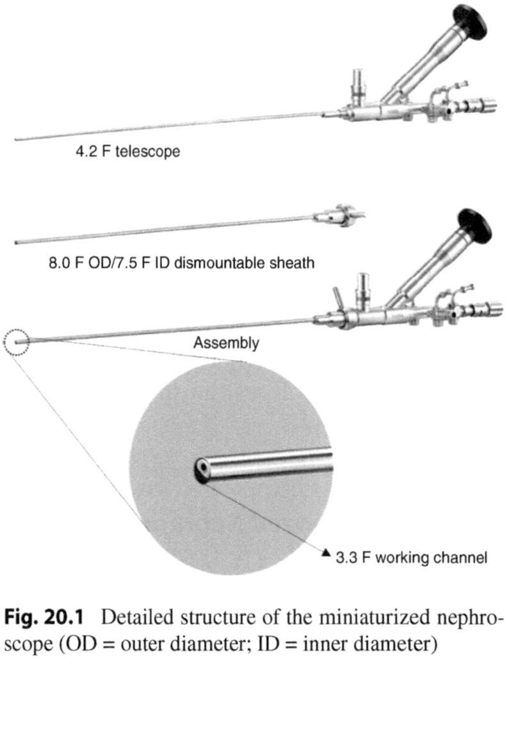


**Fig. 20.1** Detailed structure of the miniaturized nephroscope (OD = outer diameter; ID = inner diameter)

## 20.3 Indications and Contraindications

### 20.3.1 Indications

- Adult patients with stones less than 30 mm, including those who had previous unsuccessful stone clearance with SWL or ureteroscopic lithotripsy, patients with cystine calculus.

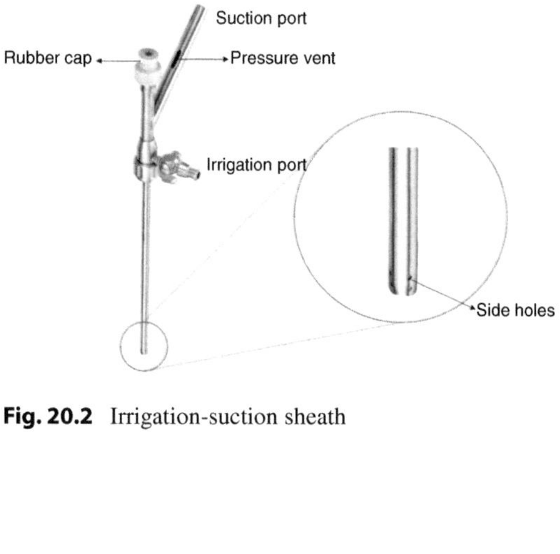


**Fig. 20.2** Irrigation-suction sheath

- Patients with unfavorable renal anatomy for RIRS such as infundibulum less than 5 mm or greater than 30 mm.
- Pediatric patients with stone size less than 25 mm who had unsuccessful treatment with SWL.

### 20.3.2 Contraindications

- Patients must suspend anticoagulant therapy before the SMP procedure.
- SMP should not be performed on patients when any of these conditions are present:
  - Untreated urinary tract infections (UTIs).
  - Pregnancy.
  - Atypical interposition of visceral organs including bowel, spleen, or liver.
  - Tumor in the probable percutaneous tract area or potential malignant renal tumor.

## 20.4 Technique

Routine preoperative preparations should be performed before any percutaneous surgery. This should include thorough evaluations of available imaging such as CTs and IVUs to assist the selection of primary calyx as the site of puncture, through which most stone bulk can be safely cleared. In patients with complex stone burden or unfavorable renal anatomy, stones located in separate calyces which are difficult to be extracted through the primary tract should also be identified. Secondary tracts could be considered preoperation in order to access these calyces safely.

In conventional SMP treatment, patients are placed in the prone position, which provides direct access to the posterior calyx. However, SMP can also be carried out in the supine position, which allows the use of endoscopic combined intrarenal surgery (ECIRS), which provides simultaneous antegrade and retrograde access to facilitate stone clearance. Supine SMP also allows easier switch from regional to general anesthesia when necessary and could be beneficial to patients with co-morbidities that may cause placing the patient in prone position anesthetically challenging. In the supine position, however, the establishment of multiple percutaneous tracks could be challenging due to space limitations.

Under general anesthesia, a 5 F ureteral catheter is first inserted in the target kidney retrogradely using a cystoscope or a ureteroscope. A Foley urethral catheter is then inserted into the bladder. Percutaneous access is carried out using an 18-gauge coaxial needle, puncturing the target calyx under fluoroscopic or ultrasonic guidance. A 0.032-inch flexible tip guidewire is then inserted through the needle. The access track can then be dilated using 10 F fascial dilators. The irrigation-suction sheath with obturator then railroads into the pelvicalyceal system following the guidewire. The guidewire is then removed together with the obturator. The handle is then mounted onto the straight sheath to create irrigation and suction channels.

The irrigation port of the handle is connected to the irrigation pump, while the suction port is connected to the aspiration unit with a specimen collection bottle attached. The pressure of the irrigation fluid should be set between 200 to 250 mmHg, while the suction pressure should be set between 100 to 150 mmHg. The miniaturized nephroscope is inserted into the access sheath through the rubber cap of the handle. Once targeted renal stones are reached, lithotripsy can be engaged using a holmium-yttrium aluminum garnet (YAG) laser or pneumatic lithotripter. Laser lithotripsy is often the preferred method in SMP, although pneumatic lithotripters could work as an alternative when laser lithotripters are not readily available. With continuous suction, small stone fragments could travel through the gap between the endoscope and the straight sheath then exit through the suction channel. The suction pressure could be modified by the surgeon pressing or releasing the pressure vent with a thumb while holding the handle. If stone fragments are unable to travel through the space between the scope and the access sheath, the scope can be gradually withdrawn to create a wider channel for those fragments to evacuate. To treat patients with greater stone sizes such as staghorn stones, secondary percutaneous tracks should be considered to assist stone clearance.

After stone clearance, a fluoroscopic image is captured to confirm the stone-free status following endoscopic assessment. Antegrade insertion of a double-J stent should be considered for patients with significant ureteric inflammatory changes associated with the stone obstructions, evidence of ureteropelvic junction obstruction, following rigid ureteroscopic treatment of ipsilateral ureteric stones, significant pyelocaliceal blood clots after the lithotripsy, or significant residual stones after SMP. Lastly, the straight sheath is removed, and the incision is either sutured or sealed with absorbable gelatin.

With smaller percutaneous tracts, the less invasive characteristic of SMP comparing to conventional PCNL makes it possible for patients to be tubeless, especially in uncomplicated cases when the patient is completely stone-free. Advantages of a tubeless procedure include better patient comfort, less postoperative pain, a shorter hospital stay, and a quicker recovery.

Nephrostomy tube placement could be considered in selected patients with significant residual stone fragments following SMP that requires auxiliary procedures, as well as in patients who developed significant pyelocaliceal blood clots or bleeding following lithotripsy.

## 20.5 Clinical Evidence

Comparative studies were conducted to analyze the advantages and disadvantages of SMP and other modalities such as RIRS and SWL. Overall, these studies demonstrate that SMP has relatively higher efficacy and a lower risk of complications.

### 20.5.1 A Comparison Between SMP and RIRS in Treating 10–20 mm Lower-Pole Renal Stones

According to available literature, stone-free rates of RIRS range from 65% to 92%, and the procedure is known for its low risk of complications when treating smaller renal stones. However, the stone-free rates of RIRS drop significantly when treating lower-pole renal stones, especially in the case of a narrow calyceal infundibulum with an acute infundibulo-pelvic angle. Additionally, RIRS has shown other disadvantages, including the need to perform multiple procedures if passive ureteral dilatation is required and if stone size or location is unfavorable, which increases the risk of ureteric damage. Temporary ureteric stenting is often required after the RIRS procedure, which may result in a higher cost for patients in comparison to SMP.

As of today, Level-1 evidence is limited when comparing SMP and RIRS for treating 10–20 mm lower calyceal calculus. To further investigate the safety and efficacy of the two modalities, we carried out a prospective, multicenter, randomized controlled trial from 2015 to 2017 [7]. The results show that SMP had a higher stone-free rate and a lower auxiliary rate comparing to those of RIRS, making it the preferred treatment method for 10–20 mm lower-pole stones. Despite that RIRS was associated with less postoperative pain, the risks of complications and duration of hospital stay between the two modalities were compatible. Therefore, the SMP technique could be a safe and effective substitute for RIRS, especially when treating smaller renal calculi in the lower calyceal.

### 20.5.2 A Comparison Between SMP and Miniperc in Treating Renal Stones Greater than 20 mm

Similar to conventional PCNL, miniperc is a multistep procedure with a smaller percutaneous tract size. When comparing SMP with miniperc, the track-size-related complication risks of SMP are expected to be lower than those of miniperc. The results from an international multicenter comparative study show that SMP is the preferred treatment option for stones less than 40 mm as compared to miniperc. For patients with 20–30 mm renal stones, SMP is more efficacious with advantages including a lower chance postoperative fever, less blood loss and pain comparing to miniperc. When treating stones larger than 40 mm, however, SMP requires a prolonged operative time which reduces its efficiency [8].

### 20.5.3 A Comparison Between SMP and SWL in Treating Pediatric Patients with Renal Stones Less than 25 mm

Although urinary stones are rarely found in children, management of urinary stones in pediatric patients poses a technical challenge. SWL has gained widespread popularity because of its conservative and non-invasive nature. However, SWL often requires multiple treatment sessions and additional auxiliary procedures to achieve desired stone clearance. A retrospective study suggests that alternatively, SMP could be a valuable substitution [9]. In selected pediatric patients, the SMP technique is able to achieve a comparatively higher stone-free rate after one single treatment session, with a higher tubeless rate, less need for auxiliary procedures, and an acceptable complication rate in the minimally invasive treatment of stones less than 25 mm. Additionally, unlike SWL, the use of SMP allows a much broader range of indications that is less limited by both stone (size, location, and density) and patient (obesity, anatomic abnormalities) related factors.

## 20.6 Summary

The notion of SMP has yet to be widely recognized. Nevertheless, both the safety and efficacy of the SMP technique have been investigated in adults and pediatric patients [8, 9]. Although SMP could be performed in treating larger stones in carefully selected patients, the procedure should be performed by a surgical team that has been properly trained and has adequate experience in using the equipment involved. Careful patient selection and thorough surgical planning pre-operation are crucial for a successful SMP procedure.

## References

1. Professionals S-O Urolithiasis. In: Uroweb. https://uroweb.org/guideline/urolithiasis/. Accessed 13 Apr 2019.
2. Desai J, Zeng G, Zhao Z, Zhong W, Chen W, Wu W. A novel technique of ultra-mini-percutaneous nephrolithotomy: introduction and an initial experience for treatment of upper urinary calculi less than 2 cm. Biomed Res Int. 2013;2013:490793.
3. Desai M, Mishra S. "Microperc" micro percutaneous nephrolithotomy: evidence to practice. Curr Opin Urol. 2012;22:134–8.
4. Zeng G, Wan S, Zhao Z, et al. Super-mini percutaneous nephrolithotomy (SMP): a new concept in technique and instrumentation. BJU International. 2016;117:655–61.
5. Zeng G, Zhu W, Liu Y, Fan J, Zhao Z, Cai C. The new generation super-mini percutaneous nephrolithotomy (SMP) system: a step-by-step guide. BJU Int. 2017. https://doi.org/10.1111/bju.13955.
6. Zeng G, Zhu W, Lam W. Miniaturised percutaneous nephrolithotomy: Its role in the treatment of urolithiasis and our experience. Asian J Urol. 2018;5:295–302.
7. Alsmadi J, Fan J, Zhu W, Wen Z, Zeng G. The Influence of Super-Mini Percutaneous Nephrolithotomy on Renal Pelvic Pressure In Vivo. J Endourol. 2018;32:819–23.
8. Liu Y, AlSmadi J, Zhu W, Liu Y, Wu W, Fan J, Lan Y, Lam W, Zhong W, Zeng G. Comparison of supermini PCNL (SMP) versus Miniperc for stones larger than 2 cm: a propensity score-matching study. World J Urol. 2018. https://doi.org/10.1007/s00345-018-2197-7.
9. Sarica K, Eryildirim B, Tuerxun A, Batuer A, Kavukoglu O, Buz A, Zeng G. Super-mini percutaneous nephrolithotomy for renal stone less than 25mm in pediatric patients: Could it be an alternative to shockwave lithotripsy? Actas Urol Esp. 2017. https://doi.org/10.1016/j.acuro.2017.08.005.

# 21 Flexible Mini Nephroscopy

Madhu S. Agrawal, R. Mukhilesh, and Dilip K. Mishra

## 21.1 Introduction

Percutaneous Nephrolithotripsy (PCNL) has been the surgical procedure of choice for moderate to large renal stones for more than thirty years now. However, the complications associated with the standard PCNL, specially bleeding and pain, have led to the miniaturization and development of Minimally-Invasive PCNL [1, 2]. Mini-PCNL has been shown to be effective in achieving stone clearance rates matching standard PCNL, with lower complication rates compared to conventional PCNL [2–4].

Flexible Ureterorenoscope (fURS) or Retrograde Intrarenal Surgery (RIRS) is the other minimally-invasive endourological procedure for upper tract urolithiasis, which has evolved in recent years. Though a minimally-invasive procedure, fURS has got the potential drawbacks of higher costs and the need for pre-stenting and staged procedures [5].

A novel flexible mini-Nephroscope has been developed to combine the benefits of minimally-invasive percutaneous approach as well as flexible instrumentation [6]. During regular mini-PCNL with rigid nephroscope, the creation of additional tracts may be required for achieving complete stone clearance in case of inaccessible calyces and multiple calyceal calculi. The flexible mini-nephroscope allows access to almost the entire pelvi-caliceal system through a single calyx, thereby avoiding the need for additional tracts to achieve complete stone clearance.

Flexible Mini-Nephroscope—Instrument:

The novel mini-nephroscope (Karl Storz, Germany) combines the features of flexible cysto-nephroscope and flexible ureteroscope. Compared to the regular cysto-nephroscope the diameter of which is 15 Fr, the size of mini-nephroscope is 7.5 Fr, which allows it to pass through the smallest mini-PCNL sheath. (Fig. 21.1).

The length of the shaft measures about 45 cm, which is considerably shorter than the

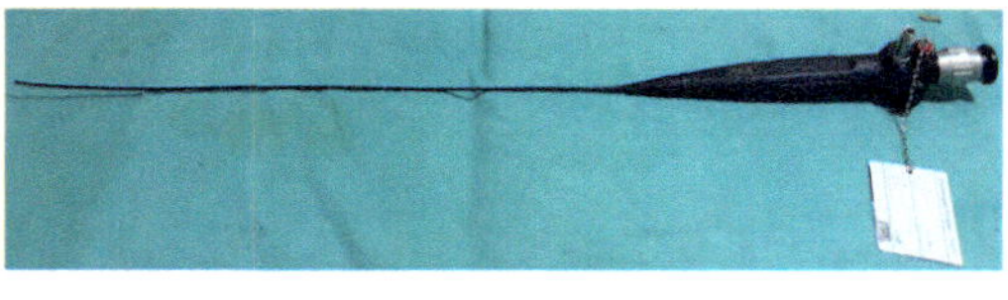

**Fig. 21.1** Flexible Mini-Nephroscope

M. S. Agrawal (✉)
Professor and Head, Department of Urology, Global Rainbow Healthcare, Agra, Uttar Pradesh, India

R. Mukhilesh
Department of Urology, KKS Hospital and Kidney Care Center, Gobichettipalayam, Erode, India

D. K. Mishra
Kasturba Medical College, Manipal, Karnataka, India

Head, Department of Urology, Pushpanjali Hospital and Research Center, Agra, Uttar Pradesh, India

Department of Urology, Center for Minimally-Invasive Endourology, Global Rainbow Healthcare, Agra, Uttar Pradesh, India


M. S. Agrawal et al. (eds.), *Minimally Invasive Percutaneous Nephrolithotomy*,
https://doi.org/10.1007/978-981-16-6001-6_21

regular flexible ureteroscope. Though the regular flexible ureteroscopes can also be utilized during mini-PCNL, the length of the scope makes it difficult to use ergonomically during mini-PCNL, besides the risk of damage to the instrument.

The flexible mini-nephroscope has a working channel of 3.6 Fr, and the tip has a deflection of about 270 degrees in both directions, similar to the flexible ureteroscope. Laser fiber and flexible basket can be used with the instrument in the same way as ureteroscope.

## 21.2 Flexible Mini Nephroscopy—Indication

The aim of any stone surgery is to achieve 100% stone-free rate, and it should be no different in the minimally-invasive techniques. Mini-PCNL has gained popularity in recent years largely because of its smaller tract size, thereby avoiding bleeding and pain. The expanding role of mini-PCNL has now led to its utilization in larger stones and multiple calculi (Fig. 21.2). However, this may require the need for additional tracts for complete clearance, especially in patients with multiple renal calculi, when the rigid nephroscope is unable to reach all calyces. Utilization of flexible mini-nephroscope helps to achieve stone clearance without increasing the number of tracts in these situations.

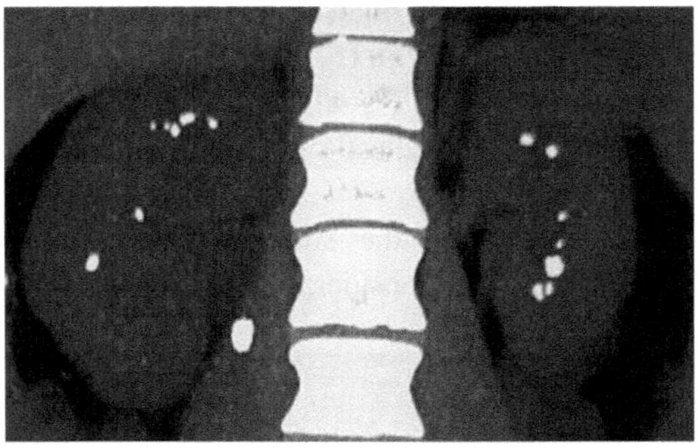

**Fig. 21.2** CT image of the kidney with multiple calyceal calculi

## 21.3 Flexible Mini Nephroscopy—Technique

The procedure is performed in the usual prone, or supine if preferred, position. Initial puncture is done in the standard fashion, under fluoroscopic or ultrasonic guidance, and single-step tract dilatation used to put in the 15–16 F mini-Amplatz sheath. The rigid mini-nephroscope(12 F) is used initially for nephroscopy and fragmentation of the main bulk of the stone. In mini-PCNL, most of the fragments can be cleared by the "whirlpool effect" without using any graspers. Following clearance of the major bulk of stone with rigid nephroscope, the flexible mini-nephroscope is introduced through the same mini-Amplatz sheath. All calyces can be inspected with the flexible nephroscope (Fig. 21.3), in a manner similar to using a flexible ureteroscope, and remaining calyceal calculi or fragments cleared with holmium laser and stone basket. The procedure can be done "tubeless" without any nephrostomy tube, leaving a DJ stent to be removed after 10–14 days. Alternatively, just an indwelling ureteric catheter can be left in at completion, to be removed the next day before discharge from the hospital.

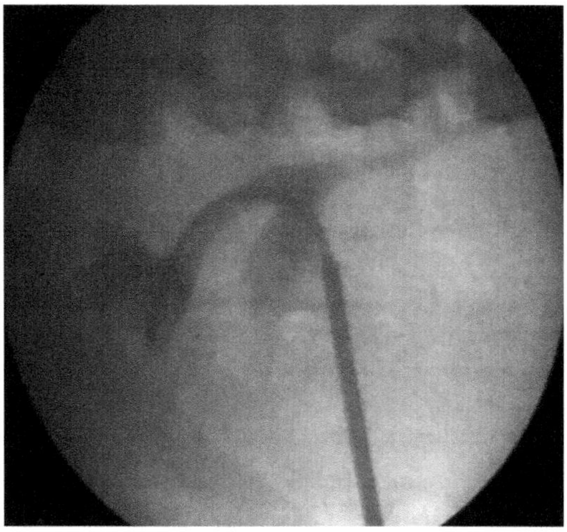

**Fig. 21.3** Fluoroscopic view of Flexible Mini-Nephroscope in use

## 21.4 RIRS Vs. Flexible Mini Nephroscopy

Flexible ureteroscopy competes with PCNL as the first line of management of renal calculus up to 2 cm depending upon the stone and anatomic factors, mainly because of its minimally-invasive nature. However, the need for pre-stenting, the need for ancillary procedures, and increased risks for sepsis are the major drawbacks of fURS. The costs for endoscopes and disposables are also high compared to mini-PCNL. There is also need for stenting postop, removal of which requires additional procedure [5]. The same can be said about combined supine mini-PCNL and flexible URS procedure (ECIRS).

Flexible cysto-nephroscope has already been shown to reduce morbidity in conventional PCNL [7, 8]. Flexible mini Nephroscopy aims to achieve the stone-free rate in minimally-invasive way. It obviates the need for additional tract in the inaccessible calyx, thereby reducing the complications. Limiting the number of tracts can limit the injury caused to the renal tissue, decrease the operative time and morbidity.

## 21.5 Flexible Mini Nephroscopy—Outcomes

Our previously published study [6] has demonstrated the utility and feasibility of flexible mini Nephroscopy in patients with renal stones up to 2 cms. The study compared the outcomes with fURS. The study showed the stone-free rate was higher in the mini-PCNL group (92% vs. 80%). The need for the ancillary procedures was also less with flexible mini-nephroscope (8%). Compared to fURS group, mini-PCNL group did not require compulsory stenting post-procedure, thus avoiding stent-related symptoms and the need for the second procedure. Flexible mini Nephroscopy helps to achieve a better stone-free rate compared to fURS in least invasive way.

## 21.6 Conclusion

Mini-PCNL has shown to be an effective treatment modality for renal stone with minimal morbidity as compared to conventional PCNL. However, in situations that warrant additional tract creation, flexible mini nephroscopy offers an effective alternative with minimum morbidity without compromising the stone-free rates. Flexible mini-nephroscope has the potential to be a useful addition to the minimally-invasive endourological armamentarium.

## References


1. Kirac M, Bozkurt ÖF, Tunc L, Guneri C, Unsal A, Biri H. Comparison of retrograde intrarenal surgery and mini-percutaneous nephrolithotomy in management of lower-pole renal stones with a diameter of smaller than 15 mm. Urolithiasis. 2013;41:241–6.
2. Sabnis RB, Ganesamoni R, Sarpal R. Miniperc: what is its current status? Curr Opin Urol. 2012;22:129–13.
3. Yamaguchi A, Skolarikos A, Buchholz NP, et al. Operating times and bleeding complications in percutaneous nephrolithotomy: a comparison of tract dilation methods in 5537 patients in the clinical research Office of the Endourological Society Percutaneous Nephrolithotomy Global Study. J Endourol. 2011;25:933–9.
4. Mishra S, Sharma R, Garg C, Kurien A, Sabnis R, Desai M. Prospective comparative study of miniperc and standard PNL for treatment of 1 to 2 cm size renal stone. BJU Int. 2011;108:896–9.
5. Schoenthaler M, Wilhelm K, Hein S, et al. Ultra-mini PCNL versus flexible ureteroscopy: a matched analysis of treatment costs (endoscopes and disposables) in patients with renal stones 10–20Â mm. World J Urol. 2015;33:1601–5.
6. Mishra DK, Agrawal MS. Use of a novel flexible mini-Nephroscope in minimally-invasive percutaneous nephrolithotomy. Urology. 2017;103:59–62. https://doi.org/10.1016/j.urology.2017.01.009.
7. Beaghler MA, Poon MW, Dushinski JW, Lingeman JE et al. Expanding role of flexible nephroscopy in the upper urinary tract. J Endourol. 1999;13(2):93–97.
8. Gücük A, Kemahlı E, Üyetürk U, Tuygun C, Yıldız M, Metin A. Routine flexible nephroscopy for percutaneous nephrolithotomy for renal stones with low density: a prospective, randomized study. J Urol. 2013;190:144–148.

# Endoscopic Combined Intrarenal Surgery (ECIRS)

# 22

Dilip K. Mishra and Karthickeyan Naganathan

## 22.1 Introduction

Percutaneous Nephrolithotomy (PCNL) has undergone various advances and modifications since it was first introduced in 1976 [1]. Since its inception, PCNL is commonly being done in prone position all over the world. There have been several advances in optics, nephroscope designs, puncture techniques and miniaturization of instruments in the past few decades resulting in better stone clearance and reduction in patient morbidity. The morbidity of PCNL is attributed to the puncturing and dilatation of the renal parenchyma which at times can lead to bleeding and also significant pain in the postoperative period. Moreover, the prone position is also responsible for the difficulty to access airway and ventilation faced by the anaesthesiologists [2]. Prone positioning is time-consuming and requires more personnel in the theatre [3].

In the year 1990, Valdivia presented his work on PCNL in the supine position for the first time in world literature. It took more than two decades for a more widespread acceptance of the supine position for PCNL after various modifications in patient positioning. With the advent of the supine position and the Galdakao-modified supine Valdivia (GMSV) position [4, 5], the simultaneous access to the kidney both from below and above became less cumbersome. This has evolved beautifully in the technique of Endoscopic Combined Intrarenal Surgery (ECIRS) [6].

ECIRS is a very versatile technique wherein PCNL is combined with flexible ureteroscopy to achieve maximal stone clearance in minimal time duration. The disadvantages of additional time for prone positioning and restricted or no access from below are transformed to advantages in the supine position. ECIRS not only helps in the reduction of the number of access tracts, but also in complete clearance of large stone bulk in a single session in a short time thereby reducing the chances of bleeding [7].

## 22.2 Evolution of Mini ECIRS

Performing PCNL in the prone position gives us a large surface area for obtaining access. It is not so in the supine position, wherein there is a small window to obtain access. The advances in miniaturization of access tract with the advent of mini PCNL have been very fruitful as the smaller sheaths can be easily guided into the pelvicalyceal system (PCS) even from a small window as

D. K. Mishra (✉)
Kasturba Medical College, Manipal, Karnataka, India

Head, Department of Urology, Pushpanjali Hospital and Research Center, Agra, Uttar Pradesh, India

Department of Urology & Center for Minimally-Invasive Endourology, Global Rainbow Healthcare, Agra, Uttar Pradesh, India

K. Naganathan
Frontline Hospital, Trichy, Tamil Nadu, India


M. S. Agrawal et al. (eds.), *Minimally Invasive Percutaneous Nephrolithotomy*,
https://doi.org/10.1007/978-981-16-6001-6_22

is available in the supine position [8]. Traditionally, ECIRS has been performed with flexible ureteroscopy from below using the modern flexible scopes and a standard PCNL (>20 F) for the percutaneous tract. Flexible ureteroscopy helps to assess the pelvicalyceal system anatomy, stone size, location and its configuration before making the renal access. Furthermore, the renal access can be guided under vision making a perfect papillary puncture through the papilla. In mini ECIRS, the renal access tract is small (<20F) which can be easily created from the limited window available. The dilation process can be a single step in all cases of mini PCNL thereby minimizing the time to create the tract. Most of the stone fragmentation is done through the nephroscope and the renal tract is used for egress of the fragments. There is minimal chance of raised intra-pelvic pressure as the renal tract offers a low-pressure outlet [9].

## 22.3 Indications

The various indications of mini ECIRS include the following situations.

1. Partial staghorn stone with secondary stones in other calyces.
2. Large bulk impacted upper ureteric stones.
3. Multiple stones in various calyces.
4. Stone at PUJ with suspected PUJ obstruction.
5. Large compound/multiple necrosed detached papilla in the PCS.

## 22.4 Armamentarium

Mini ECIRS is a versatile technique but it needs more armamentarium than conventional PCNL or flexible ureteroscopy. It requires

(i) Standard or large operation theatre to accommodate two operating teams simultaneously.
(ii) Two Endourology operating teams (2 Urologists and 2 Operating assistants).
(iii) Two camera units.
(iv) Fluoroscopy unit.
(v) Ultrasonogram.
(vi) Flexible ureteroscopy with its accessories.
(vii) Mini PERC nephroscope set.
(viii) Lithotripsy devices (LASER/Pneumatic/Trilogy).

This enormous amount of armamentarium needs planning to avoid clutter in the operating room. Positioning of endoscopy and fluoroscopy monitors should be in such a way that both the renal and ureteral surgeons should have direct visual access to their corresponding monitors as well as the fluoroscopy screen. There are various schemes described for the accommodation of the equipment. We prefer to arrange this equipment as shown in Fig. 22.1.

## 22.5 Technical Considerations

### 22.5.1 Anaesthesia

Traditionally PCNL has been done under general anaesthesia in the prone position for several decades. Restricted access to the upper airway, changes in the key cardio respiratory parameters and neurological damages are some of the well-known complications of the prone position. Supine position eliminates most of these disadvantages and access to the upper airway is readily available to the anaesthetist. The safety of PCNL under regional anaesthesia is well established in many recent studies [10, 11]. Mini ECIRS can be safely performed under regional or general anaesthesia depending on the preference of the operating team, stone burden, patient's comorbidities and patient's choice.

### 22.5.2 Positioning

The standard Galdakao-Modified Supine Valdivia (GMSV) position works very well for all cases of ECIRS giving excellent access to renal as well as the ureteric surgeon [6]. The patient is positioned under anaesthesia at the edge of the table with the ipsilateral side tilted 15 to 20 degrees to the

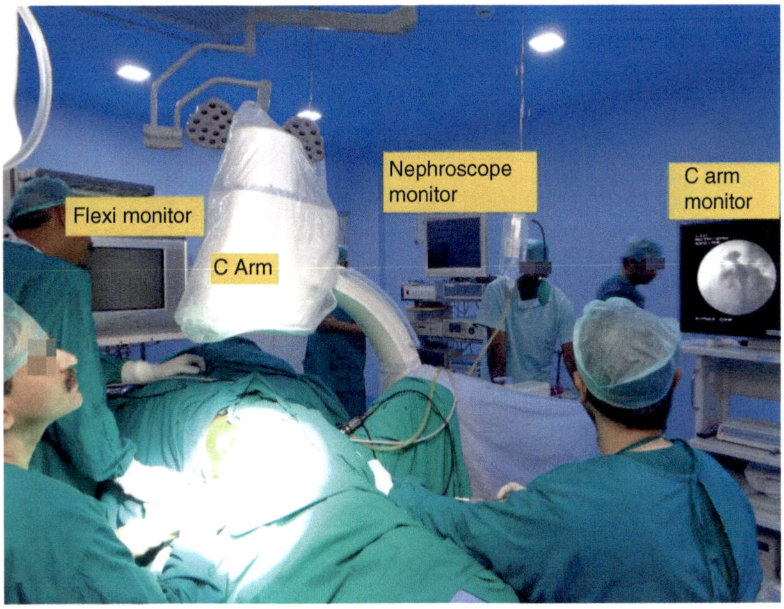


**Fig. 22.1** Operation room set-up. Note the endoscopy and fluoroscopy monitor positions

opposite side. The ipsilateral knee is extended and the contralateral thigh flexed and abducted. The ipsilateral hand is rested over the thorax appropriately while the contralateral hand is extended for easy access to the anaesthesia team. This position gives the renal surgeon comfortable access to the kidney percutaneously allowing simultaneous retrograde access to the ureteric surgeon. Retrograde access to the contralateral unit is also possible in this position to perform simultaneous bilateral endoscopic surgery [12]. At times the angulation can be difficult to negotiate a rigid ureteroscope into the upper ureter due to the pushing effect by the renal surgeon but the same renal tract can be used to push the kidney cranially to straighten the ureter.

### 22.5.3 Retrograde Access

The initial access is almost always retrograde in a mini ECIRS procedure [13]. The upper ureter is visualized directly using a 6/7.5-Fr semi-rigid ureteroscope (Wolf™; Richard Wolf GmBH, Knittlingen, Germany) which paves the way for the insertion of a suitable Ureteral Access sheath (UAS). The initial rigid ureteroscopy assesses the ureter for any strictures or any stones which might have been missed. It also assesses the ureteric orifice and may obviate the dilation of the orifice with a balloon if required to allow placement of suitable UAS (11/13-Fr or 13/15-Fr). A smaller UAS always suffices as the aim is to facilitate passage of the flexible scope and not retrieval of stone fragments which is usually done via renal access.

The flexible scope is used to create a roadmap of the whole PCS and access the calyces for a suitable puncture site for renal access. The flexible scope can be used to direct the renal access for a completely end vision guided puncture [13].

We have been using mini ECIRS for the treatment of large upper ureteric stones which are always in the dilemma group on the selection of suitable modality. The rigid ureteroscope works very well in this setting as it can be used to fragment and disimpact the stone and renal access can be used to clear the fragments.

### 22.5.4 Renal Access

The renal access is created mostly using ultrasonography for the initial puncture. The access can also be guided with the help of flexible scope which visualizes the target calyx and can fine-tune

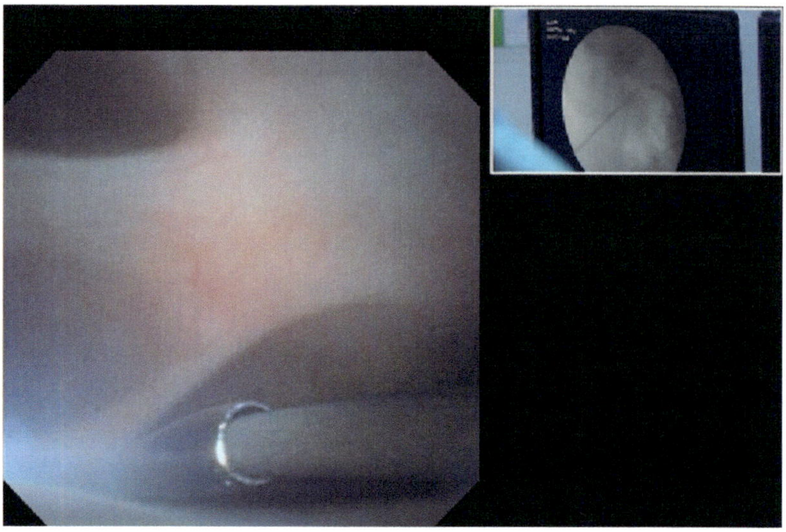

Fig. 22.2 Endovision assisted renal puncture. The flexible scope will guide the puncture through desired calyx

the entry of the puncture needle (Fig. 22.2). With the needle in place, a hydrophilic Terumo guide wire can be passed into the system down the ureter followed by a single step dilator. Mostly the inferior or middle calyx is used to create the renal access followed by insertion of a 16 or 18F renal access sheath depending on the stone burden. As the damage to the flexible scope is significantly higher for lower polar stones especially when the infundibulopelvic angle is less than or equal to 60 degrees [14], it is prudent to clear the lower calyceal stone burden with the percutaneous access. The renal access quickly clears the turbid urine or clot formed following which both the scopes can work in tandem to clear the stone. The nephroscope used in this access can be a standard 12–15F scope.

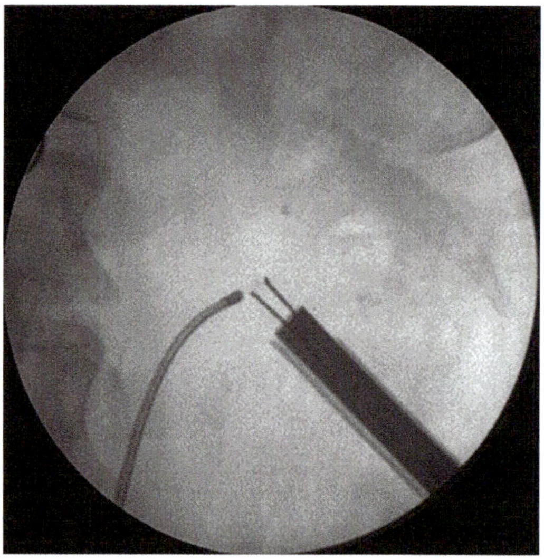

Fig. 22.3 Passing the ball technique. The stone fragment is passed from the flexible ureteroscope to the nephroscope which will be removed through the percutaneous tract

## 22.5.5 Stone Fragmentation and Retrieval

Most of the times, renal access is used for fragmentation and retrieval of stone fragments. Laser energy (VersaPulse PowerSuite 100 W Lumenis, San Jose, CA, USA) or a Swiss mini LithoClast probe (EMS Electro Medical Systems SA, Nyon, Switzerland) can be utilized for stone fragmentation with the mini nephroscope. The stone fragments are curated to a size appropriate to pass through the renal access sheath. The flexible scope is used just to collect any peripherally lying stones and to deliver them to the nephroscope using 1.5-Fr tipless nitinol baskets (NCircle/Ngage; Cook Medical) by the technique of "Passing the ball" (Fig. 22.3). Sometimes for an impacted calyceal stone inaccessible by nephroscope, the flexible scope is used to fragment the stone and wash it out of the calyx which can then be picked up by the nephroscope and cleared through the percutaneous tract.

### 22.5.6 Exit Strategy

Once all stone fragments have been cleared, both scopes are used to relook into the PCS to clear any leftover fragments and clots. Flexible ureteroscopy is very helpful in identifying any residual fragments in the calyx of nephroscope entry as well as in any of its parallel calyx. A nephrostomy tube is seldom required following mini PCNL [15]. Nephrostomy tube (8–14 Fr) insertion is required rarely in complicated cases having uncontrolled bleeding, prolonged operating time of more than 2 hours, perforation of the renal pelvis and the presence of residual stones. A double J stent is inserted routinely and removed after 10–14 days. In some uncomplicated cases, a 5/6 Fr Ureteric catheter is left in situ and is removed on the first postoperative day. It is also possible to be totally tubeless following uncomplicated mini ECIRS when the stone burden and the operating time are less without any excessive bleeding and/or pelvis perforation.

## 22.6 Follow-up

Plain radiograph of the KUB region is done after 24–48 h to confirm stone clearance. Ultrasonogram is a good modality for follow-up following mini ECIRS without any radiation exposure. But the artefact created by the indwelling double J stent may be misleading in some cases. Follow-up computed tomography is rarely required unless they are radiolucent stones.

## 22.7 Complications

The complications following mini ECIRS may be related to either flexible ureteroscopy or mini-PCNL or both. Fever and urosepsis are the most dreadful complications of flexible ureteroscopy which are less frequent in mini ECIRS owing to less intrarenal pressure during the procedure. With the advent of miniaturization of flexible scopes and hence the small size of ureteric access sheath used, ureteric injury due to access sheath use is uncommon in the current era. Bleeding, drop in haemoglobin, blood transfusion and pelvic perforation are statistically less in miniPCNL when compared to conventional PCNL [16].

## 22.8 Conclusion

Mini ECIRS is a versatile endourology technique for complex upper tract stones. It has the advantage of maximal stone clearance with minimal nephron loss. The overall stone free rate is comparable to conventional PCNL with reduced risk of bleeding and other complications. The need for two operating teams with various equipment may be a rate limiting step in the widespread adaptation of mini ECIRS.

## 22.9 Future Considerations

With the recent widespread adaptation of mini PCNL and ECIRS, there is a compelling need for more RCTs in this topic.

## References


1. Fernstroem I, Johansson B. Percutaneous pyelolithotomy, a new extraction technique. Scand J Urol Nephrol. 1976;10:257–9.
2. Ibarluzea G, Scoffone CM, Cracco CM, et al. Supine Valdivia and modified lithotomy position for simultaneous anterograde and retrograde endourological access. BJU Int. 2007;100:233–6.
3. Valdivia Urı'a JG, Valle GJ, Villarroya S. Why is percutaneous nephroscopy still performed with patient prone? J Endourol. 1990;4:269–72.
4. Valdivia Urıa JG, Valle GJ, Lopez Lopez JA, et al. Technique and complications of percutaneous nephroscopy: experience with 557 patients in the supine position. J Urol. 1998;160:1975–8.
5. Shoma AM, Erakay I, El-Kenawy MR, El-Kappany HA. Percutaneous nephrolithotomy in the supine position. Technical aspects and functional outcome compared with the prone technique. Urology. 2002;60:388–92.
6. Scoffone CM, Cracco CM, Cossu M, Grande S, Poggio M, Scarpa RM. Endoscopic combined intrarenal surgery in Galdakao-modified supine Valdivia position: a new standard for percutaneous nephrolithotomy? Eur Urol. 2008;54:1393–403.
7. Scoffone CM, Cracco CM, Poggio M, Scarpa RM. Endoscopic combined intrarenal surgery for

high burden renal stones. Arch Ital UrolAndrol. 2010;82:41–2.
8. Ruhayel Y, Tepeler A, Dabestani S, et al. Tract sizes in miniaturized percutaneous nephrolithotomy: a systematic review from the European Association of Urology. Urolithiasis Guidelines Panel. Eur Urol. 2017;72:220–35. https://doi.org/10.1016/j.eururo.2017.01.046.
9. Doizi S, Uzan A, Keller EX, et al. Comparison of intrapelvic pressures during flexible ureteroscopy, mini-percutaneous nephrolithotomy, standard percutaneous nephrolithotomy, and endoscopic combined intrarenal surgery in a kidney model. World J Urol. 2020;39(7):2709–17.
10. Movasseghi G, Hassani V, Mohaghegh MR, Safaeian R, Safari S, Zamani MM, Nabizadeh R. Comparison between spinal and general anesthesia in percutaneous nephrolithotomy. Anesthesiol Pain Med. 2014;4(1):e13871.
11. Cicek T, Gonulalan U, Dogan R, Kosan M, Istanbulluoglu O, Gonen M, Ozturk B, Ozkardes H. Spinal anesthesia is an efficient and safe anesthetic method for percutaneous nephrolithotomy. Urology. 2014;83(1):50–5.
12. Giusti G, Proietti S, Rodríguez-Socarrás ME, Eisner BH, Saitta G, Mantica G, Villa L, Salonia A, Montorsi F, Gaboardi F. Simultaneous bilateral endoscopic surgery (SBES) for patients with bilateral upper tract urolithiasis: technique and outcomes. Eur Urol. 2018;74(6):810–5.
13. Cracco CM, Scoffone CM. Endoscopic combined intrarenal surgery (ECIRS)-tips and tricks to improve outcomes: a systematic review. Turk J Urol. 2020;46(Suppl 1):S46.
14. Ozimek T, Cordes J, Wiessmeyer JR, Schneider MH, Hupe MC, Gilbert N, Merseburger AS, Kramer MW. Steep infundibulopelvic angle as a new risk factor for flexible ureteroscope damage and complicated postoperative course. J Endourol. 2018;32(7):597–602.
15. Lahme S. Miniaturisation of PCNL. Urolithiasis. 2018 Feb;46(1):99–106.
16. Huusmann S, Nagele U, Herrmann TR. Miniaturization of percutaneous nephrolithotomy smaller, but better? Curr Opin Urol. 2017;27(2):161–9.

# Part VII

# Special Situations

# Failed Access and Secondary Puncture

# 23

Evangelos Liatsikos, Panagiotis Kallidonis,
Arman Tsaturyan, and Despoina Liourdi

## 23.1 Introduction

Percutaneous nephrolithotomy (PCNL) is the standard of care treatment modality for renal stones >2 cm. It is also recommended for 1–2 cm renal stones located in the lower calyces [1]. Since its introduction, surgical approaches and instrumentation of PCNL have undergone continuous improvement decreasing the complications and improving the outcomes. Nevertheless, the procedure is associated with several intra and postoperative complications ranging from 4 to 50.8% according to different authors. Most of the complications are minor, serious complications occurring in approximately 5% of cases [2].

No PCNL procedure is possible without an appropriate puncture of the renal collecting system. The puncture and establishment of a working access tract are critical steps for PCNL. As such the puncture can be successfully obtained using papillary and non-papillary approaches [3]. Tract dilation can be achieved with different dilators [4]. As for the positioning of the patient supine and prone approaches can be utilized [5]. Finally, single or multiple tracts can be required to reach stone-free status [6].

Ideal renal access allows achievement of a stone-free rate (SFR) at the shortest operative time with minimal perioperative complications. An inappropriate puncture can increase the risk of intraoperative and postoperative complications. On the other hand, the development of intraoperative complications could result in significant difficulty for the surgeon and may lead to the displacement of the already existing tract and further failure of the procedure [7, 8].

In fact, the failure of PCNL access is not rare. According to different authors, its prevalence can range from 1.7% to 9% [9, 10]. Several factors including anatomic target restricted vision, difficulties of handling of instruments and hand-eye coordination, an atomic structure deformations, and movement of organs are reported to impact the puncture quality and obscure its proper performance [11]. Knowledge of those factors and specific tricks can allow the surgeon to diminish the failure rate and associated complications.

Failure of establishment of the initial PCNL tract may lead to additional punctures. Overall, secondary puncture can be required in clinical scenarios such as multiple tract procedures, lack of scope maneuverability, displacement of stone fragments, loss of initial access, doubt of the puncture of vessel or other adjacent organs.

E. Liatsikos (✉) · P. Kallidonis · A. Tsaturyan
Department of Urology, University of Patras, Patras, Greece

D. Liourdi
Department of Internal Medicine, General Hospital of Patras "Ag. Andreas", Patras, Greece



M. S. Agrawal et al. (eds.), *Minimally Invasive Percutaneous Nephrolithotomy*,
https://doi.org/10.1007/978-981-16-6001-6_23

## 23.2 Determinants of Successful Puncture

### 23.2.1 Surgeon's Expertise

Surgeon's experience is a crucial factor for achieving successful outcomes. According to de la Rosette et al., obtaining renal access is responsible for the steep learning curve of PCNL [12]. It is, therefore, recommended, that a minimum of 24 PCNL are required during residency period for good surgical proficiency. Surgeons competency is reached after 60 procedures and >100 procedures are required for excellency [12]. To achieve successful dilation of tract fluoroscopic and ultrasound guidance or a combination of approaches can be used [13]. In addition, new technologies including robotics, augmented reality, or electromagnetic navigation have been proposed [14]. Fluoroscopic-guided PCNL is widely accepted among urologists [13]. The limitations of the approach are radiation exposure and additional difficulties in positions other than prone [13, 15]. In a single surgeon analysis, it was shown that the fluoroscopy time significantly decreases from a mean time of 17.5 min during the first 15 cases to 8.9 min for the cases 46–60. An additional decrease in fluoroscopy time was observed thereafter, though the difference failed to show statistical significance [16]. Therefore, it was concluded that surgeons learning curve for fluoroscopic-guided PCNL was 60 surgeries. In addition, the learning curve for obtaining PCNL access with only ultrasound guidance was evaluated by Yu et al. [17]. The authors similarly reported improved competency after 60 surgeries with a significantly decreased mean puncture duration time of 4.4 min and excellency after 120 surgeries with a further 1.3 min mean time decrease [17]. It seems that the puncture approach does not change the learning curve and the puncture success required for PCNL for competency and proficiency. In a direct comparison of ultrasound- and fluoroscopic-guided PCNL approaches of trainees with experience <25 PCNL, ultrasound guidance was associated with less radiation exposure. However, 6 out of 32 patients in the ultrasound guidance group required fluoroscopic adjustment. Therefore, it was recommended for a beginner to have expertise in fluoroscopic-guided access to effectively handle all possible situations [18]. Factors such as obesity, presence of stag horn calculi, and hydronephrosis might pose additional risk for change from ultrasound to fluoroscopic guidance [19, 20].

In terms of safety for the patients none of the approaches was found to be superior over the other. According to meta-analyses of 8 randomized controlled trials, lower complications in the ultrasound-guided group were reported only in one study. Other studies found similar overall complication rates in 2 groups. Moreover, the pooled data showed no differences in terms of success rate, surgery duration, hospital stay, drop in hemoglobin after the surgery, and auxiliary-procedure rate [13]. Nevertheless, the ultrasound-guided PCNL could be easier performed in the supine position.

Electromagnetic (EM) guidance kidney puncture is the recent advancement of technology. The feasibility for obtaining renal puncture was evaluated in the porcine model among specialists with different levels of expertise [21]. The authors observed higher success rates, fewer attempts, and shorter access time when comparing EM with fluoroscopy, even for beginners. For sure the new method is appealing in regard to no radiation and effectiveness, however, new studies are required before any conclusion can be drawn.

### 23.2.2 Standardization and Preoperative Planning

PCNL represents a difficult endourological procedure with several essential steps for its performance. Therefore, standardization of each surgical step is essential for obtaining good results, limiting the complications, and evaluating the sources of complications. We recommend a standardized approach for every PCNL procedure.

For preoperative planning of the surgery imaging with computer tomography (CT) and meticulous examination of the CT images should be performed. Significant information extracted from the CT is the size and exact location of the stone, the vascular and collecting system anatomy of the renal system, and relationship of the kidney to the adjacent anatomic structures [2]. Based on the aforementioned the site and number of the punctures should be decided. Subsequently, the occurrence of serious complications such as colon, liver, and spleen injury can be avoided.

In cases of big and complicated stones where a multiple tract surgery is planned, the punctures should be performed at the initial step before proceeding to the dilation of the tract. Exudation, bleeding, contrast extravasation, and presence of the working tract may hinder the visibility of the collecting system negatively affecting the success of the puncture. Regardless of the puncture-guidance approach (ultrasound or fluoroscopic) neglecting this simple but important strategy can lead to difficulties and failure of the second puncture, increased operative time, and a higher rate of perioperative complications. Ding et al. evaluated the effect of the pre-puncture of collecting system at the time of double-tract PCNL [7]. In 63 out of 178 patients, the puncture for obtaining the second PCNL tract was performed after the first tract dilation (non-pre-puncture technique). In the remaining 115 patients pre-puncture approach was applied. The reported instant and final SFR was similar in both of the groups. Nevertheless, the non-pre-puncture double-tract PCNL approach was associated with higher rates of blood transfusion and longer operative time compared to pre-punctured technique.

## 23.3 Puncture Site and Secondary Puncture

After initial puncture failure obtaining a secondary puncture can be more challenging. Depending on the nature of failure (staghorn stone, horseshoe kidney, and contrast extravasation) the subsequent site of the puncture should be decided accordingly.

It is widely accepted that the puncture for the establishment of the percutaneous tract should be performed through the fornix of the calyceal papilla with an attempt to reduce the possibility of vascular injury. The current beliefs are based on existing anatomical studies evaluating the correlation of vascular network to the collecting system in unaffected cadaveric kidneys [22–24]. Their results indicated that the puncture to renal papilla carried 7–8% probability of vessel injury, whereas punctures to the upper, middle, or lower infundibulum were associated with 67.6%, 61.5%, and 68.2% vessel injuries, respectively [23]. However, the performance of papillary puncture due to individual anatomical particularities is not always possible in clinical practice. A more medial puncture of the collecting system could provide a solution for successful completion of surgery.

The technique for a non-papillary PCNL has been well-described in the literature [3, 25, 26]. In general, there is no exact indication or contra-indication for performance of papillary or non-papillary puncture. In fact, the non-papillary approach can be utilized in all clinical scenarios of prone PCNL, where papillary puncture is possible. For specialists practicing papillary technique, non-papillary alternative could be an option in patients with small calyces and narrow infundibula, staghorn stones and stones impacting the anterior and posterior lower calyces. It could be advocated that in any challenging case that the papillary access fails, the non-papillary approach could be performed with safety.

In terms of safety, the non-papillary technique was not associated with an increased rate of overall complications compared to papillary PCNL [3]. Moreover, tract dilation was not associated with significant differences in vascularization irrespectively of the puncture site [26]. Importantly, the non-papillary approach has been correlated to several advantages [3, 25, 26]. Specifically, entering the collecting system of the kidney more medially provides a wider range of movements of the nephroscope. Thus, more locations of the pelvicalyceal system could be accessed reducing the number of additional punctures in comparison to the papillary technique. The given advantages can result in a reduction of the operative time and overall radiation exposure when using the non-papillary technique

[3, 25, 26]. In addition, the non-papillary technique provides an easier passage of the guide wire down to the ureter which is a well-established safety step for PCNL. Nevertheless, the current technique was only described in prone PCNL. Whether this approach is an option for supine PCNL needs to be proven.

## 23.4 Failed Access

A wide variety of factors can affect the success of the percutaneous puncture and subsequent tract dilation. Although difficulties of obtaining PCNL access are present in the practice of every urologist, little is documented in the literature. We tried to summarize our experience and the available literature and present factors and specific recommendations for reducing the possibility of failure of the access. In an attempt to have easier classification, patient-related and surgery-related factors were considered.

### 23.4.1 Patient-related Factors

Several patient-related factors might increase the risk of access failure. These factors include anatomical malformations of the kidneys, transplanted kidneys, renal surgery prior to PCNL, presence of staghorn and impacted stones, as well as obesity [9, 19, 27, 28].

PCNL can be safely performed in most of the patients with anatomical malformations. However, their presence makes the access establishment more difficult. Horseshoe, ectopic kidneys, and malrotation of the kidney represent the most often observed anatomical anomalies in the PCNL population [9]. The presence of those anomalies was associated with significantly higher rates of failed procedures (5.0%) compared to the general population (1.7%). In most of these cases, prone PCNL was the preferred approach. Nevertheless, patients with ectopic and malrotation of the kidneys more often required supine procedures [9]. Autosomal dominant polycystic kidney disease (ADPKD) represents another renal malformation affecting the success of the PCNL tract establishment [28]. It results in compression and elongation of the collecting system. Several techniques may ease the puncture of the latter kidneys including methylene blue injection via retrograde ureteral catheter or aspiration of the cyst along the access tract [28].

The stone disease of the transplanted kidney is found in 0.4–1% [28]. PCNL procedure is feasible in transplanted kidneys, though it can be associated with increased bleeding [29]. Due to the specific location of the kidney in the pelvis, supine PCNL should be performed. Although it is located anteriorly, post-implantation scarring and formation of the tough fibrous capsule surrounding the kidney pose a threat for PCNL failure [29].

The presence of prior renal surgery increases the number of puncture attempts, and the risk of access failure in non-transplanted kidneys [27]. Margel et al. reported a 2-times higher mean of puncture attempts, longer operative time, and a significantly higher rate of secondary procedures in patients with open nephrolithotomy prior to PCNL [8, 27]. Falahatkar et al. documented a longer guide wire insertion and tract dilation time in individuals with prior renal surgeries [30]. Nonetheless, this prolongation did not increase the rate of perioperative complications. The impact of prior renal surgery on the success of the access establishment may be more pronounced with the presence of additional confounding factors.

Obesity and the presence of staghorn stones might also complicate the puncture and tract dilation during PCNL. A longer learning curve for successful puncture with ultrasound guidance was documented in a recent study [19]. It was proposed that the increased skin to stone distance as well as the absorption of ultrasound waves by the fatty tissue contributed to poor ultrasound image resulting in puncture failure [19]. On the other hand, staghorn stones may impact appropriate tract dilation and the safety step of guide wire insertion in the ureter may not be possible [31].

### 23.4.2 Surgery-related Factors

The puncture site and the course of the needle are decisive for subsequent dilation of the tract.

During PCNL procedures accurate navigation is confounded with continuous movement of the kidney. Depending on anatomical differences, the kidney can be located at 5 to 10 cm depth from the skin. Nevertheless, the needle trajectory cannot be corrected after the advancement of more than 2 cm, although the deflection of the needle from its initial course may occur. The parameters influencing the deflection are needle diameter, depth of the target, the shape of the needle tip, insertion force, and speed, as well as mechanical properties of the tissue [11]. Hing et al. documented reduced tissue deformation with the slower advancement of the needle as a result of reduced force generated on the tip of the needle [32].

After successful puncture of collecting system tract dilation is initiated. The standard instruments proposed for dilation include Amplatz fascial dilators, Alken metal dilators, and balloon dilators. In a recent randomized controlled trial, none of the dilation instruments was superior over the other in terms of success [4]. It was additionally found that dilation technique did not affect the renal displacement. Patient's characteristics such as female gender, body mass index (BMI), and previous flank scar were the reported determinants of significant renal displacement [33]. In contrast, Joel et al. described 17% of total failure with the use of balloon dilation [8]. A higher rate of failure comprising 25% was reported in patients with prior renal surgery. The failed cases were successfully managed with the Amplatz dilators in 15 patients, whereas Alken metal dilators were used in the remaining 2 patients [8].

## 23.5 Minimizing the Failure: Recommendations from Practice

An individual approach to overcome intraoperative issues during PCNL surgery is mostly required. Nevertheless, some general rules should be followed to obtain a safe PCNL tract while minimizing the failure rate.

As a general rule, the subcostal puncture should be preferred to decrease the risk of pleural complications [2]. Regardless of the used puncture approach (papillary or non-papillary), the puncture should be performed at posterolateral surface of the kidney at 20–30 degrees from the vertical axis, known as Brodel's avascular line. In case of a suspect of vessel penetration, the needle should be withdrawn and additional puncture should be performed in another site (Fig. 23.1).

As already discussed, when multiple tracts are planned, initial puncture and passage of the hydrophilic guide wire is essential. The guide wire is left in the collecting system, preferentially in the ureter, till the subsequent dilation. If no dilation is intended, the guide wire can be removed in the end of the procedure (Fig. 23.2a and b).

In most of the cases, the PCNL procedures are performed with a retrograde ureteral catheter in place. Care must be taken to adequately dilate the renal collecting system with contrast instillation allowing easier puncture and tract establishment. Ureteral catheters with an incorporated balloon on their tips can successfully block the outflow of the injected fluid keeping the system distended. When normal ureteral catheters (without balloon) are utilized, a continuous fluid injection should be performed at specified steps. The injection should be initiated during the puncture and at the time of tract dilation when the tip of the dilator reaches the kidney. This maneuver prevents contrast extravasation and preserves unchanged visualization during the whole

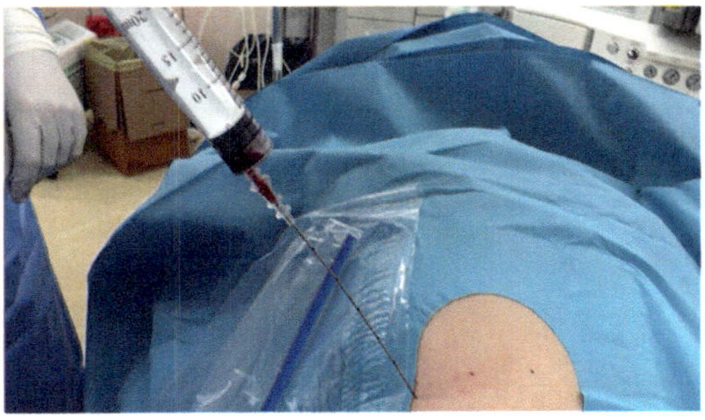

**Fig. 23.1** Blood aspiration

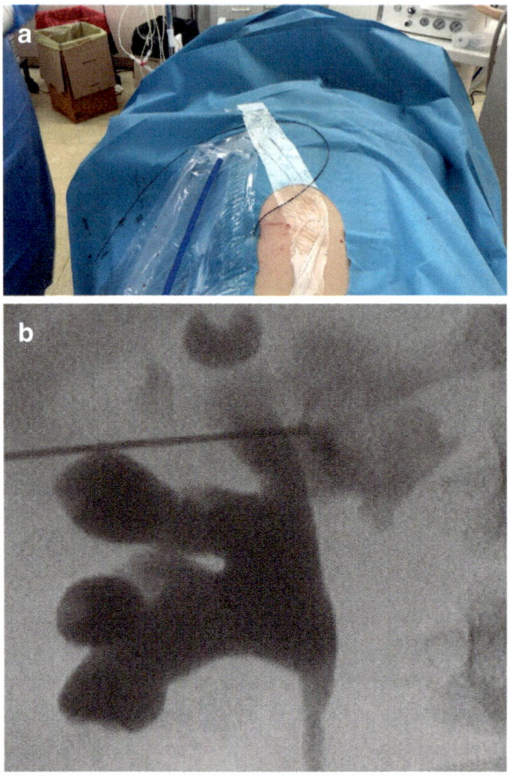


**Fig. 23.2** (a) Guidewire fixed outside view. (b) 2 Guidewires_X-ray view

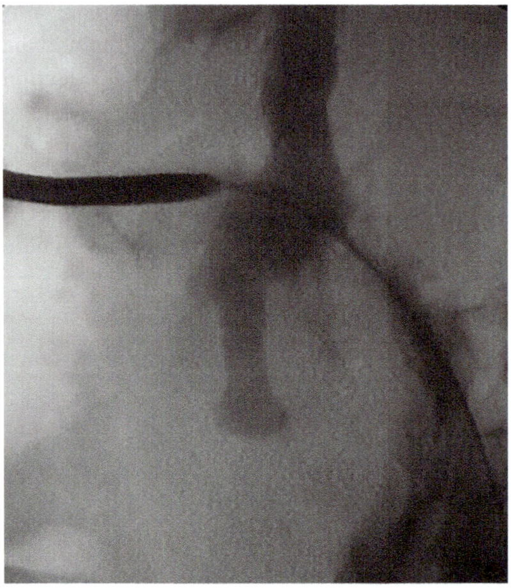

**Fig. 23.3** X-ray image dilation

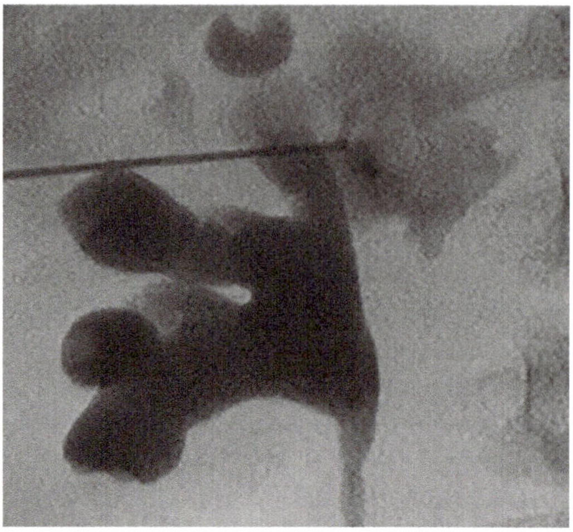

**Fig. 23.4** Do not inject contrast

dilation step (Fig. 23.3). Moreover, contrast injection through the puncture needle should be omitted (Fig. 23.4). To check the correct position of the needle aspiration rather than injection should be performed.

An adequate initial skin incision is another important rule for successful tract dilation. It should be kept in mind that increased friction between skin and dilators can increase the force applied to the dilator. The latter could turn the dilation to a cumbersome procedure resulting in injury of the collecting system or even the major blood vessels of the kidney. During balloon dilation, smaller skin incision can limit the full expansion of the balloon. Additional injury of the balloon and spillage of the contrast medium can occur with extension of skin incision with the dilated balloon in place.

One of the main considerations is to establish the PCNL tract over a stiff guide wire. A safety maneuver of passing the guide wire down the ureter diminishes the unexpected damage of the collecting system or hilar structures since the forces of dilation are directed towards the ureter. Care should be taken to advance the dilator according to the course of the guide wire without bending it. If still a bending of a guide wire occurs, it should be exchanged with the new one to enable successful dilation (Fig. 23.5). When

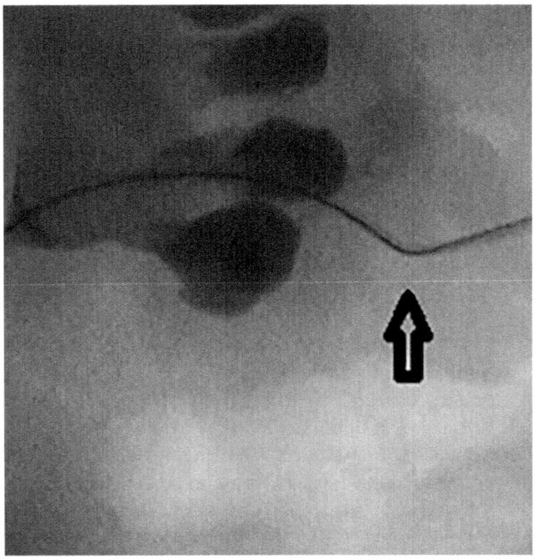

**Fig. 23.5** Bending of the guide wire

passage of the guide wire down the ureter is not possible, usage of stiff guide wire with short, floppy J tip is recommended. The guide wire will be coiled inside the collecting system.

In some cases, the dilation is not easily achieved and the access sheath remains inside the renal parenchyma requiring reinsertion of dilators and their further advancement. Alternatively, the advancement of the access sheath can be performed endoscopically (under direct vision) over the grasper or lithotripter probe.

Putting patients with general anesthesia in selective apnea can be required for hyper mobile kidneys and punctures of difficult locations. The latter trick limits the movements of the kidneys due to breathing and eases the targeting of the preferred area of the collective system.

## 23.6 Conclusion

The puncture and dilation of the tract remain the critical steps in the successful performance of PCNL. The surgery is associated with a steep learning curve. A wide variety of patient and surgery-related factors including anatomical anomalies, presence of prior surgery, presence of staghorn and impacted stones, high BMI, and surgeon's experience may impact renal access leading to its failure. High expertise, deep knowledge, and standardization of each step could improve the clinical outcome.

## References


1. Turk C, Petrik A, Sarica K, Seitz C, Skolarikos A, Straub M, Knoll T. EAU guidelines on interventional treatment for urolithiasis. Eur Urol. 2016;69(3):475–82. https://doi.org/10.1016/j.eururo.2015.07.041.
2. Kallidonis P, Panagopoulos V, Kyriazis I, Liatsikos E. Complications of percutaneous nephrolithotomy: classification, management, and prevention. Curr Opin Urol. 2016;26(1):88–94. https://doi.org/10.1097/MOU.0000000000000232.
3. Kallidonis P, Kyriazis I, Kotsiris D, Koutava A, Kamal W, Liatsikos E. Papillary vs Nonpapillary puncture in percutaneous nephrolithotomy: a prospective randomized trial. J Endourol. 2017;31(S1):S4–9. https://doi.org/10.1089/end.2016.0571.
4. Srivastava A, Singh S, Dhayal IR, Rai P. A prospective randomized study comparing the four tract dilation methods of percutaneous nephrolithotomy. World J Urol. 2017;35(5):803–7. https://doi.org/10.1007/s00345-016-1929-9.
5. Li J, Gao L, Li Q, Zhang Y, Jiang Q. Supine versus prone position for percutaneous nephrolithotripsy: a meta-analysis of randomized controlled trials. Int J Surg. 2019;66:62–71. https://doi.org/10.1016/j.ijsu.2019.04.016.
6. Aron M, Yadav R, Goel R, Kolla SB, Gautam G, Hemal AK, Gupta NP. Multi-tract percutaneous nephrolithotomy for large complete staghorn calculi. Urol Int. 2005;75(4):327–32. https://doi.org/10.1159/000089168.
7. Ding X, Wu W, Hou Y, Wang C, Wang Y. Application of prepuncture on the double-tract percutaneous nephrolithotomy under ultrasound guidance for renal staghorn calculi: first experience. Urology. 2018;114:56–9. https://doi.org/10.1016/j.urology.2018.01.011.
8. Joel AB, Rubenstein JN, Hsieh MH, Chi T, Meng MV, Stoller ML. Failed percutaneous balloon dilation for renal access: incidence and risk factors. Urology. 2005;66(1):29–32. https://doi.org/10.1016/j.urology.2005.02.018.
9. Osther PJ, Razvi H, Liatsikos E, Averch T, Crisci A, Garcia JL, Mandal A, de la Rosette J, Croes PSG. Percutaneous nephrolithotomy among patients with renal anomalies: patient characteristics and outcomes; a subgroup analysis of the clinical research office of the endourological society global percutaneous nephrolithotomy study. J Endourol. 2011;25(10):1627–32. https://doi.org/10.1089/end.2011.0146.

10. Srirangam SJ, Darling R, Stopford M, Neilson D. Contemporary practice of percutaneous nephrolithotomy: review of practice in a single region of the UK. Ann R Coll Surg Engl. 2008;90(1):40–4. https://doi.org/10.1308/003588408X242240.
11. Rodrigues PL, Rodrigues NF, Fonseca J, Lima E, Vilaca JL. Kidney targeting and puncturing during percutaneous nephrolithotomy: recent advances and future perspectives. J Endourol. 2013;27(7):826–34. https://doi.org/10.1089/end.2012.0740.
12. de la Rosette JJ, Laguna MP, Rassweiler JJ, Conort P. Training in percutaneous nephrolithotomy—a critical review. Eur Urol. 2008;54(5):994–1001. https://doi.org/10.1016/j.eururo.2008.03.052.
13. Yang YH, Wen YC, Chen KC, Chen C. Ultrasound-guided versus fluoroscopy-guided percutaneous nephrolithotomy: a systematic review and meta-analysis. World J Urol. 2019;37(5):777–88. https://doi.org/10.1007/s00345-018-2443-z.
14. Rassweiler J, Rassweiler MC, Klein J. New technology in ureteroscopy and percutaneous nephrolithotomy. Curr Opin Urol. 2016;26(1):95–106. https://doi.org/10.1097/MOU.0000000000000240.
15. Galonnier F, Traxer O, Rosec M, Terrasa JB, Gouezel P, Celier D, Bassinet C, Ruffion A, Paparel P, Fiard G, Terrier JE. Surgical staff radiation protection during fluoroscopy-guided urologic interventions. J Endourol. 2016;30(6):638–43. https://doi.org/10.1089/end.2016.0022.
16. Tanriverdi O, Boylu U, Kendirci M, Kadihasanoglu M, Horasanli K, Miroglu C. The learning curve in the training of percutaneous nephrolithotomy. Eur Urol. 2007;52(1):206–11. https://doi.org/10.1016/j.eururo.2007.01.001.
17. Yu W, Rao T, Li X, Ruan Y, Yuan R, Li C, Li H, Cheng F. The learning curve for access creation in solo ultrasonography-guided percutaneous nephrolithotomy and the associated skills. Int Urol Nephrol. 2017;49(3):419–24. https://doi.org/10.1007/s11255-016-1492-8.
18. Jagtap J, Mishra S, Bhattu A, Ganpule A, Sabnis R, Desai MR. Which is the preferred modality of renal access for a trainee urologist: ultrasonography or fluoroscopy? Results of a prospective randomized trial. J Endourol. 2014;28(12):1464–9. https://doi.org/10.1089/end.2014.0229.
19. Bayne DB, Usawachintachit M, Tzou D, Taguchi K, Shindel A, Chi TL. Increasing body mass index steepens the learning curve for ultrasound-guided percutaneous nephrolithotomy. Urology. 2018;120:68–73. https://doi.org/10.1016/j.urology.2018.07.033.
20. Usawachintachit M, Tzou DT, Hu W, Li J, Chi T. X-ray-free ultrasound-guided percutaneous nephrolithotomy: how to select the right patient? Urology. 2017;100:38–44. https://doi.org/10.1016/j.urology.2016.09.031.
21. Borofsky MS, Rivera ME, Dauw CA, Krambeck AE, Lingeman JE. Electromagnetic guided percutaneous renal access outcomes among surgeons and trainees of different experience levels: a pilot study. Urology. 2020;136:266–71. https://doi.org/10.1016/j.urology.2019.08.060.
22. Sampaio FJ. Renal collecting system anatomy: its possible role in the effectiveness of renal stone treatment. Curr Opin Urol. 2001;11(4):359–66. https://doi.org/10.1097/00042307-200107000-00004.
23. Sampaio FJ, Aragao AH. Anatomical relationship between the intrarenal arteries and the kidney collecting system. J Urol. 1990;143(4):679–81. https://doi.org/10.1016/s0022-5347(17)40056-5.
24. Sampaio FJ, Passos MA. Renal arteries: anatomic study for surgical and radiological practice. Surg Radiol Anat. 1992;14(2):113–7. https://doi.org/10.1007/bf01794885.
25. Kyriazis I, Kallidonis P, Vasilas M, Panagopoulos V, Kamal W, Liatsikos E. Challenging the wisdom of puncture at the calyceal fornix in percutaneous nephrolithotripsy: feasibility and safety study with 137 patients operated via a non-calyceal percutaneous track. World J Urol. 2017;35(5):795–801. https://doi.org/10.1007/s00345-016-1919-y.
26. Kallidonis P, Kalogeropoulou C, Kyriazis I, Apostolopoulos D, Kitrou P, Kotsiris D, Ntasiotis P, Liatsikos E. Percutaneous nephrolithotomy puncture and tract dilation: evidence on the safety of approaches to the infundibulum of the middle renal calyx. Urology. 2017;107:43–8. https://doi.org/10.1016/j.urology.2017.05.038.
27. Margel D, Lifshitz DA, Kugel V, Dorfmann D, Lask D, Livne PM. Percutaneous nephrolithotomy in patients who previously underwent open nephrolithotomy. J Endourol. 2005;19(10):1161–4. https://doi.org/10.1089/end.2005.19.1161.
28. Tan YK, Cha DY, Gupta M. Management of stones in abnormal situations. Urol Clin North Am. 2013;40(1):79–97. https://doi.org/10.1016/j.ucl.2012.10.001.
29. Crook TJ, Keoghane SR. Renal transplant lithiasis: rare but time-consuming. BJU Int. 2005;95(7):931–3. https://doi.org/10.1111/j.1464-410X.2005.05481.x.
30. Falahatkar S, Panahandeh Z, Ashoori E, Akbarpour M, Khaki N. What is the difference between percutaneous nephrolithotomy in patients with and without previous open renal surgery? J Endourol. 2009;23(7):1107–10. https://doi.org/10.1089/end.2008.0630.
31. Zagoria RJ, Dyer RB. Do's and don't's of percutaneous nephrostomy. Acad Radiol. 1999;6(6):370–7. https://doi.org/10.1016/s1076-6332(99)80233-5.
32. Hing JT, Brooks AD, Desai JP. A biplanar fluoroscopic approach for the measurement, modeling, and simulation of needle and soft-tissue interaction. Med Image Anal. 2007;11(1):62–78. https://doi.org/10.1016/j.media.2006.09.005.
33. Aminsharifi A, Haghpanah R, Haghpanah S. Predictors of excessive renal displacement during access in percutaneous nephrolithotomy: a randomized clinical trial. Urolithiasis. 2014;42(1):61–5. https://doi.org/10.1007/s00240-013-0600-9.

# Simultaneous Bilateral Mini PCNL

# 24

Rajeev TP, Karthickeyan Naganathan, and B. M. Zeeshan Hameed

## 24.1 Introduction

The incidence of kidney stone disease shows an increasing trend globally [1]. The prevalence of urolithiasis is between 1% to 15% worldwide and in the Asian continent it ranges between 1% to 5% [2]. Nearly a quarter of patients present with multiple stones. Over a period, 33% of the stone patients without symptoms end up with an intervention [3].

Percutaneous nephrolithotomy (PCNL) is the standard of care for large renal stones. Over the past few decades, various innovations in the field of instruments pertaining to size, endoscopic lens and design; the emergence of powerful laser machines and accessories have led to miniaturization of this procedure. Mini PCNL has gained popularity owing to smaller access tract, less pain, shorter hospital stay and faster post-operative recovery.

In cases with symptomatic bilateral renal stone disease, there has always been a reluctance in performing PCNL in a simultaneous approach when compared to staged PCNL. Simultaneous surgeries can be both synchronous and asynchronous depending on the case selection and surgical team's proficiency. Although there were concerns regarding the risk of morbidity and complications, it was proven otherwise by many recent studies including a randomized control trial by Wang et al. [4] The documented safety and efficacy of bilateral simultaneous standard PCNL (BS-spinal) has garnered interests among experienced Endo Urologists to adopt this procedure for bilateral renal stones [5, 6]. While there are no studies reported in the literature regarding the practice of bilateral simultaneous mini PCNL (BS-mPCNL), we discuss the various intricacies and technical aspects involved in performing this procedure for bilateral renal stone disease.

## 24.2 Causes of Bilateral Urolithiasis

The occurrence of bilateral urinary tract stones has always been a source of grave danger to the patient and the Urologist is faced with dilemmas and difficulties concerning treatment strategies. In patients with bilateral nephrolithiasis, it is imperative to know the presence of any metabolic abnormality, stone burden, presence of infection, the function of the kidney and anomalies in the urinary system to plan the procedure. The presence of anuria and infection are the tell-tale signs for immediate interventions such as diversion in

R. TP (✉)
Department of Urology, Gauhati Medical College Hospital, Guwahati, India

K. Naganathan
Frontline Hospital, Trichy, Tamil Nadu, India

B. M. Zeeshan Hameed
Department of Urology, Kasturba Medical College, Manipal, Karnataka, India


M. S. Agrawal et al. (eds.), *Minimally Invasive Percutaneous Nephrolithotomy*,
https://doi.org/10.1007/978-981-16-6001-6_24

the form of nephrostomies or double J stenting, but may not be a candidate for bilateral simultaneous stone clearance [7]. Amaro et al. detected the presence of the following metabolic disorders—hypercalciuria (74%), hypocitraturia (37.3%), hyperoxaluria (24.1%), hypomagnesuria (21%), hyperuricosuria (20.2%), primary hyperparathyroidism (1.8%), secondary hyperparathyroidism (0.6%) and renal tubular acidosis (0.6) in a cohort of 158 patients. Further, 95.5% of these patients with urinary lithiasis showed metabolic changes [7].

## 24.3 Treatment Options for Bilateral Renal Stones

The treatment options for bilateral renal disease include both simultaneous and staged procedures. The simultaneous intervention for bilateral renal stones remains an uphill task for Endo Urologists and demands expertise along with the availability of multiple armamentaria. Hence they pose a tough challenge and are usually performed at high volume centres. With the careful patient selection and competence of surgeon, the outcomes of simultaneous procedures are favourable, cost-effective and have improved the quality of life [8]. An adequate pre-operative counselling which includes the other surgical options such as shock-wave lithotripsy (SWL), Percutaneous Nephrolithotomy (PCNL), Retrograde Intrarenal Surgery (RIRS), open/laparoscopic/robotic-assisted pyelolithotomy, their stone-free rates and complications rates should be made available by the surgical team. The patient should be made aware of the possibility of deferring the contralateral procedure if warranted.

## 24.4 Evolution of Simultaneous Bilateral mini PCNL

Since the first description of percutaneous surgical removal of renal stones by Fernstrom and Johansson in 1976, PCNL has undergone multiple technical modifications and innovations. It has even replaced open surgeries for complex renal stones and staghorn calculi. Although PCNL is technically challenging, it is one of the commonest procedures performed by the endourologist for stone disease. The availability of PCNL simulators and other training models along with the vast knowledge of experts in this field of endourology have drastically upgraded the resident training at a global level. Prone PCNL practised for decades is being reconsidered in cases suitable for the supine position and ECIRS [9–11]. The traditional practice of leaving a nephrostomy tube is replaced by tubeless PCNL (only double J stent, no nephrostomy) and totally tubeless PCNL (no double J stent, no nephrostomy) with better patient tolerance, recovery rates and similar outcome [12–14].

Colón-Pérez et al. reported a case series of three simultaneous bilateral PCNL in 1987 [15]. There is always a debate regarding the performance of bilateral simultaneous vs staged PCNL for bilateral renal stones. Though there is a theoretical risk of renal injury and morbidity, recent studies have proven bilateral simultaneous standard PCNL to be safe and with better outcomes [16–18]. Smaller instruments, technical advancements in optics and introduction of robust laser machines have led to miniaturization of PCNL. The exact definition of mini PCNL is debatable, but it is commonly defined as a renal tract size less than or equal to 22 Fr [19]. Anything beyond 22 Fr is considered as standard PCNL. The indications for mini PCNL are more or less the same as the standard PCNL. The minimization of invasiveness has broadened the indications for mini PCNL in smaller renal stones less than 2 cm, which includes adult lower pole kidney stones; failed ureteroscopy due to narrow infundibulum, inaccessible calyx; stones in calyceal diverticulum; paediatric renal stones and secondary access to residual fragments [20–22]. This low morbid procedure has also been recently performed for staghorn calculus and proximal ureteric stones [23, 24]. There are no direct studies comparing BS-standard to BS-mPCNL, but for all practical purposes, we assume mini PCNL to be at least as efficacious as standard PCNL for bilateral small medium-sized stones.

## 24.5 Bilateral Simultaneous vs Staged PCNL

Traditionally, staged PCNL is being preferred due to concerns of higher complication rate, injury to both renal units and fear of acute renal insufficiency. In a comparative study by Kadlec et al, involving 47 bilateral vs 78 unilateral PCNL, there was an overall higher complication rate in the bilateral PCNL group when compared to unilateral PCNL [25]. Subsequent studies [26–30] including a survey [31] regarding the surgeon preference for bilateral renal stones did not show any difference in complication rates. Indeed, these studies have published favourable outcomes of BS-PCNL concerning procedure time, overall anaesthesia time, stone-free rate, procedure cost and patient recovery. It is evident that with careful patient selection and counselling, BS-PCNL offers the same advantages as staged PCNL. In Synchronous BS-PCNL, two surgical teams will be working in tandem whereas in asynchronous approach the second side is operated after the completion of the first side by the same or another team. The following is the comparison between bilateral simultaneous PCNL and staged PCNL concerning indications, procedure, armamentarium, complications, hospital stay, recovery and cost efficiency (Table 24.1).

**Table 24.1** A comparison between bilateral Simultaneous vs Staged PCNL

| Variables | Bilateral simultaneous | Bilateral staged |
|---|---|---|
| *Indications* | *Synchronous:*<br>Simple anatomy, small and medium-sized stones<br>Nil comorbidities<br>*Asynchronous:*<br>Symptomatic first, Simple anatomy, small and medium-sized stones<br>Nil comorbidities | Most symptomatic side first.<br>Large stones, staghorn calculus<br>Complex anatomy<br>Patient comorbidities<br>Patient preference |
| Blood investigations and imaging | Once | Twice |
| *Procedure* | | |
| Personnel | Synchronous PCNL—Two teams<br>Asynchronous—One team | One team |
| Armamentarium | Two sets (Nephroscope, Laser machine/lithotripters, Monitors) | One set |
| Experience of surgeon | Experienced surgeon | Novice |
| Anaesthesia time | Short | Longer |
| Duration of procedures | Short | Longer |
| Operation Room (OR) space | Larger OR | Regular OR |
| Ancillary procedures | May require | May not require |
| *Complications* | | |
| Renal injury | Similar | Similar |
| Blood transfusion rate | Similar | Similar |
| Analgesia requirement | Same as a single unit | Cumulative—Higher |
| Stone-free rate | Similar | Similar |
| Hospital stay | Shorter | Cumulative—Longer |
| Costing | | |
| Procedure | + | ++ |
| Social | + | ++ |
| Reimbursement to doctor/hospital | + | ++ |
| Patient recovery | Early | Cumulative—Delayed |

## 24.6 Advantages of Bilateral Simultaneous Mini PCNL

Lingeman et Al. conducted a survey of members of Endourological Society regarding surgical management in bilateral renal stone disease [31]. Of the 153 respondents, only 38% performed bilateral PCNL under anaesthesia, indicating the general trend among endourologists in embarking bilateral PCNL. However, the safety and efficacy of BS-PCNL were well established in many studies [4, 5]. Reduction in cumulative operative time, overall hospital stay, avoidance of multiple anaesthesia are some of the advantages of performing bilateral simultaneous PCNL [4, 16]. Bagrodia et al. have reported at least 30% reduction in the overall cost when PCNL was done simultaneously on both sides. [30] Blood investigations and imaging need not be repeated if both sides are dealt with in the same sitting. Limited use of disposables, reduced use of pharmaceuticals and its associated cost and short cumulative hospital stay all contribute to the overall reduction in the total expenditure to the patient [5, 16].

## 24.7 Disadvantages of Bilateral Simultaneous Mini PCNL

Prolonged operative time, hypothermia, slightly increased risk of bleeding are some of the major concerns in doing bilateral PCNL simultaneously. Need for repositioning the fluoroscopy and other Urological armamentarium including monitors, lithoclast and laser machines are time consuming and requires more theatre personnel. If bilateral PCNL is contemplated in the supine position, then the patient also needs to be repositioned at the end of the first side procedure.

One major disadvantage to the operating surgeon is the financial disincentive for performing bilateral PCNL in one sitting. Globally, all health insurance companies reimburse only half of the authorised amount for the second procedure if done in the same sitting [4, 16, 30].

## 24.8 Technical Considerations

Technically there is no major difference between simultaneous and staged bilateral PCNL except for the need for two sets of instruments. However, due considerations should be given to case selection, patient positioning and OR set up.

## 24.9 Importance of Case Selection

The most important step in successful bilateral simultaneous mini PCNL is proper case selection. After establishing enough experience and expertise in various forms of PCNL like standard PCNL and mini PCNL endourologists should attempt bilateral mini PCNL simultaneously. Initially, clinicians should select young patients with good renal function with favourable calyceal anatomy and without large stone burden (Fig. 24.1). Any anatomy requiring more than one tract on one side should not be selected for simultaneous procedure initially.

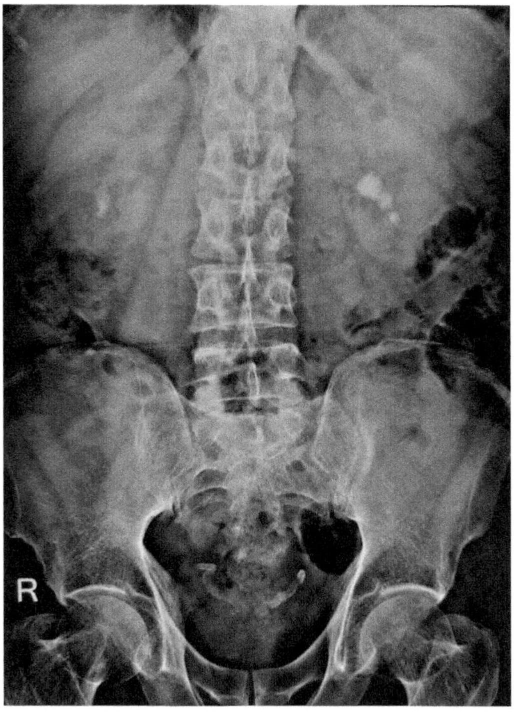


**Fig. 24.1** X-ray KUB showing bilateral renal calculus ideally suited for BS-mini PCNL

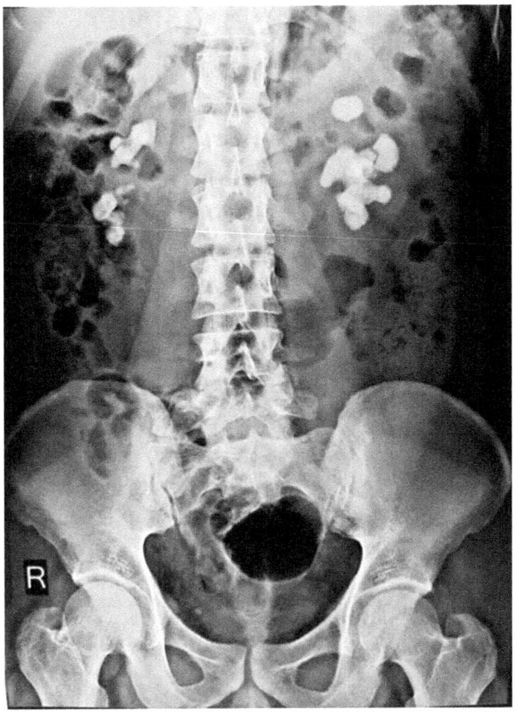


**Fig. 24.2** X-ray KUB showing bilateral large staghorn calculus requiring more than two tracts on each side, not an ideal case for BS-mini PCNL

As one grows with experience and confidence more complex anatomy, young patients with limited comorbidities and elderly patients can be included. Patients with complex stone and calyceal anatomy with anticipated more than two tracts on one side should not be selected for bilateral PCNL simultaneously (Fig. 24.2).

Case selection should be tailored according to patient demography, comorbidities, stone and calyceal anatomy, surgeon and anaesthetist experience [1]. Other complications of PCNL like bleeding, sepsis, perforation of the renal pelvis, extravasation and residual fragments should also be discussed.

## 24.10 Prone vs Supine Position

Bilateral PCNL can be done simultaneously in both prone and supine positions depending on the surgeon's preference. However, the prone position is more suitable for bilateral mini PCNL as there is no need to change the patient position for the contralateral side. The availability of large working space in the prone position is another advantage.

PCNL in the modified supine lithotomy position allows access to both upper and lower tracts at the same time. After successful completion of unilateral side, the patient has to be repositioned to allow access to the contralateral side to perform supine PCNL.

## 24.11 Operation Room (OR) Set-up

OR set up including the position of instrument trolley, fluoroscopy and lithotripsy equipment vary according to the patient position. The side with maximal stone load, complex anatomy, or more symptomatic side is operated first. After placing retrograde catheters on both sides, the patient is repositioned to prone. The operating surgeon stands on the ipsilateral side with a monitor and fluoroscopy positioned on the opposite side. A Pneumatic/Ultrasonic lithotripter/Laser machine is positioned behind or to the side of the operating surgeon. After successful completion of the ipsilateral side, everything needs to be repositioned to the opposite side to allow contralateral PCNL. Some experienced endourologists might be able to complete PCNL with fluoroscopy in the ipsilateral side itself.

For supine PCNL, the patient is positioned in the modified supine lithotomy position with ipsilateral side brought to the edge of the table with slight 15 to 20-degree torso tilt to the opposite side and the ipsilateral arm is adequately supported. The same side thigh and knee extended and slightly lowered (Fig. 24.3). Standard landmarks for supine PCNL like posterior axillary line, 12$^{th}$ rib and iliac crest are marked for better orientation.

## 24.12 Armamentarium for Bilateral Simultaneous Mini PCNL

Two sets of

Standard miniperc nephroscope (Wolf/Karl Storz/Olympus)

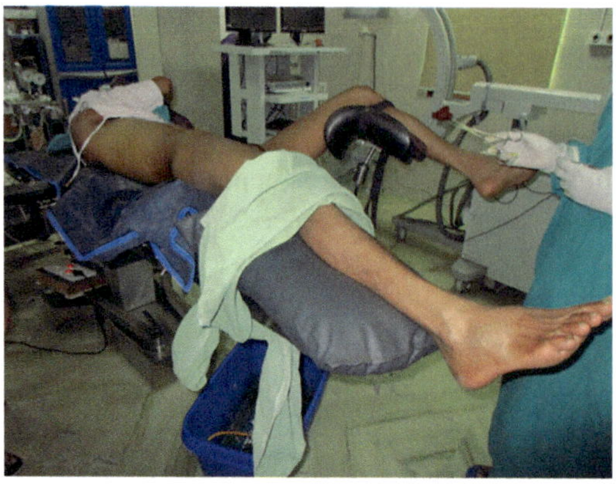

**Fig. 24.3** Patient positioned for supine PCNL, note the position of right thigh and knee

Amplatz sheath of variable sizes
Two-part puncture needle
Guide wires and retrograde catheters
Fascial dilators
Pneumatic/Ultrasonic lithotripsy/Laser machine
Graspers and baskets
Double J stents

## 24.13 Access and Dilatation

Renal access can be achieved by ultrasound or fluoroscopy-guided depending on surgeon's experience and preference. Ultrasound guided access has the advantage of less radiation exposure and it also helps in avoiding adjacent organ injury during puncture and dilatation. After puncturing the desired calyx, a hydrophilic floppy tip guide wire (0.032/0.035 inch) is placed through the puncture cannula into the ureter or the renal pelvis or the desired calyx. Tract dilatation over the guide wire should be done with metal dilator or balloon dilator monitored under fluoroscopy. Single-step dilatation saves time and reduces radiation exposure to the patient as well as the operating team. The tract should be secured with Amplatz sheath of appropriate size using the Seldinger technique over the guide wire under fluoroscopy guidance.

## 24.14 Nephroscopy and Stone Clearance

The standard mini nephroscope ranges from 12 F to 18 F (Karl Storz, Olympus, Wolf). With adequate irrigation ensuring clear vision, thorough nephroscopy should be done to assess the pelvicalyceal anatomy and stone localisation. Lithotripsy can be performed with laser, pneumatic or ultrasonic lithotripters. The need for stone graspers is greatly reduced in miniperc as the stone fragments are passively cleared due to the whirlpool effect created by the flow of irrigation fluid. Because of the rapid passive stone clearance by the whirlpool effect, the operative time is comparable to standard PCNL [1].

## 24.15 Exit Strategy

Weld and Wake, first performed tubeless bilateral simultaneous PCNL in the year 2000 [32]. Since then several successful series with tubeless BS-PCNL were published [16, 26]. Exit strategy following bilateral simultaneous PCNL should be tailored for each individual case [5]. Tubeless or totally tubeless should be dependent on the amount of intraoperative bleeding, any perforation, residual fragments, subsequent plan to re-look, surgeon's preference and other features. For miniperc tracts, there is no need for the routine placement of nephrostomy tubes [33]. Thapa found 75–80% of miniperc are tubeless in his series [34]. It is always safe to place at least double J stent on one side as post-operative anuria, though rare is one dreadful complication following bilateral PCNL [16].

## 24.16 Follow-up

Post-operative X-ray of kidney, ureter and bladder region needs to be taken after 24 hours to assess any residual fragment and stent position. Hemogram and renal function tests should be repeated after 24–48 hours to identify any significant blood loss and renal function impairment. CT KUB may be more precise in identifying residual fragments, especially in radiolucent stones.

## 24.17 Complications

Any complication inherent to PCNL is theoretically doubled in bilateral simultaneous PCNL. But in practice, most studies have found the complications rates are similar to or at least comparable to single side or staged PCNL [17, 35]. Fever is the most common complication after simultaneous bilateral PCNL in the majority of studies [36, 37]. The release of bacteria and bacterial endotoxins during stone fragmentation and manipulation is responsible for postoperative fever and sepsis [38]. Even when the pre-operative urine culture is negative, pyrexia and systemic inflammatory response can occur as preoperative urine culture does not represent stone culture in a significant number of cases. Korets et al. prospectively evaluated the correlation between preoperative urine culture, renal pelvic urine culture and stone culture in 198 patients who underwent PCNL. He found that 48.5% of cases with positive stone culture had negative pre-operative bladder urine culture indicating the poor correlation between the two [39]. Maintaining a low-pressure system intraoperatively is paramount in preventing sepsis and fever [40].

Haematuria, delayed bleeding requiring blood transfusion, persistent urine leak through the tract site, bowel injury and pulmonary complications occur in a similar frequency to single-sided PCNL if each unit is considered individually rather than the number of patients [5]. In a randomised control study conducted by Li et al., the rate of blood transfusion is much lesser in mini PCNL (1.1%) when compared to standard PCNL (6.9%).

## 24.18 Conclusion

Bilateral simultaneous mini PCNL is feasible and safe for small bilateral renal stones. The procedure can be done both simultaneous or staged depending on the case, consent of the patient and the availability of armamentarium and personnel. However, the morbidity of the procedure can be reduced by careful case selection and experience of the surgeon.

## References


1. Geraghty RM, Jones P, Somani BK. Simultaneous bilateral endoscopic surgery (SBES) for bilateral urolithiasis: the future? Evidence from a systematic review. Curr Urol Rep. 2019;20(3):1–11. https://doi.org/10.1007/s11934-019-0877-5.
2. Sorokin I, Mamoulakis C, Miyazawa K, Rodgers A, Talati J, Lotan Y. Epidemiology of stone disease across the world. World J Urol. 2017;35:1301–20. https://doi.org/10.1007/s00345-017-2008-6.
3. Scales CD, Smith AC, Hanley JM, Saigal CS. Prevalence of kidney stones in the United States. Eur Urol. 2012;62(1):160–5. https://doi.org/10.1016/j.eururo.2012.03.052.
4. Wang CJ, Chang CH, Huang SW. Simultaneous bilateral tubeless percutaneous nephrolithotomy of staghorn stones: A prospective randomized controlled study. Urol Res. 2011;39(4):289–94. https://doi.org/10.1007/s00240-010-0342-x.
5. Jones P, Dhliwayo B, Rai BP, et al. Safety, feasibility, and efficacy of bilateral synchronous percutaneous nephrolithotomy for bilateral stone disease: Evidence from a systematic review. J Endourol. 2017;31(4):334–40. https://doi.org/10.1089/end.2016.0851.
6. Conort P, Bah OR, Tostivint I, et al. Simultaneous bilateral percutaneous nephrolithotomy: Series of 60 cases. Prog Urol. 2010;20(13):1194–9. https://doi.org/10.1016/j.purol.2010.04.001.
7. Cobb KD, Gomella PT, DiBianco JM, Batter TH, Eisner BH, Mufarrij PW. Are emergently placed nephrostomy tubes suitable for subsequent percutaneous endoscopic renal surgery? Urology. 2019;126:45–8. https://doi.org/10.1016/j.urology.2019.01.006.
8. Desai M, Grover R, Manohar T, Ganpule A. Simultaneous bilateral percutaneous nephrolithotomy: A single-center experience. J Endourol. 2007;21(5):508–14. https://doi.org/10.1089/end.2006.0401.
9. Uria JGV, Gerhold JV, Lopez JAL, et al. Technique and complications of percutaneous nephroscopy: experience with 557 patients in the supine position. J Urol. 1998;160(6 Part 1):1975–8. https://doi.org/10.1016/S0022-5347(01)62217-1.
10. Valdivia JG, Scarpa RM, Duvdevani M, et al. Supine versus prone position during percutaneous nephrolithotomy: A report from the clinical research office of the endourological society percutaneous nephrolithot-

omy global study. J Endourol. 2011;25(10):1619–25. https://doi.org/10.1089/end.2011.0110.
11. Scoffone CM, Cracco CM, Cossu M, Grande S, Poggio M, Scarpa RM. Endoscopic combined intrarenal surgery in Galdakao-modified supine valdivia position: a new standard for percutaneous nephrolithotomy? Eur Urol. 2008;54(6):1393–403. https://doi.org/10.1016/j.eururo.2008.07.073.
12. Marchant F, Recabal P, Fernández MI, Osorio F, Benavides J. Postoperative morbidity of tubeless versus conventional percutaneous nephrolithotomy: A prospective comparative study. Urol Res. 2011;39(6):477–81. https://doi.org/10.1007/s00240-011-0367-9.
13. Istanbulluoglu MO, Cicek T, Ozturk B, Gonen M, Ozkardes H. Percutaneous nephrolithotomy: nephrostomy or tubeless or totally tubeless? Urology. 2010;75(5):1043–6. https://doi.org/10.1016/j.urology.2009.06.104.
14. Agrawal MS, Sharma M, Agarwal K. Tubeless percutaneous nephrolithotomy using antegrade tether: a randomized study. J Endourol. 2014;28(6):644–8. https://doi.org/10.1089/end.2013.0693.
15. Colón-pérez B, Canto RJ, Ramos ME. Simultaneous bilateral nephrostolithotomies: immediate results in three cases. J Endourol. 1987;1(3):209–13. https://doi.org/10.1089/end.1987.1.209.
16. Pillai S, Mishra D, Sharma P, et al. Tubeless simultaneous bilateral percutaneous nephrolithotomy: Safety, feasibility and efficacy in an Indian setting. Int J Urol. 2014;21(5):497–502. https://doi.org/10.1111/iju.12352.
17. Angerri O, Mayordomo O, Kanashiro AK, et al. Simultaneous and synchronous bilateral endoscopic treatment of urolithiasis: A multicentric study. Cent Eur J Urol. 2019;72(2):178–82. https://doi.org/10.5173/ceju.2019.1862.
18. Proietti S, Sortino G, Giannantoni A, et al. Single-session supine bilateral percutaneous nephrolithotomy. Urology. 2015;85(2):304–10. https://doi.org/10.1016/j.urology.2014.10.036.
19. Ruhayel Y, Tepeler A, Dabestani S, et al. Tract sizes in miniaturized percutaneous nephrolithotomy: a systematic review from the European association of urology urolithiasis guidelines panel [Figure presented]. Eur Urol. 2017;72(2):220–35. https://doi.org/10.1016/j.eururo.2017.01.046.
20. Li X, He Z, Wu K, et al. Chinese minimally invasive percutaneous nephrolithotomy: the guangzhou experience. J Endourol. 2009;23(10):1693–7. https://doi.org/10.1089/end.2009.1537.
21. Ganpule AP, Bhattu AS, Desai M. PCNL in the twenty-first century: role of Microperc, Miniperc, and Ultraminiperc. World J Urol. 2014;33(2):235–40. https://doi.org/10.1007/s00345-014-1415-1.
22. Jackman SV, Docimo SG, Cadeddu JA, Bishoff JT, Kavoussi LR, Jarrett TW. The "mini-perc" technique: A less invasive alternative to percutaneous nephrolithotomy. World J Urol. 1998;16(6):371–4. https://doi.org/10.1007/s003450050083.
23. Cheng F, Yu W, Zhang X, Yang S, Xia Y, Ruan Y. Minimally invasive tract in percutaneous nephrolithotomy for renal stones. J Endourol. 2010;24(10):1579–82. https://doi.org/10.1089/end.2009.0581.
24. Long Q, Guo J, Xu Z, et al. Experience of mini-percutaneous nephrolithotomy in the treatment of large impacted proximal ureteral stones. Urol Int. 2013;90(4):384–8. https://doi.org/10.1159/000343668.
25. Kadlec AO, Greco KA, Fridirici ZC, Hart ST, Vellos TG, Turk TM. Comparison of complication rates for unilateral and bilateral percutaneous nephrolithotomy (PCNL) using a modified Clavien grading system. BJU Int. 2013;111(4 B):243–8. https://doi.org/10.1111/j.1464-410X.2012.11589.x.
26. Chang CWC. Simultaneous bilateral tubeless percutaneous nephrolithotomy of staghorn stones: a prospective randomized controlled study. Urol Res. 2011;39(4):289–94. https://doi.org/10.1007/s00240-010-0342-x.
27. Mason BM, Koi PT, Hafron J, Milhoua P, Hoenig DM. Safety and efficacy of synchronous percutaneous nephrostolithotomy and contralateral ureterorenoscopy for bilateral calculi. J Endourol. 2008;22(5):889–94. https://doi.org/10.1089/end.2007.0306.
28. Silverstein AD, Terranova SA, Auge BK, et al. Bilateral renal calculi: assessment of staged v synchronous percutaneous nephrolithotomy. J Endourol. 2004;18(2):145–51. https://doi.org/10.1089/089277904322959770.
29. Williams SK, Hoenig DM. Synchronous bilateral percutaneous nephrostolithotomy. J Endourol. 2009;23(10):1707–12. https://doi.org/10.1089/end.2009.1538.
30. Bagrodia A, Raman JD, Bensalah K, Pearle MS, Lotan Y. Synchronous bilateral percutaneous nephrostolithotomy: analysis of clinical outcomes, cost and surgeon reimbursement. J Urol. 2009;181(1):149–53. https://doi.org/10.1016/j.juro.2008.09.011.
31. Rivera ME, Bhojani N, Heinsimer K, et al. A survey regarding preference in the management of bilateral stone disease and a comparison of clavien complication rates in bilateral vs unilateral percutaneous nephrolithotomy. Urology. 2018;111:48–53. https://doi.org/10.1016/j.urology.2017.09.020.
32. Weld KJ, Wake RW. Simultaneous bilateral tubeless percutaneous nephrolithotomy. Urology. 2000;56(6):1057. https://doi.org/10.1016/s0090-4295(00)00817-7.
33. Lahme S. Miniaturisation of PCNL. Urolithiasis. 2018;46(1):99–106. https://doi.org/10.1007/s00240-017-1029-3.
34. Thapa BB, Niranjan V. Mini PCNL over standard PCNL: What makes it better? Surg J. 2020;06(01):e19–23. https://doi.org/10.1055/s-0040-1701225.
35. ElSheemy MS, Ghoneima W, Elmarakbi AA, et al. Bilateral single-session vs staged mini-percutaneous

nephrolithotomy for renal stones: a comparative study. Urology. 2018;120:62–7. https://doi.org/10.1016/j.urology.2018.07.015.
36. Proietti S, Sortino G, Giannantoni A, et al. Single-session supine bilateral percutaneous nephrolithotomy. Urology. 2020;85(2):304–10. https://doi.org/10.1016/j.urology.2014.10.036.
37. Dushinski JW, Lingeman JE. Simultaneous bilateral percutaneous nephrolithotomy. J Urol. 1997 Dec;158(6):2065–8.
38. Mcaleer IM, Kaplan GW, Bradley JS, Carroll SF, Griffith DP. Endotoxin content in renal calculi. J Urol. 2003;169:1813–4. https://doi.org/10.1097/01.ju.0000061965.51478.79.
39. Korets R, Graversen JA, Kates M, Mues AC, Gupta M. Post-percutaneous nephrolithotomy systemic inflammatory response: a prospective analysis of preoperative urine, renal pelvic urine and stone cultures. J Urol. 2011;186(5):1899–903. https://doi.org/10.1016/j.juro.2011.06.064.
40. Tokas T, Herrmann TRW, Skolarikos A, Nagele U. Pressure matters: intrarenal pressures during normal and pathological conditions, and impact of increased values to renal physiology. World J Urol. 2019;37(1):125–31. https://doi.org/10.1007/s00345-018-2378-4.

# Special Situations Stone with PUJO, Calyceal Diverticulum

# 25

C. Mallikarjuna and Mohammed Taif Bendigeri

## 25.1 Mini-PCNL in Stone with Calyceal Diverticulum

Calyceal diverticulum is the outpouching of the calyx which is lined with urothelium and drained by the neck of the diverticulum. It presents special challenges to clear the stone present in this diverticulum. Caution at every step is essential for a smooth procedure in these patients.

### 25.1.1 Work-up

Proper evaluation of the patient with regards to defining the anatomy of the pelvicalyceal system is of paramount importance in these situations. Non-contrast CT-KUB is usually the preferred investigation for renal stone disease, but sometimes it can miss the delineation of diverticulum. Patients with calyceal diverticulum stones need a contrast-based delineation of the pelvicalyceal system for better pick-up of the calyceal diverticulum. One can opt for intravenous pyelogram or contrast-enhanced computed tomography (CT-IVU/CT urography). Figures 25.1 and 25.2 show examples of imaging for the calyceal diverticular stone. The clinching feature would be the isolated presence of the diverticulum away from the calyx and connected through a neck. The neck of diverticulum is often not delineated clearly in the pre-operative evaluation. The stone in the diverticulum would appear as being present in the parenchyma and away from the calyx. This should alarm the surgeon about the presence of stone in a diverticulum and not a regular calyceal stone. If it is missed pre-operatively, then the surgeon would be in for an unexpected surprise intra-operatively.

### 25.1.2 Considerations About Diverticulum

When the stone is detected to be present in a calyceal diverticulum pre-operatively, one can plan to obtain the maximum possible information about the diverticulum. The important aspects of diverticulum that one needs to note are:

1. Location of the diverticulum
2. Neck of diverticulum
3. Stone in diverticulum

The location of the diverticulum bears an enormous impact on the difficulty of the procedure. The location can be polar in the form of an upper polar or lower polar diverticulum or it can be in the mid-zone. It should also be noted whether the diverticulum is anterior or posterior to the calyx. One should obtain a thorough

C. Mallikarjuna (✉) · M. T. Bendigeri
Asian Institute of Nephro-Urology (AINU), Hyderabad, India


M. S. Agrawal et al. (eds.), *Minimally Invasive Percutaneous Nephrolithotomy*,
https://doi.org/10.1007/978-981-16-6001-6_25

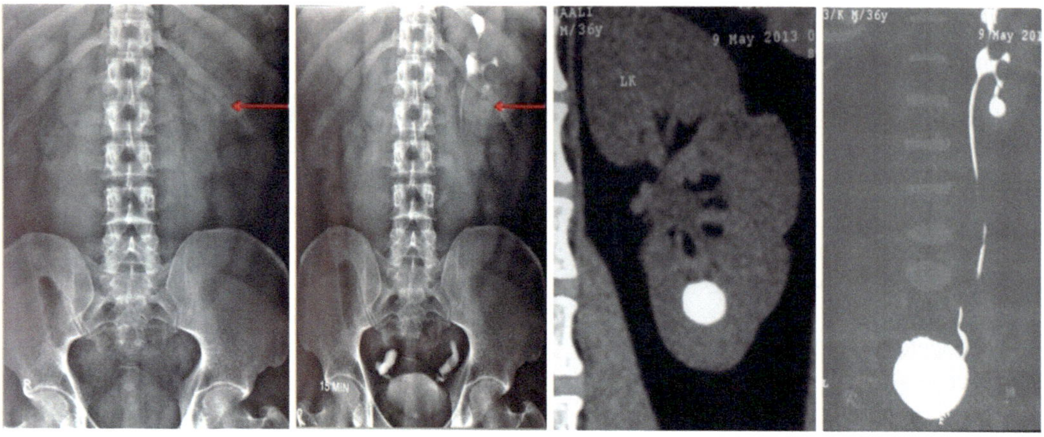

**Fig. 25.1** Imaging of a patient with left renal lower pole calyceal diverticular stone with X-ray KUB and plain CT

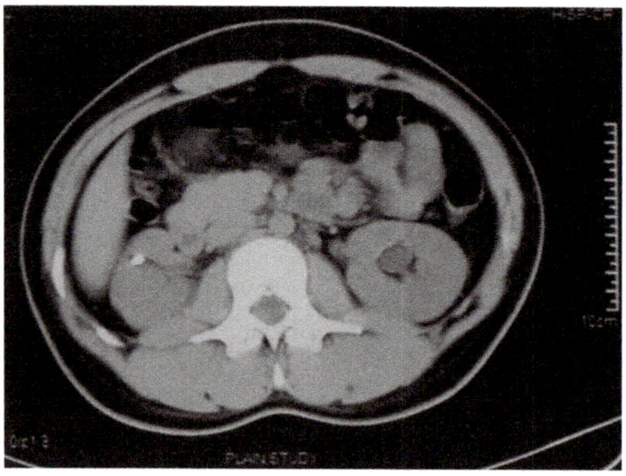

**Fig. 25.2** Anterior calyceal diverticular stone in interpolar region of right kidney on plain CT scan

orientation of the relation of the diverticulum with respect to the pelvicalyceal system. Three-dimensional computed tomography reconstruction would be of great help in simplifying this. The location determines the difficulty level in accessing the diverticulum. For example, a diverticulum that is located in the mid-zone of kidney and posterior to the middle calyx would be lot more simpler to access in conventional prone mini-PCNL than a diverticulum that is located in the lower pole on the medial aspect of the lower calyx.

Another aspect of diverticulum that needs to be looked at is the neck of the diverticulum. Most often it is not defined clearly in pre-operative evaluation. The only indirect information that can be obtained is the length of the neck. The length can be assessed by noting the distance of the diverticulum from the nearest calyx. Closer the diverticulum to the calyx, shorter is the neck. This would make it easy for incising the neck of the diverticulum to drain it into the calyx. If the diverticulum with stone is located significantly away from the wall of the calyx, it indicates that the neck would be long and incising the neck for drainage would be difficult. Longer neck also tends to be narrower in calibre and hence identification intra-operatively would be lot more challenging. The longer necks also pose a challenge in terms of incising and widening it. There are higher chances of encountering vessels in the thick parenchyma adjoining it, which can lead to significant bleeding.

The stone in the diverticulum has to be carefully assessed as well. The size and density of the stone are essential to be noted. The size of stone may dictate the size of the access sheath that one might consider using. The density of the stone would make one cautious of the type of energy opted for lithotripsy. Often the diverticular stone tends to be a bunch of small secondary calculi instead of a single stone. This might be picked up in the imaging if they tend to form a horizontal level of stone density in the diverticulum or if there is significant non-uniform stone density. The presence of bunch of small stones will have a bearing on the intra-operative improvisations needed.

- *Intra-operative considerations*:

Tackling calyceal diverticular stone needs improvisation in every step of the procedure. The challenges in each step need to be pre-empted in order to prevent complications.

1. Puncture: The biggest challenge in doing mini-PCNL for calyceal diverticular stone would be obtaining proper access to the diverticulum. The first step of doing a proper puncture often presents the biggest hurdle. The step becomes difficult if the neck of the diverticulum is narrow enough to preclude delineation of the diverticulum on the retrograde pyelography (RGP). Often one might succeed in getting a little bit of contrast across with usage of extra pressure albeit at risk of intravasation and sepsis. However, if the diverticulum gets delineated on RGP the procedure would be similar to puncturing a calyx. Figure 25.3 shows an example of RGP of left lower pole calyceal diverticular stone. If the delineation of diverticulum does not happen on RGP, then the next option would be to consider a stone-guided puncture. This would be based on the feel of touching the stone with the puncture needle. The stone-guided puncture works well when the diverticular stone is a single stone. However, when the diverticular stone is actually a bunch of small secondary stones instead of a single stone, the sensation of feeling the stone with a puncture needle becomes challenging. In such scenarios one has to look for other signs for confirmation of presence of the tip of needle inside the diverticulum such as movement of the stones on passage of guide wire, aspiration of urine from the needle, injecting saline and watching for stone movement, antegrade injection of dilute contrast to delineate diverticulum, confirmation on rotating the fluoroscopy in second axis as part of triangulation technique, usage of ultrasonography to puncture the diverticulum and demonstrate the needle tip inside the diverticular cavity. The aspiration of urine might not be helpful if there is a blood clot in the cavity due to previous puncture attempts. In this case, in spite of being inside the cavity one may not be able to aspirate. Antegrade instillation of dilute contrast can be helpful in such a situation but carries a high risk of impairing the fluoroscopy image if there is extravasation happening. The extravasated contrast would make further attempts extremely challenging. Considering these risks, one might be better off using guide wire to look for signs of confirmation such as stone movement with the wire and the guide wire curling inside the diverticulum taking the shape of the cavity. This can be repeated without risk of spoiling the image on fluoroscopy and works well even if blood clots are present in cavity. However, if previous multiple puncture attempts have failed, the guide wire might tend to repeatedly take the false passage of prior puncture instead of coiling inside the cavity. A combination of all the improvisation possible would help in negotiating our way out of difficulty.

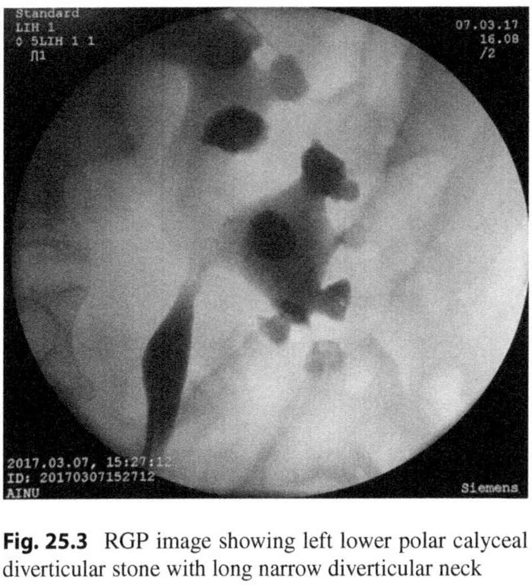


**Fig. 25.3** RGP image showing left lower polar calyceal diverticular stone with long narrow diverticular neck

2. Dilatation: The dilatation is tricky in the sense that the guide wire would almost always be coiled up in the diverticulum itself and hence the chances of error during dilatation are higher. There can be over-dilatation due to lack of stability, under-dilatation or tangential dilatation. These will make the subsequent procedure difficult as the bleeding will impair

the visibility during mini-PCNL significantly. The errors during dilatation are higher due to the instability of the guide wire, which can be coiled up only in the diverticulum. The length of wire that can be coiled up will also be marginal in some cases due to inadequate space. This would increase the chances of slippage of guide wire during dilatation. Hence, utmost care has to be taken during dilatation in diverticular stones. As the mini-PCNL usually follows single-step dilatation, the chances of errors can be minimised as compared to the multi-step dilatation of conventional PCNL. Overcautious dilatation can be often an under-dilatation which is a better bargain than having an aggressive over-dilatation scenario. Figure 25.4 gives an example of pre-operative imaging and the various steps of the procedure.

3. Stone clearance: If the diverticulum is containing multiple secondary stones that are usually small in size, the clearance can be

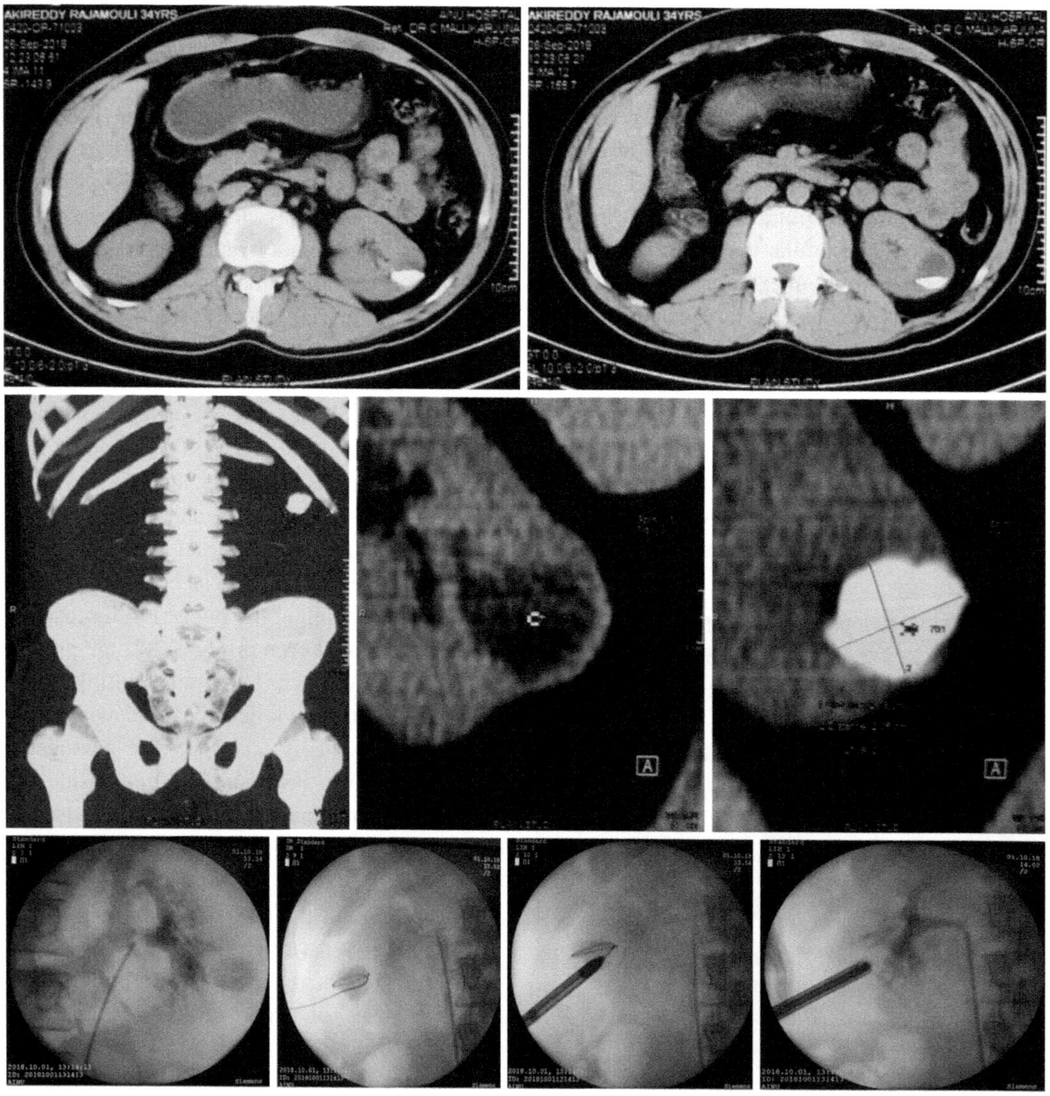

Fig. 25.4 Left lower polar calyceal diverticulum with pre-operative imaging, RGP and intra-operative steps of mini-PCNL

easily accomplished with the vacuum cleaner effect of the mini-PCNL. If the stone is large and needs lithotripsy, care has to be taken regarding selection of energy used. Pneumatic lithotripsy can have risk of injuring the parenchyma and extrusion of the stone fragments into the parenchyma and beyond it. This can happen more often if the stone is very hard in nature and the underlying parenchyma is of inadequate thickness to provide adequate counter support. The risk is higher in the medially located diverticulae and especially the polar ones. Injury to the underlying parenchyma and extrusion of stone fragments will lead to incomplete stone clearance and extravasation of irrigation fluid intra-operatively. The bleeding from the parenchymal injury would obscure the vision significantly and one might have to even terminate the procedure prematurely. To avoid this scenario, one would be better off using Laser energy for lithotripsy in diverticular stones as the preferred energy source.

4. Exit strategy: After the clearance of stone is over, one needs to decide about the exit strategy for the case. Multiple options are available for this. The safest would be to identify the neck of the diverticulum and negotiate across it and place a stent across the neck of the diverticulum. This would ensure drainage of urine antegradely and minimal chances of peri-nephric collection. Identification of neck of diverticulum can be accomplished with injecting contrast mixed with a colouring agent such as dilute povidone iodine or methylene blue from the ureteric catheter and identifying the location of the neck. Once the location of neck is identified, a guide wire can be negotiated across it. In case the neck is too narrow for the wire to be negotiated across it, one has to consider incising the neck with help of Laser to widen the calibre of the neck. One has to be careful to avoid too deep incision into the parenchyma in order to prevent bleeding. Multiple radial cuts can be given to widen the neck adequately in order to pass the wire across it. The longer length of the neck makes it more challenging to achieve this incision due to the larger thickness of intervening parenchyma. Sometimes the neck might not be visible at all. In such scenarios, one has to create a neo-infundibulum of the diverticulum by puncturing across the wall of diverticulum with the initial puncture needle and then dilating the track. One might encounter increased chances of bleeding in this step. Once neo-infundibulum is created, it is required to place a nephrostomy tube across it. Another option would be to ablate the surface of the diverticulum so that urine extravasation does not happen from the surface. This can be achieved with help of Laser in mini-PCNL. This would reduce the chances of post-operative peri-nephric urinoma formation significantly. The obliteration of the cavity is found to improve recurrence-free rates. One can place a nephrostomy tube at the exit time; however, the chances of its slippage are high due to inadequate space in the diverticulum. Placing a stent across the neck of diverticulum and ablation of surface of the diverticular cavity would be a safe play at the time of exit.

### 25.1.3 Post-operative Considerations

Post-operative care for mini-PCNL for diverticular stone would be almost the same as any other case barring a concern for the probability of peri-nephric collection. One has to be cautious to pick it up at the earliest to avoid further complications. Urinoma can happen if the antegrade drainage of the diverticulum is inadequate and the overlying parenchymal covering is thin. If in such cases scenarios, the ablation of surface is not performed there can be possibility of urinoma formation, which can lead to fistula formation as well if not picked up early enough. Injury to the parenchyma during improper dilatation can lead to bleeding post-operatively as well which can manifest as peri-nephric collection. Since the communication with pelvicalyceal system is not very broad, there might not be a significant haematuria even if there is a large peri-nephric hematoma. If the collection is large, one will have to consider an intervention to treat it accordingly.

## 25.2 Mini-PCNL in Stone with PUJO

Presence of stone and PUJO can present to us in a varied manner. The scenarios differ and this needs proper evaluation and planning of both the ailments in order to provide complete care for the patient.

- *Work-up and Various Situations*

Some of the situations that we encounter the presence of stone and PUJO are as follows:

(a) PUJO with secondary stone in calyx
(b) Stone at PUJ with suspected PUJO
(c) Stone with ballooned pelvis suspicious of PUJO
(d) Residual stone after pyeloplasty
(e) Recurrent stone after pyeloplasty

The principles of evaluation for these settings would be the same as dictated by the principles of endourology. The suspicion of PUJO should always be clarified with a renogram study preferably. The presence of PUJO and secondary stone in calyx can be treated simultaneously with stone extraction during the pyeloplasty procedure. Presence of a stone impacted at PUJ with suspicious PUJO would need stone clearance and then re-assessment for the adequacy of PUJ drainage later on. Figure 25.5 shows one such example of this tricky situation. The other scenarios will need a similar approach of stone clearance and confirmation of PUJ adequacy. Figure 25.6 shows an example of left renal calculus with ballooned-out pelvis suspicious of PUJO. We would need a regular work-up for stone and the only additional evaluation required would be for the PUJ patency. Contrast-based study to delineate the pelvicalyceal system would be helpful in giving a clue on the patency of PUJ as well.

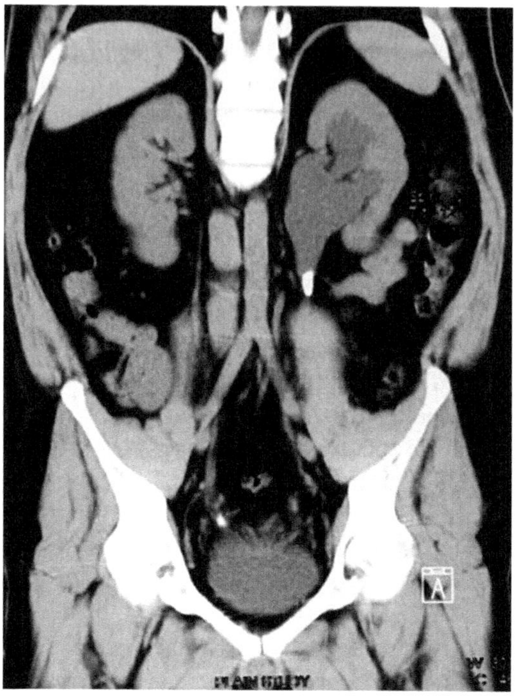


**Fig. 25.5** Plain CT KUB showing stone impacted at left PUJ. Stone impacted at PUJ is always a tricky situation wherein ruling out the presence of PUJO is not possible with surety without clearing the stone

### 25.2.1 Special Considerations

There would be several special considerations to be looked at in the setting of PUJO and stone before one proceeds with surgery. If the patient has a PUJO and a secondary stone, one needs to address whether to proceed with simultaneous clearance in same sitting versus sequencing of stone clearance and pyeloplasty. Majority of times the attempt would be to do simultaneous clearance of stone during pyeloplasty, however, often we end up facing the challenge of confirming the complete clearance intra-operatively and tackling the residual stone later on. Patient has to be informed pre-operatively about this possibility. One might also face a difficult situation post-operatively in patients who undergo clearance of impacted stone at PUJ or patients with PUJO and secondary stones that opt for clearance of only the secondary stones and without opting for a pyeloplasty. It has got significant medico-legal importance. If these patients are not counselled clearly about the nature of the PUJ, then one might have to face the blame of PUJO being a complication that has risen from the stone clearance procedure.

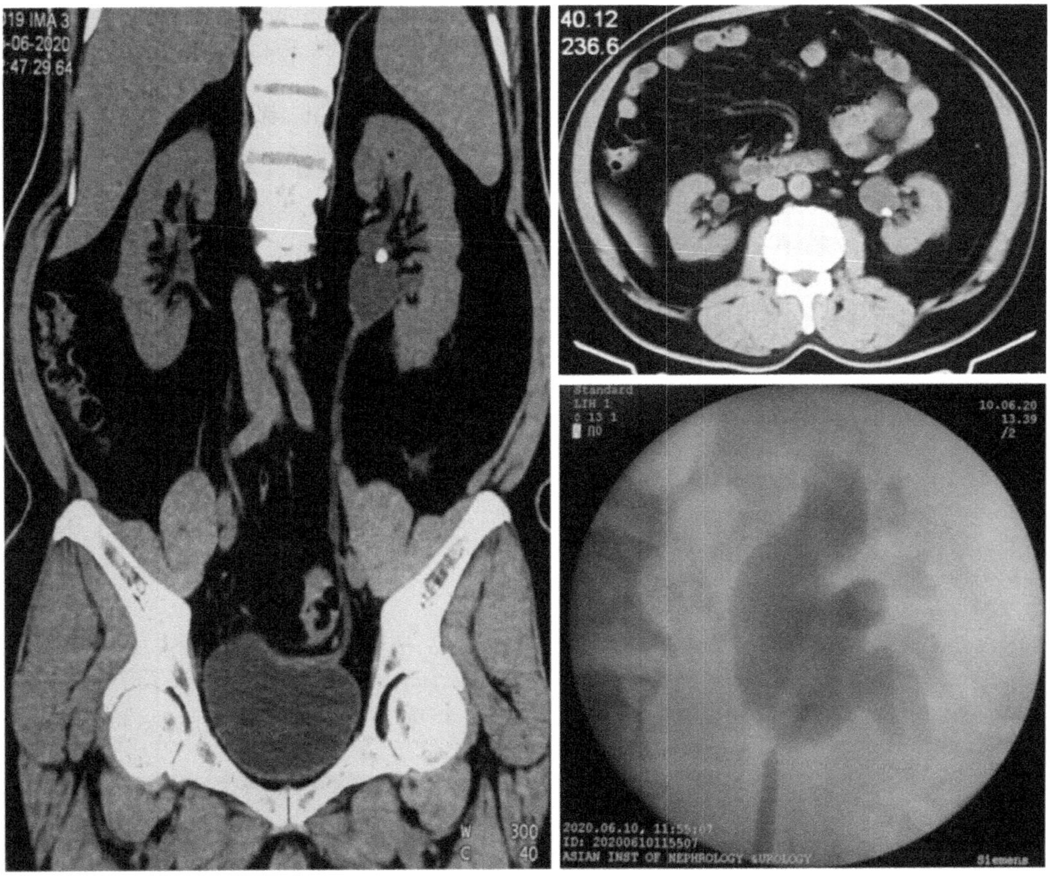


**Fig. 25.6** Plain CT KUB and RGP showing left renal calculi apparently secondary to suspected left PUJO

### 25.2.2 Endopyelotomy Consideration

There can also be a consideration for combining an endopyelotomy procedure. This would give the benefit of solving both issues in the same sitting. There have been mixed opinions about the role of endopyelotomy and the initial enthusiasm for the procedure has considerably waned off. Primary endopyelotomy has not been the favoured approach from a long-term success point of view. However, endopyelotomy might be considered in the setting of recurrent stones with previous pyeloplasty that is having a doubtful or an overtly obstructive pattern of drainage. One can consider endopyelotomy as a salvage procedure for the recurrent PUJO in these settings. Patients will have to be counselled about the advantage of a single sitting endoscopic procedure versus the possibility of recurrence later on.

The advantages that mini-PCNL provides in the setting of performing endopyelotomy is the miniaturised instruments that can easily negotiate the narrow calibre of the PUJ. Performing percutaneous endopyelotomy would be lot more comfortable when we can negotiate the nephroscope across the PUJ. This ensures the endopyelotomy incision can be done in a controlled way while retracting back the scope from the upper ureter into the pelvis. However, if the calibre of PUJ is too narrow then performing endopyelotomy would be challenging because negotiating the conventional nephroscope might not be possible in all cases. The miniaturised instrument solves this issue to a great extent. Negotiating the PUJ can be done lot more easily with the miniaturised instruments. The incision with mini-PCNL has to be performed with Laser energy. This adds to the precision of the endopyelotomy further.

The principles of performing the endopyelotomy remain the same. The site of incision has to be selected. Incision is made over the lateral aspect of the upper ureter, the lower part of the PUJ and the inferior aspect of the renal pelvis. The cut has to be deep across all the layers of the ureter and pelvis. Figure 25.7 shows the steps of laser endopyelotomy. One can confirm the adequacy of the incision depth by the visualisation of fat around the ureter and pelvis. The dye instillation would show a free extravasation outside the walls. Placing of wide calibre endopyelotomy stent would help in healing over it with epithelialisation of the defect. The stent would need to be placed for an adequately long duration of time to cover this healing phase, usually about 6–12 weeks. Some of these patients might need a re-insertion of the stent as well.

Post-operative complications due to extravasation of irrigation fluid would be expectedly lesser compared to conventional nephroscope usage since the flow rates would be lot less and the amount extravasating would be proportionately less. The post-operative pain due to this would be comparatively lesser. Nevertheless, endopyelotomy is incomplete if the incision is not deep enough to demonstrate extravasation intra-operatively. The risk of the extravasated fluid getting infected remains. Adequate coverage with antibiotics and proper drainage of the pelvicalyceal system remains extremely essential for smooth post-operative recovery.

### 25.2.3 Intra-operative Considerations

Doing a mini-PCNL in the setting of a pelvicalyceal system that bears the impact of PUJO poses few challenges. One has to be wary of the fact

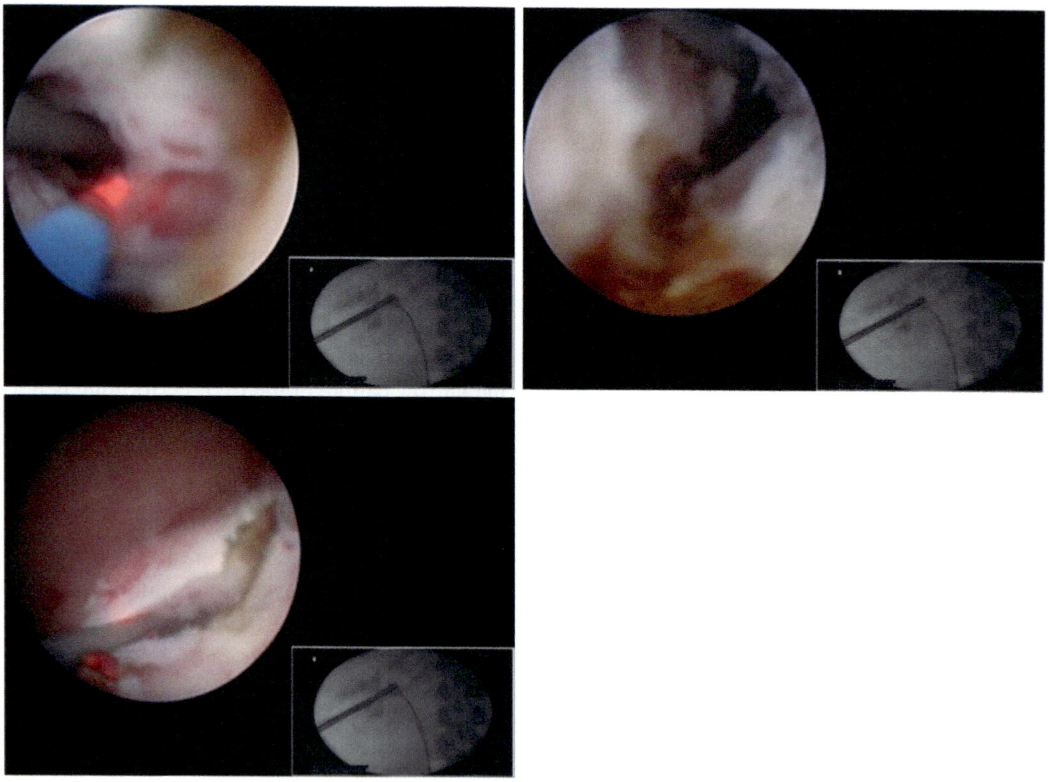

**Fig. 25.7** Left laser endopyelotomy done with mini-PCNL for secondary PUJO with stone

that a dilated system need not always be the easiest system to perform a mini-PCNL.

1. Puncture: Obtaining a puncture per se would not be a challenge in the dilated pelvicalyceal system. However, one has to be careful in not to get carried away with a dilated system. One has to be careful to make sure that the entry is not through a flattened infundibulum in the dilated pelvicalyceal system. The calyx of entry might not make a significant impact in a dilated pelvicalyceal system due to the ease of manoeuvrability.
2. Dilatation: There might be a few issues during dilatation due to the dilated pelvicalyceal system. There can be buckling of the guide wire during dilatation due to the minimal resistance of the dilated pelvicalyceal system and thinned out parenchyma. This buckling would make entry into the calyx difficult with a single-step dilatation. One might have to opt for a sequential multi-step dilatation in such situations. The other difficulty that one might face is in cases that have undergone pyeloplasty previously. The fibrosis in the peri-nephric plane would create a lot of resistance during dilatation and again makes a single step dilatation difficult.
3. Stone clearance: The challenges of clearing stones during mini-PCNL in a PUJO pelvicalyceal system are unique. A grossly dilated pelvicalyceal system is counter-productive to stone clearance by the vacuum cleaner effect of Eddy currents in mini-PCNL. One might end up struggling to clear the fragments that keep floating around in a baggy pelvicalyceal system. Keeping the pelvis semi-distended by controlling the inflow of the irrigation fluid might reduce the effective size of the pelvicalyceal system and aid in clearing stones. Another problem that one can face is finding a large dilated pelvis that is filled up with large blood clots due to infundibular entry or a troubled dilatation in the prior step. Blood clots are the biggest enemy of mini-PCNL. Clearing the clots would need a lot of patience or one might have to even consider converting it to a conventional PCNL. Usage of a suction probe might be of some help in clearing the clots. Stone clearance cannot be performed efficiently unless the clots are cleared. The chances of leaving residual fragments are higher if the clots are not cleared completely and the entire pelvicalyceal system is checked for stone clearance. Since the drainage of the PUJ is circumspect in this set of cases, one has to make sure that the clearance of stone fragments is complete. Relying on the natural passage of small residual fragments would not be an ideal proposition in these kidneys. One has to put extra effort to clear even the minimal amount of "stone dust" also from the pelvicalyceal system intra-operatively.
4. Exit strategy: The exit strategy in cases with doubtful PUJ would need to be considered separately from a regular case. Proceeding with a tubeless or a totally tubeless strategy might not be the safest approach. There can be an increased risk of urinary extravasation from the access track if the PUJ does not drain adequately. Since these patients have compromised and doubtful PUJ, it would make sense to opt for stenting in these cases at the end of procedure.

### 25.2.4 Post-operative Considerations

There could be higher chances of urinary extravasation in patients with PUJO who undergo mini-PCNL and have a tubeless or totally tubeless exit. One needs to be careful in avoiding this scenario which might lead to risk of urinoma formation and getting infected to form an abscess with septic complications. The other aspects of post-operative care would be similar to any regular mini-PCNL.

## Suggested Reading

1. Krambeck AE, Lingeman JE. Percutaneous management of calyceal diverticuli. J Endourol. 2009;23:1723–9.

2. Bellman GC, Silverstein JI, Blickensderfer S, Smith AD. Technique and follow-up of percutaneous management of caliceal diverticula. Urology. 1993;42:21–5.
3. Lancini V, Liatsikos EN, Bernardo NO, Dinlenc CZ, Kapoor R, Smith AD. Percutaneous treatment of calculosis in caliceal diverticulosis: 13-year experience. Arch Ital Urol Androl. 2000;72:59–63.
4. Hulbert JC, Reddy PK, Hunter DW, Castaneda-Zuniga W, Amplatz K, Lange PH. Percutaneous techniques for the management of calyceal diverticula containing calculi. J Urol. 1986;135:225–7.
5. Landry JL, Colombel M, Rouviere O, Lezrek M, Gelet A, Dubernard JM, et al. Long term results of percutaneous treatment of caliceal diverticular calculi. Eur Urol. 2002;41:474–7.
6. Ndez-Probst CE, Fuller A, Nott L, Denstedt JD, Razvi H. Percutaneous nephrolithotomy of caliceal diverticular calculi: A single center experience. J Endourol. 2011;25:1741–5.
7. Srivastava A, Chipde SS, Mandhani A, Kapoor R, Ansari MS. Percutaneous management of renal caliceal diverticular stones: Ten-year experience of a tertiary care center with different techniques to deal with diverticula after stone extraction. Indian J Urol. 2013;29:273–6.
8. Donnellan SM, Harewood LM, Webb DR. Percutaneous management of caliceal diverticular calculi: Technique and outcome. J Endourol. 1999;13:83–8.
9. Matlaga BR, Kim SC, Watkins SL, Munch LC, Chan BW, Lingeman JE. Pre-percutaneous nephrolithotomy opacification for caliceal diverticular calculi. J Endourol. 2006;20:175–8.

# 26 PCNL in Complex Situations: Obese Patients and Spinal Deformities, Ectopic, and Pelvic Kidneys

Pankaj N. Maheshwari, Venkat Arjunrao Gite, Amandeep M. Arora, and Mayank Agrawal

## 26.1 Introduction

PCNL is a standard of care for large and complex renal calculi. Although most percutaneous access are safe to make, in some clinical situations, making access can be a huge challenge. The challenge could be related to patient factors like morbid obesity or spinal deformities, or renal factors like un-ascended pelvic ectopic kidney or polycystic kidney disease. Here, the intra- or peri-renal anatomy and anatomical relations change making the PCNL procedure difficult. Such patients should be treated only by a very experienced endourologist who is backed by a complete gamut of equipment and technology.

P. N. Maheshwari (✉)
Fortis Hospital Mulund, Mumbai, Maharashtra, India

Department of Urology, Grant Government Medical College and Sir JJ Group of Hospitals, Mumbai, Maharashtra, India

V. A. Gite · M. Agrawal
Department of Urology, Grant Government Medical College and Sir JJ Group of Hospitals, Mumbai, Maharashtra, India

A. M. Arora
Tata Memorial Hospital, Mumbai, Maharashtra, India

## 26.2 PCNL in Morbid Obesity

### 26.2.1 Introduction

The World Health Organization defines obesity as "abnormal or excessive accumulation of fat that may impair health." For adults, a body mass index (BMI) of 18.5 to 24.9 kg/m$^2$ is considered normal. "Overweight," "obesity," and "severe obesity" are defined as BMI of 25–29.9 kg/m$^2$, >30 kg/m$^2$, and >40 kg/m$^2$, respectively. Worldwide, the incidence of obesity has tripled since 1980 with more than 650 million adults classified as obese in 2016.

Obesity leads to metabolic alterations, most notably, insulin resistance which leads to lowered urine pH on account of decreased excretion of ammonia. This urinary milieu is conducive to uric acid stone formation. Obesity has been identified as an independent risk factor for formation of renal stones and also for stone recurrence. Percutaneous management of urolithiasis in obese patients poses distinct anesthetic and surgical challenges, which require certain modifications in the standard procedure of percutaneous nephrolithotomy (PCNL).

### 26.2.2 Anesthesia Considerations

Obesity presents a triad of challenges to the anesthetist. There could be a difficulty for intubation


M. S. Agrawal et al. (eds.), *Minimally Invasive Percutaneous Nephrolithotomy*,
https://doi.org/10.1007/978-981-16-6001-6_26

that can be reduced by "ramped" position instead of the "sniff" position while intubating. Severe obesity is associated with decreased compliance of the respiratory system, reduction in lung volumes and oxygenation, and an increase in the work of breathing. Also, obesity hardly ever exists alone and is almost always associated with other comorbidities like hypertension, diabetes, and cardiac disease as a spectrum of the metabolic syndrome, and these conditions increase the overall anesthesia risk.

### 26.2.3 Positioning

Prone position continues to remain the traditional and most commonly used position in which PCNL is performed across the world. Extra precaution and personnel are required while turning an obese patient from the supine to the prone position. This needs to be done with utmost care to prevent any kind of spine or skeletal injury. The patient needs to be positioned with bolsters under the chest and the pelvis to allow the abdominal wall to move freely. This reduces splinting of the diaphragm and inferior vena cava compression and helps reduce the burden on the cardiopulmonary system.

To circumvent the challenge associated with turning an anesthetized obese patient from supine to prone, Wu and colleagues described the technique of awake intubation and prone patient self-positioning [1]. This problem can be completely avoided by supine PCNL. Mazzucchi and colleagues compared the supine and prone positions for PCNL in obese patients [2]. They reported similar stone-free rates for both positions and shorter operating times and hospital stays in the supine position group. However, it must be remembered that supine positioning is associated with a longer access tract and reduced nephroscope maneuverability, both of which are anyways existing concerns in obese patients.

### 26.2.4 Challenges in the PCNL Technique and their Solutions

While performing a PCNL in an obese patient, difficulties might be encountered at various steps: puncturing the desired calyx, maintaining the established tract, and maneuvering the nephroscope in the pelvicalyceal system. The underlying problem here is the excess abdominal fat which increases the "skin to calyx distance."

While excess body fat may not prove to be a problem in visualizing the collecting system under fluoroscopy, it can lead to poor quality of ultrasound images and a steep learning curve for ultrasound guided PCNL. Visualization of deep-seated kidneys can be improved by using lower frequency ultrasound probes and by optimizing the brightness, gain, and focal zone.

The increased skin-to-calyx distance can prove to be too long for instruments and accessories of standard length. This calls for use of "extra-long" equipment. The standard Amplatz sheath is 17 cm long while the extra-long one has a length of 20 cm. This long sheath may also require the use of an extra-long nephroscope and stone grasping forceps. To prevent an on-table surprise, the skin to calyx distance should be estimated using the pre-operative CT scan and one should be ready with the necessary instruments. In centers that have facilities for holmium laser enucleation of prostate, the morcelloscope can be utilized as an extra-long nephroscope. A flexible nephroscope, if available, may also be used if the length of the rigid nephroscope proves to be short in reaching stones in different calyces.

On certain occasions, even the extra-long sheath may prove inadequate then the skin and subcutaneous tissue can be incised down to the thoracolumbar fascia so that the tract begins at the level of the back muscles. If the skin and subcutaneous tissue has not been incised, there is a risk that the access sheath may be advanced too far and get lost under the level of the skin. Nguyen and Belis described tying long sutures to the access sheath (Fig. 26.1), using which the sheath could be pulled out at the end of the procedure even if it had advanced below the skin [3]. Another technique includes opening the stone grasping forceps beyond the sheath and then retracting the forceps along with the sheath. Also, a Foley catheter may be passed into the collecting system via the sheath. The balloon is inflated with radiocontrast and the catheter is then withdrawn under fluoroscopic guidance along with the sheath.

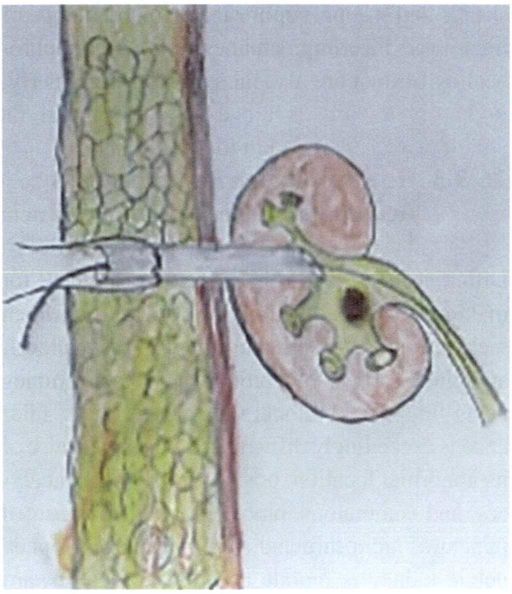

**Fig. 26.1** Sutures placed through the amplatz sheath that can be used at the end of the procedure to pull out the sheath from inside the abdominal wall

Anatomically, we are aware that in prone position the upper calyx is more superficial as compared to lower calyx. Whenever feasible, an upper calyx tract would be shorter than the lower calyx tract and hence may be appropriate in obese patients.

### 26.2.5 Results with PCNL in Obese Patients

Multiple series have described the efficacy of PCNL in the setting of obesity. The largest review from the CROES (Clinical Research Office of the Endourological Society) database reported on the results of PCNL in more than 3700 patients stratified as normal weight, overweight, obese, and super-obese [4]. The study concluded that PCNL can be safely performed in obese patients, albeit with longer operative times and an inferior stone-free rate. Studies have also noted no difference in perioperative complications in super obese patients compared to patients with normal BMI. Credibility to evidence for safety and efficacy of PCNL in obese patients is also provided by a recently reported meta-analysis, which analyzed outcomes in close to 2000 patients with obesity [5].

The use of miniaturized scopes has also been evaluated in obese patients. Akbulut et al. reported mini-PCNL with 18 Fr sheath size in 50 patients with a mean stone size of 25 mm [6]. They noted no significant increase in complications or duration of hospital stay and comparable stone-free rates (70%) as compared to mini-PCNL in nonobese patients. Super mini-PCNL with 12/14 Fr access sheath has also been compared to retrograde intra-renal surgery (RIRS) in obese patients [7]. In a study for stone size between 20–30 mm, no difference was noted in the efficacy of the 2 approaches. However, the super mini-PCNL group had a shorter operating time and lower total cost and rates of reintervention.

While the ideal exit strategy following PCNL is debatable, researchers have reported on the safety and feasibility of the totally tubeless technique of PCNL in obese and severely obese patients [8]. It was associated with lower requirement of postoperative analgesics and faster return to routine activity. However, whenever a nephrostomy tube is placed following a PCNL, there is a higher chance of tube dislodgement in an obese patient. Thus, it would be prudent to use a nephro-ureteral tube that has a coil in the renal pelvis with a further extension down the ureter.

### 26.2.6 Urolithiasis Following Bariatric Surgery

Obesity increases the risk of stone formation due to associated metabolic alterations as previously outlined. Even the surgical treatment of obesity poses its own metabolic problems. Bariatric surgery, especially Roux-en-Y gastric bypass causes alterations in 24-h urine profile in the form of increase in urinary oxalate, decreased urine volume, and urinary citrate levels. This leads to the development of calcium oxalate stones that can be recurrent. PCNL in a patient who has undergone bariatric surgery would not be expected to pose any special challenges of its own except that there is an increased risk of retro-renal colon in these patients [9].

### 26.2.7 Conclusion

PCNL is safe, feasible, and effective in obese patients with no risk of increased perioperative complications compared to patients with normal BMI. Obesity should not lead one to avoid PCNL if it is clinically indicated. However, it is important to be aware of the challenges posed by the long access tract and be prepared with technical modifications to provide optimum results in this special cohort of patients.

## 26.3 PCNL in Patients with Pelvic Kidney Disease

### 26.3.1 Introduction

The pelvic ectopic kidney (PEK) is a common renal anomaly where the kidney fails to ascend to its normal location and remains positioned in the pelvis anterior to the sacrum. Pelvic kidney usually has anomalous blood supply with a short tortuous ureter with high insertion, leading to poor drainage and hence predisposition to the formation of renal calculi. The options of treatment depending on the stone characteristics could be ESWL, RIRS, PCNL, or open surgery.

### 26.3.2 Issues in Patients with Pelvic Kidney Disease

PEK has abnormal calyceal orientation and anomalous vascular patterns and is surrounded by bowel anteriorly and sacrum posteriorly hence the percutaneous transperitoneal approach to the pelvic kidney would be a big challenge. Risk of injury to the surrounding bowel, abnormal vasculature resulting in bleeding from tract dilatation, and spillage of urine into peritoneal cavity are major concerns during PCNL. The deeply located pelvic kidney necessitates a longer amplatz sheath and a long nephroscope. The chances of tract loss, bleeding, and a prolonged time for healing of tract are also theoretically higher [10].

### 26.3.3 How to Make a Percutaneous Access in These Patients

Different approaches have been described for making the initial puncture safely in a PEK, which includes guidance by laparoscopy, ultrasound, CT, and fluoroscopy. Puncture in an ectopic kidney using fluoroscopy alone, without any other guidance is exceedingly difficult and unsafe because of its abnormal location, position of pelvis and calyces and anomalous blood supply. USG-guided punctures are a safe and effective approach when pelvic kidney is mobile and displaceable toward the abdominal wall [11]. In supine oblique position, the kidney must be elevated by placing a small bolster behind the pelvis. This maneuver displaces the bowel overlying the kidney. The main limitation of the USG access is its learning curve and potential risk of injury to bowel, if bowel is collapsed or fixed, so this approach is suitable only for highly selected thin individuals with large hydronephrotic kidney [12].

Laparoscopy-guided PCNL is the safest access to PEK [13–15]. There are two teams, the laparoscopy team keeps the bowel away from the PCNL tract, while the PCNL team makes a fluoroscopy and laparoscopy-guided tract (Fig. 26.2). This is a versatile technique that can be used in most patients even who are obese or have adhesions related to prior surgery. The kidney is usually very easily visible on laparoscopy and most often mobilizing the bowel and the overlying mesentery is not needed.

Mini PCNL offers advantages in reducing the size of the puncture tract with Laser fragmentation of the stone which reduces the morbidity of standard PCNL.

### 26.3.4 How to Prevent Bowel Injury?

Bowel injury is the biggest concern during PCNL for PEK. This could be prevented by:

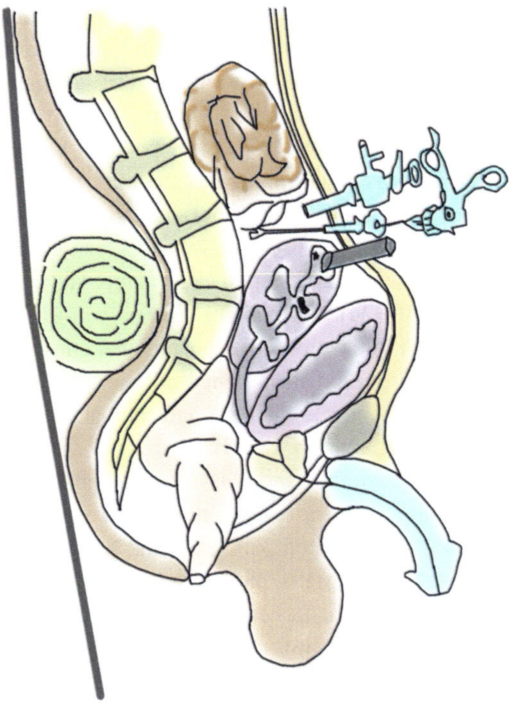

**Fig. 26.2** Laparoscopy-assisted PCNL: A versatile technique that can be used in most patients with pelvic ectopic kidney, even those who are obese and have adhesions related to prior surgery

A. Proper positioning (Trendelenburg) which shifts the bowel upward.
B. Peripheral puncture under ultrasound guidance.
C. Puncture and tract placement under direct visual control (laparoscopy guidance).

### 26.3.5 Post-op Care and Complications

**Urine Spillage**—Use of an Amplatz sheath gives a stable and secure tract to the kidney and helps maintain a low intrarenal pressure thus reducing the risk of intraperitoneal spillage. Occurrence and morbidity of spillage can be avoided using intraperitoneal drain, double J stent without any external drainage or both. At the end of the procedure extravasated fluid in the abdomen can be aspirated along with any stone fragments. Zafar et al. [16] modified the laparoscopic technique to include intracorporeal suturing of the nephrotomy site and ureteral stent placement allowing elimination of a transperitoneal nephrostomy tube.

**Paralytic ileus**—Extravasation of fluid into the abdominal cavity, even a small amount, is enough to irritate the peritoneal surface to cause ileus. Meticulous care at the end of laparoscopy procedure to aspirate all extravasated fluid can reduce this complication.

**Prolonged postoperative leak**—Any obstruction in the tract due to migrated stone down the ureter, obstructed stent or associated comorbidity/impaired renal function can delay healing.

**Bleeding**—One must watch for postoperative bleeding and manage accordingly.

### 26.3.6 Literature Review

Eshghi and coworkers [13] were the first to report a method of PCNL in a pelvic kidney by a combination of retrograde nephrostomy and laparoscopic retrieval of the guide wire. Toth and colleagues [17] described an antegrade transperitoneal approach. The puncture was controlled both fluoroscopically and laparoscopically. Both techniques depended on the laparoscope for observation and displacement of bowel. Holman et al. reported 15 patients treated with laparoscopic-assisted transperitoneal PCNL [14]. With the patient in the Trendelenburg position under laparoscopic control, the bowel was dislodged until the kidney became visible, allowing percutaneous access. Troxel et al. described extraperitoneal laparoscopy-assisted percutaneous approach to access the lower-pole calyx of a pelvic kidney for PCNL [18].

USG-guided PCNL has also been adopted in many centers. Otano et al. performed PCNL in 26 patients with USG-guided punctures [19]. They concluded that USG-guided puncture was a safe and effective approach to the collecting system even in renal anomalies like in pelvic ectopic kidneys.

Monga et al. used prone supra-iliac approach. However, postoperative incomplete femoral neuropathy was observed probably due to direct trauma to dorsal divisions of the lumbar plexus [20]. Watterson et al. described the approach through the greater sciatic foramen under fluoroscopic control [21].

Due to problems associated with other approaches PCNL with assistance of laparoscopic/sonography supine and oblique position is the favored approach.

## 26.4 PCNL in Patients with Spinal Deformity

Management of upper urinary tract calculi in patients with severe spinal deformity becomes a huge challenge. Spinal deformities lead to alterations in the curvature of the spine, mainly caused by congenital and neuromuscular diseases. Stone disease (carbonate apatite and struvite) is common with spinal deformities due to its associated restricted mobilization, voiding dysfunction, metabolic disorders such as hypercalcemia and chronic recurrent urinary infections.

Stone management in the presence of spinal deformity, however, can be a challenge. The issues with spinal deformity are that not only the person becomes more prone to stone formation and recurrence, but due to difficulty in positioning and altered anatomy, the treatment also becomes difficult. All standard modes of stone treatment have been attempted with difficulties and poor results. Extracorporeal shock wave lithotripsy is possible and safe (in patients who can be positioned), but stone-free rates are poor and need for ancillary procedures is higher [22]. Rigid ureteroscopy may be difficult as even lithotomy position may be awkward. Small renal and upper ureteric calculi can be treated using flexible ureteroscopy, while larger stone burden still requires PCNL. [23]

Spinal deformities could be a combination of scoliosis with lordoscoliosis or kyphoscoliosis. Such curvatures lead to a three-dimensional deformity in the thorax or pelvis leading to altered internal anatomy and restriction of lung ventilation and consequent respiratory dysfunction. The changed internal relations could increase the risk of injuring neighboring organs during PCNL. The severity of deformity is diagnosed by measurement by Cobb angle. When Cobb angle is above 45°, most patients would have impaired pulmonary function reserve. Especially for those with thoracic spinal deformity, pulmonary compliance would decrease dramatically because of a small chest cavity and stiff chest wall [24]. Pulmonary issues would be amplified if the patient is under regional anesthesia or in prone position hence all such patients need a pulmonary evaluation and intubated general anesthesia before PCNL.

One more important consideration for PCNL is appropriate positioning. In view of extreme curvatures, associated pelvic tilt and hip alkaloses, even placing the patient on the operation table may be difficult hence positioning needs to be individualized. Soft cushions and holders can help steady the patient and cover the pressure points. All positions like prone, lateral, supine, and other unconventional positions have been described. Supine position may have an advantage of easier airway control, less ventilation problems, and possibility to perform a simultaneous retrograde ureteroscopy (ECRIS). Prone position is still preferred if feasible with the patient's body habitus, because it provides enough space for access establishment and endoscopic instruments.

The key determinant of the complexity of the procedure is which side of the curvature the affected kidney is; the kidney on the convex side of the spine would have ample space while access making would be difficult on the concave side as the kidney is squeezed by internal organs.

Puncture can be made under the guidance of ultrasound, fluoroscopy, or CT scan. Ultrasound provides advantages like proper visualization of the kidney and its surrounding structures, clear delineation of the anterior and posterior calices, detection of radiolucent calculi, and identification of blood vessels so that injury can be avoided. Fluoroscopy may be difficult in view of severe body distortion, the abnormal relationship between kidney and surrounding structures also increases the risk of visceral injury during fluoroscopy-guided puncture. CT-guided access may be the safest but it increases the radiation exposure to the patient. One important precaution is that the treating surgeon should monitor CT-guided access so that the choice of calyx and the direction of the tract is appropriate for further PCNL and lithotripsy. For anteriorly pushed kidneys with larger burden in anterior calyces, laparoscopic assistance for PCNL has also been described. After a proper and safe tract is made, having access to ECIRS, flexible nephroscopy and laser lithotripsy would improve access to the stones and hence improve overall stone-free rates.

Apart from surrounding organ injury and pulmonary complications, infection and sepsis are the most common perioperative events. Appropriate antibiotic prophylaxis and intraoperative care would help reduce these events. Infection remains one of the important causes for stone recurrence in these patients. Overall there is a higher rate of minor complications reported in patients with spinal deformity. Considering the higher recurrence rate in this subgroup and the possibility of needing surgery in the future, these surgeries should be performed in centers with experienced surgeons so that every attempt should be made to achieve complete stone-free status. Post-procedure aggressive treatment of infection and stringent follow-up is very vital.

## 26.5 PCNL in Autosomal Dominant Polycystic Kidney Disease

### 26.5.1 Introduction

Incidence of nephrolithiasis in patients with autosomal dominant polycystic kidney disease (ADPKD) is 20–28% which is 5–10 times more than in the general population. About 50% are symptomatic and 20% ultimately require intervention. Occurrence of stone (uric acid and calcium oxalate) in ADPKD may be due to anatomic and metabolic factors which include hypocitraturia, aciduria or low urinary pH, abnormal transport of ammonia, and distal acidification defects. All four management options (RIRS, ECIRS, ESWL, and PCNL) can be offered as per the standard stone and patient characteristics. PCNL is the ideal method for the larger stones and in failed cases of ESWL.

### 26.5.2 Anesthesia and Surgical Consideration

Majority of the patients with ADPKD have decreased renal reserves hence, nephrotoxic drugs like NSAIDS and aminoglycosides need to be avoided. Although PCNL can be done under general or regional anesthesia, general with controlled ventilation is the technique of choice for PCNL. The position of the patient can be supine or prone. Prone position in patients with large cysts carries a risk of compression of the diaphragm with ventilation difficulty or at times rupture of these cysts.

**Preoperative issues**—Every case should receive preoperative nephrological consultation as majority have decreased renal reserve. Preoperative management of urinary tract infection, correction of electrolyte imbalance, coagulation defects, and de-obstruction of obstructed-infected system is advisable.

**Issues with the diagnosis of stone**—Wherever possible, a contrast-enhanced computed tomography (CECT) with excretory films is preferred over sonography or NCCT. It helps in differentiating cyst wall or parenchymal calcification from the stone, dilated PCS from cyst, and better delineation of length of the infundibula of the calyces.

### 26.5.3 Issues with the Puncture and Dilatation

Distorted PCS in ADPKD can lead to difficulty in puncture, dilatation, or may result in cyst puncture, cyst bleeding, cyst infection. The calyceal spaces are often narrow and long due to the compressive effects of the parenchymal cysts leading to difficulty in puncture and subsequent tract dilatation which necessitates the use of a special smaller caliber and longer instruments.

### 26.5.4 How to Make the Initial Puncture?

The cysts can come in the way of the puncture and, in some cases, might need to be aspirated before a puncture or use of ultrasound guidance may be required. Ultrasound-guided puncture could be difficult owing to the presence of multiple cysts that could interfere with accurate localization of the compressed calices. To overcome this, ultrasonography guidance along with fluoroscopy control, should be used.

**Confirmation of the correct puncture**—Jet of urine seen emerging from initial puncture needle, after flushing sterile normal saline through ureteric catheter, is enough evidence of right puncture. Al-Kandari and Ahmad et al. alludes contrast material mixed with methylthioninium chloride (methylene blue) during retrograde pyelogram to confirm the correct puncture [25]. Any coloring fluid-like betadine or methylene blue can be used. Once proper tract is made access to flexible nephroscopy and ECIRS would improve your reach and hence increase the overall stone-free status.

### 26.5.5 Complications and Post-Op care

In postoperative period one must watch for complications such as bleeding, fever, paralytic ileus, inadequate stone clearance, and worsening of preexisting renal failure.

**Bleeding**—Causes:

1. Tendency to over dilate as the parenchyma is not as dense as a normal kidney.
2. Trans-calyceal puncture can result in infundibular injury.
3. Preexisting renal failure and associated coagulopathy.
4. Cyst rupture in PCS.

### 26.5.6 Literature Review

Umbreit et al. found PCNL to be safe and efficacious for patients of ADPKD with a large stone burden, despite increased operative complexity, need for multiple punctures, and repeat endoscopy [26]. In a case series of 19 patients with ADPKD and upper-tract nephrolithiasis, PCNL achieved stone clearance in 89.4%. Another case series by Srivastava et al. of 25 such patients achieved stone clearance in 88% [27]. Despite the distorted calyceal anatomy and associated chronic kidney disease, PCNL is safe and effective in managing nephrolithiasis in ADPKD. Proper identification of the targeted calyx and access to flexible nephroscope and laser lithotripsy can make this safe and effective [28].

## 26.6 Conclusion

PCNL is a versatile procedure for large and complex renal calculi. Although the risks and complications in these difficult situations are higher than when the kidney that is normally placed and oriented, with experience, proper planning by radiology, backup of long nephroscopes, flexible nephroscopes, ultrasound puncture, and laser lithotripsy, it is possible to surmount the difficulty posed by these anatomical variations.

**Acknowledgments:** A sincere thanks to Mr. Ramkhilavan Aditya, MSc (PA) for making the figures for this manuscript.

## References

1. Wu SD, Yilmaz M, Tamul PC, Meeks JJ, Nadler RB. Awake endotracheal intubation and prone patient self-positioning: anesthetic and positioning considerations during percutaneous nephrolithotomy in obese patients. J Endourol. 2009;23:1599–602.
2. Mazzucchi E, Vicentini FC, Marchini GS, Danilovic A, Brito AH, Srougi M. Percutaneous nephrolithotomy in obese patients: comparison between the prone and total supine position. J Endourol. 2012;26:1437–42.
3. Nguyen TA, Belis JA. Endoscopic management of urolithiasis in the morbidly obese patient. J Endourol. 1998;12(1):33–5.

4. Fuller A, Razvi H, Denstedt JD, Nott L, Pearle M, Cauda F, et al. The CROES percutaneous nephrolithotomy global study: the influence of body mass index on outcome. J Urol. 2012;188:138–44.
5. Zhou X, Sun X, Chen X, Gong X, Yang Y, Chen C, Yao Q. Effect of obesity on outcomes of percutaneous nephrolithotomy in renal stone management: a systematic review and meta-analysis. Urol Int. 2017;98:382–90.
6. Akbulut F, Kucuktopcu O, Kandemir E, Ucpinar B, Ozgor F, Simsek A, Arslan B, Erbin A, Yanaral F, Binbay M, Gurbuz G. Efficacy and safety of mini percutaneous nephrolithotomy in obese patients. Springerplus. 2016;5:1148.
7. Xu C, Song R, Lu P, Jiang M, Zeng G, Zhang W. A retrospective study comparing super-mini percutaneous nephrolithotomy and flexible ureteroscopy for the treatment of 20–30 mm renal stones in obese patients. Peer J. 2020;8:e8532.
8. Aghamir SMK, Mohseni MG, Hosseini SR, Salavati A, Ganjali H, Fallah MA, Rezaei H, Modaresi SS. Totally tubeless percutaneous nephrolithotomy is feasible in morbidly obese patients. Turk J Urol. 2017 Jun;43(2):162–4.
9. Maheshwari PN. Retrorenal colon: is it an acquired anomaly. J Endourol. 2011;25(1):A16.
10. Singh AG, Jairath A, Balaji SS, Tak G, Ganpule AP, Vijayakumar M, Sabnis RB, Desai MR. Changing trends in the endourological management of urolithiasis in anomalous kidneys. BJU Int. 2019;123:318–27.
11. Ganesamoni R, Sabnis RB, Mishra S, Desai MR. Microperc for the management of renal calculi in pelvic ectopic kidneys. Ind J Urol. 2013;29:257–9.
12. Maheshwari PN, Saple AL. Percutaneous stone removal from ectopic kidneys. J Endourol. 2001;15:649.
13. Eshghi AM, Roth JS, Smith AD. Percutaneous transperitoneal approach to a pelvic kidney for endourological removal of staghorn calculus. J Urol. 1985;134:525–7.
14. Holman E, Toth C. Laparoscopically assisted percutaneous transperitoneal nephrolithotomy in pelvic dystopic kidneys: experience in 15 successful cases. J Laparoendosc Adv Tech. 1998;8:431–5.
15. Maheshwari PN, Bhandarkar DS, Andankar MG, Shah RS. Laparoscopically guided transperitoneal percutaneous nephrolithotomy for calculi in pelvic ectopic kidneys. Surg Endosc. 2004;18:1151.
16. Zafar FS, Lingeman JE. Value of laparoscopy in the management of calculi complicating renal malformations. J Endourol. 1996;10:379–83.
17. Toth C, Holman EE, Pasztor I, Khan M. Laparoscopically controlled and assisted percutaneous transperitoneal nephrolithotomy in a pelvic dystopic kidney. J Endourol. 1993;7:303–5.
18. Troxel SA, Low RK, Das S. Extraperitoneal laparoscopy assisted percutaneous nephrolithotomy in a left pelvic kidney. J Endourol. 2002;16:655–7.
19. Otaño N, Jairath A, Mishra S, Ganpule A, Sabnis R, Desai M. Percutaneous nephrolithotomy in pelvic kidneys: is the ultrasound-guided puncture safe? Urology. 2015;85:55–8.
20. Monga M, Castaneda-Zuniga WR, Thomas R. Femoral neuropathy following percutaneous nephrolithotomy of a pelvic kidney. Urology. 1995;45:1059–61.
21. Watterson JD, Cook A, Sahajpal R, Bennett J, Denstedt JD. Percutaneous nephrolithotomy of a pelvic kidney: a posterior approach through the greater sciatic foramen. J Urol. 2001;166:209–10.
22. Niedrach WL, Davis RS, Tonetti FW, Cockett AT. Extracorporeal shock-wave lithotripsy in patients with spinal cord dysfunction. Urology. 1991;38:152–6.
23. Polat F, Yesil S. Retrograde intrarenal surgery by flexible ureteroscope in patients with spinal deformities. J Spinal Cord Med. 2017;40:26–9.
24. Wang HH, Wiener JS, Ferrandino MN, Lipkin ME, Routh JC. Complications of surgical management of upper tract calculi in spina bifida patients: analysis of nationwide data. J Urol. 2015 Apr;193(4):1270–4.
25. Al-Kandari AM, Shoma AM, Eraky I, El-Kenawy MR, Al-Eezi H, El-Kappany HA. Percutaneous nephrolithotomy for management of upper urinary tract calculi in patients with autosomal dominant polycystic kidney disease. Urology. 2009;74:273–7.
26. Umbreit EC, Childs MA, Patterson DE, Torres VE, LeRoy AJ, Gettman MT. Percutaneous nephrolithotomy for large or multiple upper tract calculi and autosomal dominant polycystic kidney disease. J Urol. 2010;183:183–7.
27. Srivastava A, Bansal R, Srivastava A, et al. Percutaneous nephrolithotomy in polycystic kidney disease: is it safe and effective? Int Urol Nephrol. 2012;44:725–30.
28. Baishya R, Dhawan DR, Kurien A, Ganpule A, Sabnis RB, Desai MR. Management of nephrolithiasis in autosomal dominant polycystic kidney disease—A single center experience. Urol Ann. 2012;4:29–33.

# Horseshoe Kidneys, Polycystic Kidney, and Post-transplant Kidneys

27

Aneesh Srivastava and Rahul Jena

## 27.1 Introduction

Percutaneous nephrolithotomy (PCNL) is the treatment of choice for large upper urinary tract calculi and its widespread use and integration in the teaching programs across the world has made it one of the most important components of the armamentarium of a urologist dealing with urolithiasis in his/her daily practice. It has gradually been realized that miniaturization of PCNL, also called mini PCNL (mPCNL) in terms of sheath size can definitely reduce its morbidity while retaining the same efficiency. The procedure has successfully been able to replace the conventional PCNL in almost all situations barring large staghorn calculi or multiple calculi filling most of the calyces where the operative time may get significantly prolonged.

However, as useful and reproducible results of PCNL might be in normal and native kidneys, its implementation in dealing with calculi in special situations like polycystic kidneys, horseshoe kidneys (HSK), and transplant kidneys is often unfamiliar to a lot of urologists and comes with its own set of attendant challenges. HSKs are the commonest type of renal fusion anomaly and have an estimated incidence of 1 in 400–700 live births from both autopsy and radiographic data [1]. Urolithiasis is the most common complication observed in HSKs and has an incidence of 20–60% [2]. Autosomal dominant polycystic kidney disease (ADPKD) is an inherited disorder affecting 4–six million people worldwide and responsible for up to 10% of people with end-stage renal disease (ESRD) who are on renal replacement therapy (RRT) [3]. Patients with ADPKD have a 5–10 fold higher incidence of nephrolithiasis compared to the general population, affecting 20–28% of patients [4]. While kidney transplant continues to be the treatment of choice for ESRD, it has a significant incidence of urological complications. Allograft urolithiasis though, is rather uncommon and affects between 0.2 and 6% of all renal transplant recipients [5–7].

In the subsequent sections, we will describe in brief, the salient points of urolithiasis in these three special situations, including aggravating factors, indications of and the rationale behind planned interventions. We will also describe in detail the use of PCNL in dealing with such stones, including a brief history, the description of the applied surgical anatomy and technique, the advantages and disadvantages versus other available options, and the expected complications. Occasionally, these situations may need to be extrapolated from the conventional PCNL to mini PCNL where one may not get sufficient literature as the technique is relatively new.

A. Srivastava (✉) · R. Jena
Department of Urology and Renal Transplant, Sanjay Gandhi Postgraduate Institute of Medical Sciences, Lucknow, Uttar Pradesh, India


M. S. Agrawal et al. (eds.), *Minimally Invasive Percutaneous Nephrolithotomy*,
https://doi.org/10.1007/978-981-16-6001-6_27

## 27.2 Upper Tract Urolithiasis in Special Situations

### 27.2.1 Horseshoe Kidney

***Factors Predisposing to Urolithiasis*** In patients with HSKs, the upward migration of the kidneys is arrested in the embryological stage of development due to trapping of the fused lower poles under the inferior mesenteric artery. The alterations in the molecular levels responsible for the arrested ascent of the fused HSK also express themselves in abnormalities of the collecting system and the vasculature [8, 9].

Upper tracts of the HSK have great variations in structure and number in contrast to normal kidneys. Typically, the upper two-thirds of each renal moiety contain the calyces, but the isthmus may be drained by an external calyx or an independent ureter. Secondary hydronephrosis and pelvi-ureteric junction obstruction (PUJO) are a direct result of the high insertion of the ureter into the pelvis, leading to delayed drainage. Added to this is an element of malrotation present in almost all HSKs, which are typically incomplete rotations or non-rotations but can also be hyper-rotation or reverse rotation. The ureter passing over the isthmus has also been postulated to be one of the causes of obstruction. But the predisposition towards nephrolithiasis in HSKs is not just structural. Patients with HSKs have a higher incidence of metabolic abnormalities, up to 100% in some series, including hypercalciuria, hyperoxaluria, hypocitrauria, and hyperuricosuria, leading to supersaturation of urine [8]. Urinary tract infections resulting from urinary stasis also accelerate the process of stone formation. The coexistence of medullary sponge kidney with HSK is another predisposing factor for urolithiasis.

***Indications for Intervention for Urolithiasis in HSK*** Indications for treatment of calculi in HSK are similar to those in normal kidneys. European and American Urological Association guidelines are often used to determine the indications and modalities for treatment of urolithiasis in normal kidneys and these have been extrapolated onto HSKs [10, 11]. Percutaneous nephrolithotomy (PCNL) is indicated for stone burden exceeding 2 cm in HSK, nevertheless, reported stone-free rates range from 65 to 93% and there may be a need for multiple access points [12–16]. Anatomical abnormalities like PUJO and high insertion of the ureter may preclude drainage of stone fragments and therefore in the presence of such factors, even smaller stones may be best suited for PCNL, over modalities like extracorporeal shock wave lithotripsy (ESWL) and ureterorenoscopy (URS) and retrograde intrarenal surgery (RIRS). Additionally, patients who have failed to achieve stone clearance with the abovementioned procedures are also candidates for PCNL.

***Specific Anatomical Considerations for PCNL*** Familiarity with the unique anatomy of the HSK is the key to performing a safe PCNL in these patients. The malrotation of the HSK and its curtailed ascent in the retroperitoneum of the developing embryo place it in a position such that the pelvis is placed anteriorly and the posterior calyces of the upper and middle poles are angled almost directly posteriorly and more medially compared to a normal kidney. The lower pole calyces are usually directed inferiorly and laterally and are difficult to access percutaneously. Therefore, percutaneous access into a posterior superior calyx of the HSK would give easy access to the pelvis and the lateral calyces [17]. But more often than not, a single puncture does not give access to all calyces, and multiple access points are required, especially when dealing with staghorn stones or large stone burdens. Alternatively, a flexible nephroscope may be used. Due to its lower location in the retroperitoneum, the access tract is seldom supracostal in location [18]. However, the anterior and medial location of the HSK may cause the access tract to be longer than in normal kidneys and may pose a problem in obese patients. In addition, a retrorenal colon may be present along with a HSK and preoperative CT is recommended to plan the safest percutaneous access.

***Complications and Stone-free Rates*** Most studies on PCNL in normal kidneys have reported a complication rate in the range 20–40%. PCNL in HSKs has the same set of complications as in normal kidneys [19, 20].A recent multi-centric study on PCNL in HSKs showed an overall complication rate of 17.5% with majority of the complications (>75%) being Clavien Grade I/II complications [15]. The rate of transfusion was 3.8% and the mean fall in hemoglobin was 1.5 g/dl. Immediate stone-free rate (no residual fragments on CT scan) was 50% and immediate success rate (residual fragment <4 mm on CT scan) was 59.2%. Auxiliary procedures in the form of ESWL/RIRS/PCNL were required in 24.5% of the patients and the final success rate (residual fragments <4 mm) was 72.4%. Similar rates of immediate stone-free rates (65–85%) and final success rates (75–92%) were also seen in other studies [13, 16]. More contemporary studies making use of flexible nephroscopes and/or the simultaneous use of flexible URS have reported even higher rates of stone clearance compared to PCNL alone [14, 15]. So, there is enough evidence to understand that PCNL has got acceptable stone clearance rates and complication rates in HSKs, but is not without the need for auxiliary procedures to achieve final stone clearance.

***Supine Versus Prone Positioning*** The unique anatomy of the HSK has influenced traditional teaching to stress upon the fact that the upper pole calyx of the HSK is best amenable to puncture in the prone position and that it gives the best possible access to the collecting system of the kidney during PCNL. While the outcomes with this position have been good and this is an established technique, a lot many urologists around the world have explored the option of supine PCNL in HSKs, just as they have done with PCNL in normal kidneys [15, 21]. The supine position has many proposed advantages over the prone position. Firstly, turning the patient prone is unnecessary and so the operating time is reduced. The Amplatz sheath is in a horizontal or downward direction in supine PCNL, and therefore the irrigation outflow is under low pressure leading to lower chances of pyelovenous backflow and thus reduced chances of infectious postoperative sequalae [22, 23]. Also, supine position gives you the added option of using a flexible URS for combined lithotripsy if the situation arises. As a matter of fact, the only trial comparing the results of supine PCNL to prone in HSKs reported lower operating times with supine PCNL and a higher rate of Clavien Grade 2 complications with lower final stone clearance rates in the prone group. However, it was a retrospective analysis and the results merely give us a hint about the need to pursue this aspect further.

***Role of Other Modalities in the Contemporary Era of mPCNL*** The use of RIRS and ESWL in treating calculi in HSK has increased in parallel to an advancement in technology, and high success rates and low complication rates have been reported even in moderate-sized stones [16, 24]. In a recent study comparing PCNL to RIRS in HSKs with stones with a mean size greater than 2 cm, the initial and final success rates of the two modalities were not statistically different, although patients who underwent RIRS needed a significantly more number of auxiliary procedures to achieve adequate stone clearance [16]. This highlights the importance of mPCNL in this situation. The rate of complications, though not statistically significant was lower in the RIRS group compared to the PCNL group, with a fewer number of Clavien grade II/III complications. Operation time and hospital stay were significantly shorter in the RIRS group. Similar results were reported by Ding et al. [24] In their study, the mean stone size was 29 ± 8 mm and they emphasized that RIRS is better than PCNL for stones less than 3 cm in size with lower complication and comparable success rates. What we have to understand though is that the handling and deflection of the flexible ureteroscope are more difficult within the narrow space provided by the flatter pelvis and the other parts of the collecting system of the HSK. The high insertion of the ureters, the relatively long length of scope remaining outside the urethra and narrower infundibulopelvic angle contribute toward the difficulty of the procedure. Use of a ureteral access sheath helps but due to inferior location of the kidney, care must be taken to prevent mucosal injury and bleeding leading to decreased vision. mPCNL is the ideal option for <3 cm stones with much reduced complication rates as compared to the standard PCNL.

ESWL in treatment of kidney stones in HSK has generally been evaluated in smaller stones (<2 cm). A recent meta-analysis reported that RIRS has a better initial success rate, lower retreatment rate, and final success rate when compared to ESWL, even in the setting of larger stones in the URS group [25]. For now, the role of ESWL lies mainly in initial treatment of smaller stones and as an auxiliary procedure following initial PCNL/RIRS for larger stones.

***Future of mPCNL in Horseshoe Kidneys*** The use of supine PCNL in HSKs has opened up newer venues of treatment. The combined use of supine PCNL and flexible URS in the same sitting, better known as endoscopic combined intrarenal surgery or ECIRS would hopefully lead to better stone clearance rates and lesser number of sessions.

### 27.2.2 Polycystic Kidney

***Factors Predisposing to Urolithiasis*** Approximately 25% of ADPKD patients with urolithiasis are symptomatic, with flank pain and hematuria being the most common symptoms and necessitating urologic intervention [4]. The difficulty in the management of this particular group of patients starts with the diagnosis. The frequent presence of cyst wall and parenchymal calcifications necessitates the use of a non-contrast CT scan for the correct diagnosis and this is the investigation of choice [26]. The higher incidence of nephrolithiasis in ADPKD has been attributed to a combination of anatomical and metabolic factors. Enlarging cysts in the parenchyma cause distortion of the pelvicalyceal system and lead to urinary stasis, delayed washout of crystals, infections, and thus a higher chance of stone formation [27]. Higher the number of cysts and greater the cyst size, greater are the chances of stone formation [28]. A large proportion of patients with ADPKD have hypocitrauria, aciduria, distal acidification defects, defects in ammonia transport in the renal tubule along with low levels of urinary magnesium, potassium, and phosphate. 26 These metabolic abnormalities are major predisposing factors for nephrolithiasis in ADPKD patients. Uric acid and calcium oxalate are the commonest types of stones in ADPKD and low urine pH is thought to be the major contributing factor [4].

***Indications for Intervention for Urolithiasis in ADPKD*** The management of nephrolithiasis in ADPKD follows the same principles as those in the normal kidney. However, closer monitoring and a lower threshold for intervention are necessary, especially in symptomatic patients with deteriorating renal function, recurrent episodes of hematuria, flank pain, and urinary tract infections [4]. The size of the stones, location, and the presence of hydronephrosis are also important determinants of the need for surgical management. While calculi larger than 2 cm are best dealt with by PCNL, in ADPKD, the location of the stone in relation to the cysts and inside the collecting system are important determinants of the modality to be used.

***Specific Anatomical Considerations and Difficulties in Obtaining Access for PCNL*** Cysts in kidneys of ADPKD patients can be hugely enlarged. The compressive effects of these cysts can lead to distortion of the collecting system leading to narrow elongated calyces. The cysts themselves may come in the way when a tract for percutaneous access is planned and may need to be aspirated before attempting a puncture [29]. In addition, calcifications in the cyst wall may appear as radiopaque shadows under fluoroscopic guidance mimicking renal calculi. All of the above factors, including the frequent huge enlargement of the whole kidney, may present difficulties in gaining access and in dilatation of the tract. Patients with ADPKD often present with large stone burdens and multiple access tracts were required in the past. In a kidney affected by ADPKD, the number of normal nephrons is already low. Each tract created for PCNL theoretically leads to destruction of nephrons. So, more the number of tracts more is the loss of remaining viable nephrons. However, this association has not been proven. With the widespread availability of the smaller 20–22Fr size sheaths of mPCNL nephroscopes, the maneuverability inside the PCS is more. The combined use of a flexible nephroscope may also decrease the need for multiple access tracts.

***Obtaining Access: Fluoroscopic vs Ultrasound Guidance*** All reported series on PCNL in polycystic kidneys have used either fluoroscopy or ultrasound guidance or both to gain access into the collecting system [30]. The advantage of ultrasonography is that it helps to delineate the cysts that may lie in the pathway of the planned tract. It helps in the aspiration of a cyst prior to puncture if such a maneuver is planned. Contrast enhanced ultrasound may help in delineating fluid containing cyst from dilated calyx by demonstrating turbulence in the injected contrast unlike the still fluid inside the cysts. Confirmation of ultrasound-guided access can be done by demonstrating jet of saline which is injected through the ureteric catheter from below or by the efflux of methylene blue injected through the ureteric catheter. Ultrasound also helps in differentiating between calculi and cyst wall and parenchymal calcifications, which are quite common in ADPKD. However, fluoroscopy is still more commonly used for calyceal puncture. Urologists are more familiar with the use of fluoroscopy and it provides a more direct evidence of access in contrast to ultrasonography. Tract dilatation, coiling of the guide wire, and delineation of the entire collecting system and the relative position of the calculi is more conveniently achieved under fluoroscopic guidance [29]. Starting with an initial tract size of 14–16 Fr, and upgrading as per stone size and time taken, is what we would recommend.

***Complications and Stone-free Rates*** A recent systematic review reported on the safety and efficacy of PCNL in ADPKD and included 16 case series and 1 cohort study with a total of 237 patients [30]. Stone-free status after a single session ranged from 45 to 100% and 0 to 64% required a second session. The percentage of patients with complications ranged from 0 to 100% and along with the usual complications of fever, bleeding, transfusion, and infection expected after PCNL, authors also reported greater chances of postoperative urine leakage, hydro- and pneumothorax, cyst infection, perirenal hematoma, renal pelvic perforations, and worsening of renal failure. However, the largest series was of only 30 patients and it is difficult to generalize these findings to all patients of ADPKD with urolithiasis. The increased incidence of above complications is probably because of creation of tracts through the cyst and the thinned out renal parenchyma not being able to provide adequate tamponade and contain the urine leak and bleeding. Hence, it is pertinent that urologists try to get a proper access as far as possible.

We had reported on a series of 22 patients with ADPKD who underwent PCNL at our institute way back in 2012 and since then we have treated 23 patients more [29]. In our original study, we had PCNL on a total of 25 renal units. The mean stone size was 2.4 ± 0.8 cm. Multiple access tracts were required in 5 cases. The immediate success rate was 80% and 3 patients who needed auxiliary procedures (2 PCNL and 1 ESWL) achieved 100% stone clearance. The findings in our subsequent patients have been similar.

***Role of Other Modalities in Contemporary Era of mPCNL*** ESWL is very frequently used for the treatment of calculi in ADPKD. Although noninvasive and convenient for patients, there are concerns about the possible risk of hemorrhage into the cysts and traumatic loss of nephrons, although these have not been demonstrated in clinical studies. However, the anatomical distortion of the collecting system leads to decreased clearance of stones and is a reason why ESWL is not suitable for larger stones in ADPKD. Coagulopathies and uncontrolled hypertension are also contraindications to ESWL. RIRS has the advantage of being a natural orifice surgery. The flexible tip of the ureteroscope and laser fiber can negotiate the elongated and narrow spaces of the collecting system, thus providing an advantage in stones in the hard to reach areas of the kidney. Even in normal kidneys, the main advantage of RIRS over PCNL or ESWL is in stones <1.5 cm located in the lower pole. But in polycystic kidneys, this advantage holds true for small stones in all calyces.

### 27.2.3 Post-transplant Kidney

Stones are uncommon in transplanted kidneys, with an incidence of 0.2% to 6.3% [31, 32]. Because of denervation of the allograft, more than half of patients present without any symptoms of pain. Hematuria, oliguria, or anuria could be one of the presenting symptoms.

***Factors Predisposing to Urolithiasis*** Allograft stones are usually the result of new stone formation but an allograft may also contain an in situ stone which is termed as donor gifted allograft lithiasis. The predisposing factors may be urinary stress, reflux, recurrent urinary tract infections, renal tubular acidosis, supersaturated urine, decreased inhibitor activity, tertiary hyperparathyroidism, hypercalcemia, or hypercalciuria [33, 34].

***Specific Anatomical Considerations*** Since Fisher et al. reported the successful management of allograft stones with PCNL in 1982, it has been a popular approach. The superficial location of transplanted kidneys makes PCNL the best treatment option for the management of all kinds of allograft stones including those following failure of ESWL. One major reported concern is the presence of perirenal fibrosis which causes difficulty and kinking of guide wire, etc. during the tract dilatation and limited mobility of kidney during rigid nephroscopy.

The anterior and posterior calyces of an allograft kidney will be oriented differently than in a normal kidney because of the frequent practice of putting a left kidney in the right iliac fossa. Even when a right-sided kidney has been placed in the right iliac fossa, the anteroposterior, longitudinal and coronal planes will be different than in a normal kidney. Some patients who have had their renal allografts placed intraperitoneally may present unique challenges, due to close proximity of the bowel on the anterior surface of the kidney.

***Technique of mPCNL in Transplant Kidney*** The armamentarium remains the same as is used in all other situations. Sheath size ranges from 14 to 22 Fr. However, the technique differs from most of the other normal or aberrant situations. Due to the aberrant location of ureteric orifice near the dome or on the anterolateral wall, the passage of a ureteral catheter is extremely difficult despite the use of 70- or 120-degree lens or other maneuvers. As a result, the preoperative opacification of the collecting system which is the pre-requisite for the fluoroscopy-guided puncture is not attainable. A well-performed NCCT scan is traditionally used to evaluate the calyceal anatomy. A suitable calyx for percutaneous access though is identified by ultrasonography immediately prior to planning a puncture at the time of surgery.

***Initial Puncture*** *Use of Storz trocar and cannula*—as the tract is fibrotic we recommend using the central rod of the Alken dilator, which is 8 Fr over the Terumo guide wire which has already been placed after the initial puncture of the desired calyx. Subsequently, the tract is dilated one time either by a 14 or 20 Fr. Teflon dilator depending upon the need to introduce a 15Fr or the 22Fr mPCNL sheath. This facilitates the insertion of the desired sheath. A super-stiff guide wire may also be used alternatively with 18 Fr fascial dilator as suggested by Chao Wei et al. [35]

Most of the studies once again mention the experience with standard PCNL. There are very few studies where the authors used some kind of miniaturization of sheath size which has become standard of care recently. He et al. were the first to use miniaturized instruments for PCNL in the setting of a transplant kidney. They placed a 16 Fr peel away sheath as an access port and used 8.5/11.5 Fr nephroscope or a 8/9.8 Fr ureteroscope [36]. They argued that the smaller tract (16Fr) can significantly decrease the risk of bleeding and tearing of renal cortex. The data from Desai et al. for managing stones in children also support the use of mPCNL, who reported that the degree of dilation and the size of sheath introduced are the most critical considerations in reducing blood loss during PCNL [37]. Jackman et al. used an 11 Fr access sheath in pre-school children to decrease the risk of bleeding as compared to standard PCNL [38]. The mean diameter of stone was 1.7 cm and mean Hb decline was 0.51 g/dl. The stone fragmentation was 100% with no complications. Munk et al. has described the use of 15Fr nephroscopes for management of calculi in renal allografts [39].

***Combined Use of Ultrasound and Fluoroscopy for Access*** Rifaioglu et al. in 2008 reported 15 cases with a mean age of 48 years using 14 Fr to 30 Fr sheath with ultrasound along or with ultrasound and fluoroscopy for initial puncture. The mean stone diameter was 1.3 cm. The stone-free ratio was 100% with no reported complications [40].

***Role of Other Modalities in the Era of mPCNL*** ESWL and ureteroscopy (flexible or rigid) are alternative options to minimally invasive approach in a transplanted kidney. The retrograde rigid or flexible ureteroscopy is not popular due to technical difficulties in access to the upper tract via bladder. Most of the ureteric anastomosis are done either on the dome or anterior wall. Even if an anastomosis is done posterolaterally, it is difficult to pass a guide wire through the ureteric orifice and complete the procedure with safety and efficacy. Antegrade ureteroscopy has been described historically when the tailor-made mPCNL instruments were not available and a rigid ureteroscope was passed through a smaller sheath after doing ultrasound-guided punctures. ESWL similarly had been an attractive option in the past notwithstanding its several limitations in treatment of the allograft lithiasis.

First of all, locating the renal stones may be difficult due to position of the kidney over the bony pelvis. The clearance of stone fragments can be limited, especially with lower calyceal stones. Subsequently, if the steinstrasse forms, it is difficult to access the lead fragment by retrograde ureteroscopy as mentioned above and one may have to resort to mPCNL for either a residual fragment or a steinstrasse. Finally, ESWL appears to require several treatment sessions and auxiliary procedures. Chellcombe et al. reported that of the 13 patients treated by ESWL, eight required several sessions and another 8 required a ureteric stent insertion before a second procedure and 04 required a nephrostomy tube to relieve obstruction.

## 27.3 Points to Remember

- PCNL in congenital anomalies like HSKs, cystic diseases like ADPKD and in situations like renal allograft lithiasis may be more technically demanding and with lower stone clearance rates, than in normal kidneys.
- In spite of the technical challenges, it is still the procedure of choice in such situations for large renal calculi.
- mPCNL overcomes a lot of potential adverse effects of using the larger standard PCNL instruments in such situations and also has the theoretical advantage of greater stone clearance due to greater maneuverability inside the PCS.
- Modifications of patient positioning, techniques of puncture, use of combined ultrasound and fluoroscopic guidance and miniaturization of instruments allow us to overcome these challenges to a great extent.

## References

1. Glodny B, Petersen J, Hofmann KJ, Schenk C, Herwig R, Trieb T, Koppelstaetter C, Steingruber I, Rehder P. Kidney fusion anomalies revisited: clinical and radiological analysis of 209 cases of crossed fused ectopia and horseshoe kidney. BJU Int. 2009;103(2):224–35.
2. Lampel A, Hohenfellner M, Schultz-Lampel D, Lazica M, Bohnen K, Thüroff JW. Urolithiasis in horseshoe kidneys: therapeutic management. Urology. 1996;47(2):182–6.

3. Nishiura JL, Neves RF, Eloi SR, Cintra SM, Ajzen SA, Heilberg IP. Evaluation of nephrolithiasis in autosomal dominant polycystic kidney disease patients. Clin J Am Soc Nephrol. 2009;4(4):838–44.
4. Mufti UB, Nalagatla SK. Nephrolithiasis in autosomal dominant polycystic kidney disease. J Endourol. 2010;24(10):1557–61.
5. Shoskes DA, Hanbury D, Cranston D, Morris PJ. Urological complications in 1,000 consecutive renal transplant recipients. J Urol. 1995;153(1):18–21.
6. Benoit G, Blanchet P, Eschwege P, Jardin A, Charpentier B. Occurrence and treatment of kidney graft lithiasis in a series of 1500 patients. Clin Transpl. 1996;10(2):176–80.
7. Sarier M, Duman I, Yuksel Y, Tekin S, Demir M, Arslan F, Ergun O, Kosar A, Yavuz AH. Results of minimally invasive surgical treatment of allograft lithiasis in live-donor renal transplant recipients: a single-center experience of 3758 renal transplantations. Urolithiasis. 2019;47(3):273–8.
8. Balawender K, Cisek A, Cisek E, Orkisz S. Anatomical and clinical aspects of horseshoe kidney: a review of the current literature. Int J Morphol. 2019;37(1):12–6.
9. Taghavi K, Kirkpatrick J, Mirjalili SA. The horseshoe kidney: surgical anatomy and embryology. J Pediatr Urol. 2016;12(5):275–80.
10. Türk C, Petřík A, Sarica K, Seitz C, Skolarikos A, Straub M, Knoll T. EAU guidelines on diagnosis and conservative management of urolithiasis. Eur Urol. 2016;69(3):468–74.
11. Assimos D, Krambeck A, Miller NL, Monga M, Murad MH, Nelson CP, Pace KT, Pais VM, Pearle MS, Preminger GM, Razvi H. Surgical management of stones: American Urological Association/Endourological Society guideline, Part I. J Urol. 2016;196(4):1153–60.
12. Wu W, Zhao Z, Zhu H, Yang D, Ou L, Liang Y, Zhao Z, Zeng G. Safety and efficacy of minimally invasive percutaneous nephrolithotomy in treatment of calculi in horseshoe kidneys. J Endourol. 2014;28(8):926–9.
13. Etemadian M, Maghsoudi R, Abdollahpour V, Amjadi M. Percutaneous nephrolithotomy in horseshoe kidney: our 5-year experience. Urol J. 2013;10(2):856–60.
14. Blackburne AT, Rivera ME, Gettman MT, Patterson DE, Krambeck AE. Endoscopic management of urolithiasis in the horseshoe kidney. Urology. 2016;1(90):45–9.
15. Vicentini FC, Mazzucchi E, Gökçe Mİ, Sofer M, Tanidir Y, Sener TE, Melo PA, Eisner BH, Batter T, Chi T, Armas-Phan M. Percutaneous nephrolithotomy in horseshoe kidneys: results of a multicentric study. J Endourol. 2020;35(7):979–84.
16. Kartal I, Çakıcı MÇ, Selmi V, Sarı S, Özdemir H, Ersoy H. Retrograde intrarenal surgery and percutaneous nephrolithotomy for the treatment of stones in horseshoe kidney; what are the advantages and disadvantages compared to each other? Cent European J Urol. 2019;72(2):156.
17. Elliott VL, Clements T, Gettle L, et al. Management of stones in anomalous kidneys. AUA Update Series. 2010;29:210–9.
18. Shokeir AA, El-Nahas AR, Shoma AM, Eraky I, El-Kenawy M, Mokhtar A, El-Kappany H. Percutaneous nephrolithotomy in treatment of large stones within horseshoe kidneys. Urology. 2004;64(3):426–9.
19. Labate G, Modi P, Timoney A, Cormio L, Zhang X, Louie M, Grabe M, de la Rosette J, On behalf of the CROES PCNL Study Group. The percutaneous nephrolithotomy global study: classification of complications. J Endourol. 2011;25(8):1275–80.
20. Michel MS, Trojan L, Rassweiler JJ. Complications in percutaneous nephrolithotomy. Eur Urol. 2007;51(4):899–906.
21. Sohail N, Albodour A, Abdelrahman KM, Bhatti KH. Supine percutaneous nephrolithotomy in horseshoe kidney. J Taibah Univ Medical Sci. 2017;12(3):261–4.
22. Li J, Gao L, Li Q, Zhang Y, Jiang Q. Supine versus prone position for percutaneous nephrolithotripsy: a meta-analysis of randomized controlled trials. Int J Surg. 2019;1(66):62–71.
23. Vicentini FC, Perrella R, Souza VM, Hisano M, Murta CB, Claro JF. Impact of patient position on the outcomes of percutaneous neprolithotomy for complex kidney stones. Int Braz J Urol. 2018;44(5):965–71.
24. Ding J, Huang Y, Gu S, Chen Y, Peng J, Bai Q, Ye M, Qi J. Flexible ureteroscopic management of horseshoe kidney renal calculi. Int Braz J Urol. 2015;41(4):683–9.
25. Chen H, Chen G, Pan Y, Zhu Y, Xiong C, Chen H, Yang Z. No wound for stones< 2 cm in horseshoe kidney: a systematic review of comparative studies. Urol Int. 2019;103(3):249–55.
26. Gupta S, Seith A, Sud K, Kohli HS, Singh SK, Sakhuja V, Suri S. CT in the evaluation of complicated autosomal dominant polycystic kidney disease. Acta Radiol. 2000;41(3):280–4.
27. Grampsas SA, Chandhoke PS, Fan J, Glass MA, Townsend R, Johnson AM, Gabow P. Anatomic and metabolic risk factors for nephrolithiasis in patients with autosomal dominant polycystic kidney disease. Am J Kidney Dis. 2000;36(1):53–7.
28. Torres VE, Wilson DM, Hattery RR, Segura JW. Renal stone disease in autosomal dominant polycystic kidney disease. Am J Kidney Dis. 1993;22(4):513–9.
29. Srivastava A, Bansal R, Srivastava A, Chaturvedi S, Ranjan P, Ansari MS, Yadav A, Kapoor R. Percutaneous nephrolithotomy in polycystic kidney disease: is it safe and effective? Int Urol Nephrol. 2012;44(3):725–30.
30. Kalatharan V, Jandoc R, Grewal G, Nash DM, Welk B, Sarma S, Pei Y, Garg AX. Efficacy and safety of surgical kidney stone interventions in autosomal dominant polycystic kidney disease: a systematic review. Can J Kidney Health Dis. 2020;7:2054358120940433.

31. Crook TJ, Keoghane SR. Renal transplant lithiasis: rare but time-consuming. BJU Int. 2005;95(7):931–3.
32. Khositseth S, Gillingham KJ, Cook ME, Chavers BM. Urolithiasis after kidney transplantation in pediatric recipients: a single center report. Transplantation. 2004;78(9):1319–23.
33. Klingler HC, Kramer G, Lodde M, Marberger M. Urolithiasis in allograft kidneys. Urology. 2002;59(3):344–8.
34. Habbig S, Beck BB, Feldkötter M, Körber F, Laffeber C, Verkoelen C, Mihatsch MJ, Hoppe B. Renal allograft calcification–prevalence and etiology in pediatric patients. Am J Nephrol. 2009;30(3):194–200.
35. Wei C, Zhang Y, Pokhrel G, Gan J, Liu X, Ye Z, Yuan X, Guo X. Percutaneous nephrolithotomy under ultrasound guidance in treating allograft stones. Int J Clin Exp Med. 2018;11(8):8352–7.
36. He Z, Li X, Chen L, Zeng G, Yuan J. Minimally invasive percutaneous nephrolithotomy for upper urinary tract calculi in transplanted kidneys. BJU Int. 2007;99(6):1467–71.
37. Desai MR, Kukreja RA, Patel SH, Bapat SD. Percutaneous nephrolithotomy for complex pediatric renal calculus disease. J Endourol. 2004;18(1):23–7.
38. Jackman SV, Docimo SG, Cadeddu JA, Bishoff JT, Kavoussi LR, Jarrett TW. The "mini-perc" technique: a less invasive alternative to percutaneous nephrolithotomy. World J Urol. 1998;16(6):371–4.
39. Rifaioglu MM, Berger AD, Pengune W, Stoller ML. Percutaneous management of stones in transplanted kidneys. Urology. 2008;72(3):508–12.
40. Challacombe B, Dasgupta P, Tiptaft R, Glass J, Koffman G, Goldsmith D, Khan MS. Multimodal management of urolithiasis in renal transplantation. BJU Int. 2005;96(3):385–9.

# Paediatric Mini PCNL

# 28

Patrick Juliebø-Jones, Anna Brewin,
and Bhaskar Somani

## 28.1 Introduction

The incidence of paediatric kidney stone disease (KSD) is rising and recurrence rates over a 10-year period reach 50% according to studies [1, 2]. Stone composition is similar to adult KSD with majority being calcium oxalate stones. However, many cases may still be associated with a metabolic cause such as hypocitraturia and hypercalciuria [3].

The need for effective and safe surgical approaches to formally treat this condition is therefore paramount. Indications for paediatric percutaneous nephrolithotomy (PCNL) include stones larger than 2 cm, and stone(s) is refractory to shockwave lithotripsy (SWL) or likely to be unsuccessful with SWL and/or ureteroscopy (URS) [4]. The first series to describe paediatric PCNL was by Woodside et al. in 1985 [5]. In paediatric urology, the trend in minimally invasive surgical treatments is rising and this applies to PCNL as well [6]. This shift also largely reflects the uptake of miniaturised PCNL since the 'mini-perc' method was first described in paediatric setting by Jackman et al. in 1998 [7]. As outlined later in this chapter, the advantages associated with this newer generation of instruments are numerous. However, the potential and requirement for an improved safety profile hold arguably even greater relevance in the paediatric setting.

## 28.2 Pre-operative Considerations

Up to date ultrasound is the imaging modality of choice to assess stone burden albeit, evaluation of the ureter is poorer (sensitivity 44–90%) [8]. Plain X-ray also holds limitations in children due to the greater presence of bowel gas (Fig. 28.1). Plain film can be combined with US to help minimise radiation yet increase sensitivity to ureteral stones. Phleboliths are less common in children [9]. Intravenous urogram (IVU), while its application is rare in modern clinical practice, does still remains a possible alternative and its application persists in developing countries [10]. Low-dose computed tomography (CT) can be considered in select cases and older children (Fig. 28.2). An advantage of CT is the option of 3D reconstruction, which can ameliorate treatment planning, e.g. for complex vasculature [11].

P. Juliebø-Jones
Department of Urology, Haukeland University Hospital, Bergen, Norway

A. Brewin
University Hospital Southampton NHS Trust, Southampton, UK
e-mail: a.e.brewin@doctors.org.uk

B. Somani (✉)
Professor and Consultant Urological Surgeon, University Hospital Southampton, Hampshire, UK


M. S. Agrawal et al. (eds.), *Minimally Invasive Percutaneous Nephrolithotomy*,
https://doi.org/10.1007/978-981-16-6001-6_28

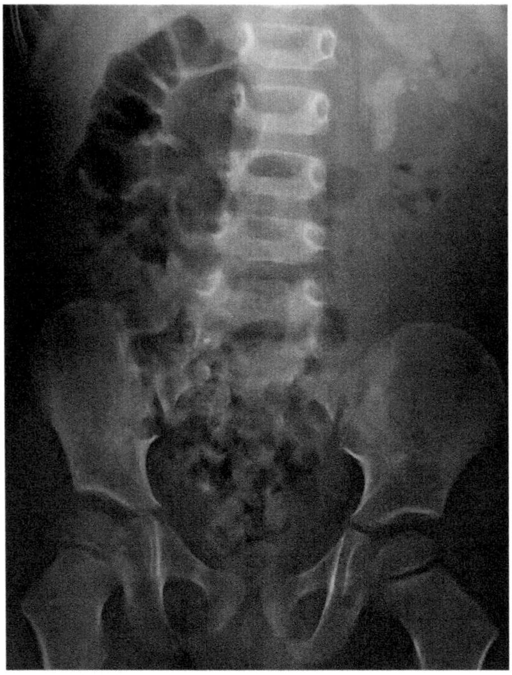

**Fig. 28.1** Plain X-ray demonstrating left side stone filling renal pelvis

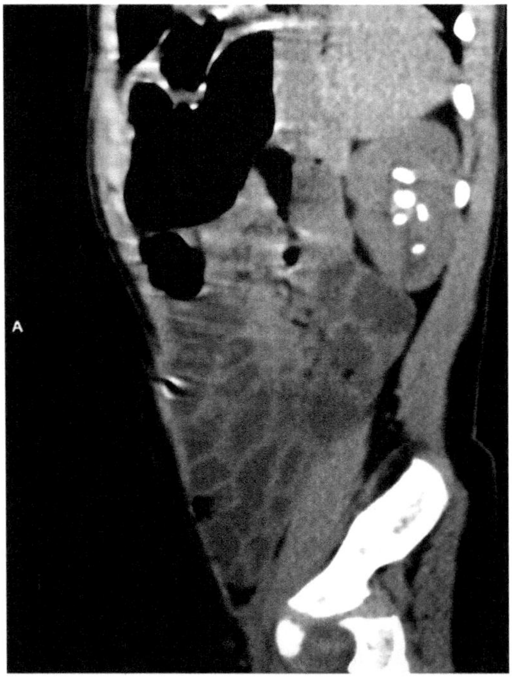

**Fig. 28.2** Sagittal view of CT showing multiple stones in the kidney

The authors encourage observing the principle of ALARA (as low as reasonably achievable) in relation to radiation dose and choice of imaging modality [12]. Each case should be discussed at a multidisciplinary meeting including paediatric urologists, nephrologists and radiologists. This can be complemented by other specialities such as dietetics for nutritional support and endocrinology for metabolic expertise. This form of planning will allow for optimisation of the patient and help long-term management after surgical intervention. In contrast to adults, the EAU guidelines recommend formal metabolic evaluation in all cases of paediatric KSD [13]. Karabacak et al. examined the metabolic profiles of all paediatric cases presenting with KSD at their institution over a 9-year period and reported 57.7% to have hypocitraturia [14]. Original studies also show that obesity does not appear to be linked to paediatric KSD unlike in the adult population [3].

As well as up-to-date imaging, obtainment of a pre-operative urine culture is considered mandatory. If there is a suggestion or proven urinary tract infection (UTI), this must be treated appropriately prior to any intervention.

## 28.3 Set-up and Positioning

Many of the operative steps remain the same as for adults [15–18]. General anaesthesia is carried out in nearly all cases. Paediatric patients are more susceptible to hypothermia and therefore close temperature monitoring should be supported by warming irrigation fluid and minimising operating time [19]. Protection of pressure points with padding should be carried out and this is of high importance in patients with conditions such as meningomyelocele. Special attention should also be paid to patients with anatomy such as spinal deformities (more common in paediatric KSD) where there is a risk of excessive flexion or joint contortion [17]. At the beginning of the surgery, the patient is positioned in lithotomy position and a retrograde pyelogram is carried out to delineate the pelvicalyceal system. The majority of cases are then carried out in prone position and bolsters should be placed to lift and support the chest and abdomen [20]. Towel rolls are preferred to the stiffer bolsters commonly used in adult cases. The surgeon should personally supervise the positioning of the patient at all times. Disadvantages related to the prone approach are the added challenges presented to the anaesthetist such as airway management with endotracheal tube and emergency situations, e.g. cardiac arrest or respiratory compromise. Additional supportive equipment may also be required, e.g. stabilising helmet, mattress, pillows and extra cost can therefore be incurred [21]. However, prone positioning does allow for the option of multiple punctures via a larger operative field. The supine position, developed more recently, overcomes these airways difficulties and provides the surgeon and anaesthetist with a more comfortable working position as well as both reduced overall time in the operating theatre and less radiation exposure [20]. It also allows for simultaneous retrograde intra-renal surgery to be performed if indicated. This is at the cost of greater kidney mobility, a more limited anatomical area that can be potentially accessed, e.g. lower calyx and the requirement for a longer percutaneous tract.

## 28.4 Accessing the Collecting System and Tract Dilatation

Either fluoroscopy or ultrasound can be used to identify the calyx of choice [22]. The latter modality eliminates the risk of radiation exposure and holds the additional ability of revealing radiolucent stones and surrounding viscera. Ultrasound also facilitates easier assessment of puncture depth. Careful attention needs to be paid to the infundibular anatomy. Accessing the collecting system is arguably the most important part of the operation. Hypermobility of a smaller kidney presents added complexity compared to adult surgery. Once the proposed site has been determined, the instrument size and number of punctures should be agreed upon.

Puncture is then gained using bull's eye or triangulation technique and aspiration of urine/contrast should follow [23]. The guide wire can then be passed into the urinary system.

Skin incision and dilators allow for placement of the auxiliary and working wire [24]. Serial dilation can be performed to secure the desired tract size. A smaller tract can be converted to a larger size during the procedure if needed. Requirement for bigger tract size(s) may be anticipated in larger stone burdens and older children.

### 28.4.1 Stone Fragmentation and Exit Strategy

While larger instruments still rely on pneumatic lithotripter, the newer generation of smaller instruments employ laser fragmentation [25]. Collection of fragments for biochemical stone analysis is important and still possible for most minimally invasive PCNL techniques.

However, in micro-PCNL (4.8F) this is not possible. Given these fragments cannot be collected, patients are also more likely to develop post-operative colic as a complication.

Historically, nephrostomy tube placement takes place at end of standard PCNL. This also allows for nephrostogram or planned relook PCNL. This is carried out less often in miniaturised PCNL, especially ultra-mini and micro PCNL. Patients will usually have a temporary ureteral catheter (78%) or double J stent (21%) [26].

## 28.5 Complications

Recent data from a national database of paediatric PCNL in the United States of America (USA) reported stone-free rates (SFR) exceeding 90% in a single sitting and reported an overall complication rate of 20.7% [27]. Post-operative bleeding rates requiring blood transfusion have been recorded as high as 24% [15]. While the efficacy of PCNL is therefore not in question, there exists margin for improvement in regard to the complication profile.

Multiple original studies and subsequent meta-analyses evaluating the outcomes associated with miniaturised PCNL have supported the theory that tract size does influence the complication profile [28, 29]. Significantly higher rates of haematuria and renal extravasation have been associated with larger tract sizes [26]. Studies employing pre- and post-surgery (12–24Fr) dimercaptosuccinic acid (DMSA) imaging reveal no detriment to the renal function [30].

## 28.6 Assessment of Stone-free Rate

In all cases, the treatment goal is to achieve the highest stone clearance in the least number of sittings [31]. This would be complete clearance in a single surgery if possible. As for pre-operative imaging, ultrasound serves as the first-line imaging modality in the majority of centres. Again, this can be selectively supplemented with low-dose CT imaging. It is widely accepted, however, that it is more difficult to reliably determine the true SFR in paediatric cases compared to adult cases with the reduced use of CT scans. Centres reporting outcomes for audit and research purposes are encouraged to adopt a standardised approach. This does represent a challenge as there still exists a lack of consensus and several classifications have been proposed [32].

## 28.7 Follow-up of Patients

As with the pre-operative assessment and treatment the follow-up pathway will adopt a tailored approach. This is based on patient's unique stone burden, age and past medical history including any special metabolic or anatomical considerations. In those patients with significant residual fragments, an auxiliary procedure will be planned. This can be in the form of repeat PCNL or an alternative such as URS or SWL. Endoscopic combined intrarenal surgery (ECIRS) has also been described in the paediatric setting and this could also serve as a possible 'sandwich therapy' [33, 34]. The multidisciplinary clinic also serves an added role in helping to identify risk factors and guide tailored recommendations for these patients, especially given the risk of recurrence is high. Education and preventive measures are of great importance given that this patient population may face a lifetime of kidney stone-related problems. Childhood obesity is a growing public health concern and is also associated with increased risk of stone formation. This represents just one area where input of dietary specialists can be invaluable.

## 28.8 Current Evidence of Mini PCNL (mPCNL)

In a recent systematic review of paediatric mPCNL, 8 studies included 384 patients with a mean age of 7.5 years [35] (Table 28.1). While the age ranged from 0.5 to 18 years, the mean stone size was 1.2 cm and ranged from 0.8 to 3.5 cm. Majority of the stone location was in the lower pole (57%) and renal pelvis (24%). The mean initial and overall stone-free rate was 87.9% and 97%, respectively. The overall complication rate was 19% with a mean transfusion rate of 3.3% with the authors concluding that mPCNL is safe and effective in the paediatric population.

## 28.9 Modifications and Further Considerations

With sufficient experience of PCNL in the adult setting, the transfer of skills to paediatric PCNL is generally considered to be very achievable. As part of the learning curve, initial surgeries are recommended to take place in older children with more optimal physical conditioning and smaller stone burdens [31]. With regards to the operating team, a twin model surgeon approach has been described and adopted by some centres [36]. This draws on the combined experience and expertise of both paediatric urologist and adult endourologist [9]. Overall, there is a paucity of original studies relating to paediatric endourology in comparison to adults [8]. Much of the international guidelines are therefore driven by lower levels of evidence such as cohort studies rather than randomised controlled trials. More RCTs are needed, especially comparing interventions, e.g. ureteroscopy versus mini PCNL.

**Table 28.1** Published paediatric papers on mini PCNL (demographics and results)

| Author (year) | Sample size (male/female ratio) | Mean age—years | Mean stone size—cm | Initial SFR (%) | Overall SFR (%) | Adverse events (n) |
|---|---|---|---|---|---|---|
| Zeng (2012) | 24 (1.6:1) | 1.92 | 2.14 | 84 | 91.3 | Fever (4) |
| Brodie (2015) | 46 (2.1:1) | 7.3 | NR | 76 | 97.9 | Anaemia (1) |
| Xiao (2015) | 68 (1.4:1) | 2.02 | 1.92 | 94 | NR | Fever (5), Pleural effusion (5) |
| Kumar (2015) | 106 (0.9:1) | 10.3 | 1.27 | NR | 94.3 | UTI (9), Pain (5), Bleeding 11 |
| D'Souza (2016) | 20 (NR) | 11.25 | 1.36 | 90 | 100 | Transfusion (2), Sepsis (1) |
| Farouk (2018) | 54 (1.7:1) | 6.48 | 1.59 | 88.9 | 92.59 | UTI (6), Bleeding (2), Extravasation (2), Perinephric haematoma (2) |
| Shrestha (2018) | 26 (3.3/1) | 10.8 | 1.92 | 84.61 | 100 | Pain (13), Extravasation (1), Haematuria—self resolution (1) Transfusion (1) |
| Jones (2020) | 40 (1.7:1) | 8.8 | 1.45 | 97.5 | 97.5 | Haematuria (3), Fever (3) |

*UTI* urinary tract infection, *NR* not reported, *SFR* stone-free rate

New areas of development include the recent preliminary reports of a newly developed technique 'the needle perc', a 4.2-Fr system. This is the smallest technique to have been established to date. Xiao et al. performed this procedure in 8 pre-school children with a mean stone size of 1.6 cm [37].

While bilateral synchronous PCNL has been described in a number of adult settings, its practice has only been very scarcely reported in the paediatric setting [38, 39]. In cases of bilateral stone disease, the authors still recommend a staged approach. Predictive nomograms such as the Guy's stone score (GSS) are now well established in adult settings but remain under-reported in paediatrics. Few studies have attempted to determine its efficacy in children and concluded that it can successfully predict SFR but not complications. This is largely because it does not hold sufficiently reflect characteristics that are particular to children such as congenital anatomical abnormalities [40]. A final area for future research is the establishment of guidelines for radiation exposure in children undergoing diagnostic and therapeutic imaging [41].

## References


1. Sharma AP, Filler G. Epidemiology of pediatric urolithiasis. Indian J Urol. 2010;26(4):516–22.
2. Rukin NJ, Siddiqui ZA, Chedgy EC, et al. Trends in upper tract stone disease in England: evidence from the hospital episodes statistics database. Urol Int. 2017;98(4):391–6.
3. Issler N, Dufek S, Kleta R, Bockenhauer D, Smeulders N, Van't Hoff W. Epidemiology of paediatric renal stone disease: a 22-year single centre experience in the UK. BMC Nephrol. 2017;18(1):136. https://doi.org/10.1186/s12882-017-0505-x.
4. Türk C, Neisius A, Petrik A, Seitz C, Skolarikos A, Tepeler A, Thomas K. Urolithiasis. Arnhem: European Association of Urology; 2017.
5. Woodside JR, Stevens GF, Stark GL, Borden TA, Ball WS. Percutaneous stone removal in children. J Urol. 1985;134(6):1166–7. https://doi.org/10.1016/s0022-5347(17)47669-5.
6. Pietropaolo A, Proietti S, Jones P, et al. Bibliometric trends of intervention for paediatric stone disease over the last two decades. Arab J Urol. 2017;15(4):306–11.
7. Jackman SV, Hedican SP, Peters CA, et al. Percutaneous nephrolithotomy in infants and preschool age children: experience with a new technique. Urology. 1998;52:697–701.
8. Grivas N, Thomas K, Drake T, et al. Imaging modalities and treatment of paediatric upper tract urolithiasis: a systematic review and update on behalf of the EAU urolithiasis guidelines panel. J Pediatr

Urol. 2020;16(5):612–24. https://doi.org/10.1016/j.jpurol.2020.07.003.
9. Marquis JR. The incidence of pelvic phleboliths in pediatric patients. Pediatr Radiol. 1977;5(4):211–2. https://doi.org/10.1007/BF00972179.
10. Marra G, Taroni F, Berrettini A, et al. Pediatric nephrolithiasis: a systematic approach from diagnosis to treatment. J Nephrol. 2019;32:199–210. https://doi.org/10.1007/s40620-018-0487-1.
11. Tailly T, Denstedt J. Innovations in percutaneous nephrolithotomy. Int J Surg. 2016;36(Pt D):665–72. https://doi.org/10.1016/j.ijsu.2016.11.007.
12. Ost MC. Radiation exposure in pediatric urology patients: how to adhere to ALARA. J Urol. 2018;199(2):351–2. https://doi.org/10.1016/j.juro.2017.11.063.
13. Tekgül S, Dogan HS, Hoebeke P, Kocvara R, Nijman JM, Radmayr C. EAU guidelines on paediatric urology. Eur Assoc Urol. 2016;40(5):589–99. Available at: https://uroweb.org/wp-content/uploads/EAU-Guidelines-Paediatric-Urology-2016-1.pdf
14. Karabacak OR, Ipek B, Ozturk U, et al. Metabolic evaluation in stone disease metabolic differences between the pediatric and adult patients with stone disease. Urology. 2010;76(1):238–41. https://doi.org/10.1016/j.urology.2010.01.036.
15. Zeren S, Satar N, Bayazit Y, Bayazit AK, Payasli K, Ozkeçeli R. Percutaneous nephrolithotomy in the management of pediatric renal calculi. J Endourol. 2002;16:75.
16. Sultan S, Aba Umer S, Ahmed B, Naqvi SAA, Rizvi SAH. Update on surgical management of pediatric urolithiasis. Front Pediatr. 2019;3(7):252. https://doi.org/10.3389/fped.2019.00252.
17. Ganpule AP, Mishra S, Desai MR. Percutaneous nephrolithotomy for pediatric urolithiasis. Indian J Urol. 2010;26:549–54.
18. Sabnis RB, Chhabra JS, Ganpule AP, Abrol S, Desai MR. Current role of PCNL in paediatric urolithiasis. Curr Urol Rep. 2014;15:423.
19. Roberts S, Bolton DM, Stoller ML. Hypothermia associated with percutaneous nephrolithotomy. Urology. 1994;44:832–5.
20. Gamal W, Moursy E, Hussein M, Mmdouh A, Hammady A, Aldahshoury M. Supine pediatric percutaneous nephrolithotomy (PCNL). J Pediatr Urol. 2015;11(2):78.e1–78.e785. https://doi.org/10.1016/j.jpurol.2014.10.012.
21. Proietti S, Rodríguez-Socarrás ME, Eisner B, De Coninck V, Sofer M, Saitta G, Rodriguez-Monsalve M, d'Orta C, Bellinzoni P, Gaboardi F, Giusti G. Supine percutaneous nephrolithotomy: tips and tricks. Transl Androl Urol. 2019;8(Suppl 4):S381–8. https://doi.org/10.21037/tau.2019.07.09.
22. Kyriazis I, Liatsikos E, Sopilidis O, Kallidonis P, Skolarikos A. European section of urotechnology educational video on fluoroscopic-guided puncture in percutaneous nephrolithotomy: all techniques step by step. BJUI Int. 2017;120(5):739–41.
23. Schuster TK, Smaldone MC, Averch TD, Ost MC. Percutanous nephrolithotomy in children. J Endourol. 2009;23(10):1699–705.
24. Sharma G, Sharma A. Determining the angle and depth of puncture for fluoroscopy-guided percutaneous renal access in the prone position. Indian J Urol. 2015;31(1):38–41. https://doi.org/10.4103/0970-1591.145291.
25. Gnessin E, Chertin L, Chertin B. Current management of paediatric urolithiasis. Pediatr Surg Int. 2012;28(7):659–65.
26. Jones P, Aboumarzouk O, Griffin S, et al. Role of minimally invasive PCNL techniques: micro and ultra-mini PCNL (15Fr) in the paediatric population – a systematic review. J Endourol. 2017;31(9):816–24.
27. Dombrovskiy V, Olweny EO. Percutaneous nephrolithotomy in children: analysis of nationwide hospitalizations and short-term outcomes for the United States, 2001-2014. J Endourol. 2018;32:912e8.
28. Wright A, Rukin N, Smith D, et al. Mini, ultra, micro - nomenclature and cost of these new minimally invasive percutaneous nephrolithotomy (PCNL) techniques. Ther Adv Urol. 2016;8(2):142–6. https://doi.org/10.1177/1756287215617674. Epub 2015 Nov 26
29. Proietti S, Giusti G, Desai M, Ganpule AP. A critical review of miniaturised percutaneous nephrolithotomy: is smaller better? Eur Urol Focus. 2017;3(1):56–61. https://doi.org/10.1016/j.euf.2017.05.001.
30. Cicekbilek I, Resorlu B, Oguz U, et al. Effect of percutaneous nephrolithotomy on renal functions in children: assessment by quantitative SPECT of (99m)Tc-DMSA uptake by the kidneys. Ren Fail. 2015;37:1118e21.
31. Önal B, Dogan HS, Satar N, Bilen CY, Güneş A, Özden E, et al. Factors affecting complication rates of percutaneous nephrolithotomy in children: results of a multi-institutional retrospective analysis by the Turkish pediatric urology society. J Urol. 2014;191:777–82. https://doi.org/10.1016/j.juro.2013.09.061.
32. Somani BK, Desai M, Traxer O, et al. Stone free rate (SFR): a new proposal for defining levels of SFR. Urolithiasis. 2014;42:95. https://doi.org/10.1007/s00240-013-0630-3.
33. Li J, Wang W, Du Y, Tian Y. Combined use of flexible ureteroscopic lithotripsy with micro-percutaneous nephrolithotomy in pediatric multiple kidney stones. J Pediatr Urol. 2018;14(281):e1–6. https://doi.org/10.1016/j.jpurol.2018.03.005.
34. Bonzo JR, Tasian GE. The emergence of kidney stone disease during childhood-impact on adults. Curr Urol Rep. 2017;18(6):44.
35. Jones P, Hawary A, Beck R, Somani BK. Role of mini-percutaneous nephrolithotomy in the Management of Pediatric Stone Disease: a systematic review of literature. J Endourol. 2020;35(5):728–35. https://doi.org/10.1089/end.2020.0743. Epub ahead of print
36. Somani BK, Griffin S. Ureteroscopy for paediatric calculi: the twin-surgeon model. J Pediatr Urol. 2018;14(1):73–4.

37. Xiao B, Diao X, Jin S, et al. A novel surgical technique for treatment of renal stones in preschool-aged patients: initial experience with needle-perc [published online ahead of print, 2020 Aug 10]. Urology. 2020;146:211–5. S0090-4295(20)30969-9. https://doi.org/10.1016/j.urology.2020.07.055.
38. Jones P, Dhliwayo B, Rai BP, et al. Safety, feasibility, and efficacy of bilateral synchronous percutaneous nephrolithotomy for bilateral stone disease: evidence from a systematic review. J Endourol. 2017;31(4):334–40. https://doi.org/10.1089/end.2016.0851.
39. Guven S, Ozturk A, Arslan M, Istanbulluoglu O, Piskin M, Kilinc M. Simultaneous bilateral percutaneous nephrolithotomy in children: no need to delay. J Endourol. 2011;25(3):437–40. https://doi.org/10.1089/end.2010.0448.
40. Kırlı EA, Erdal FS, Özman O, Özalp AU, Selçuk B, Önal B. The efficacy of Guy's stone score for predicting the stone-free and complication rates in children treated by percutaneous nephrolithotomy. J Endourol. 2020;34(2):128–33. https://doi.org/10.1089/end.2019.0127.
41. Johnson EK, Graham DA, Chow JS, Nelson CP. Nationwide emergency department imaging practices for pediatric urolithiasis: room for improvement. J Urol. 2014;192(1):200–6. https://doi.org/10.1016/j.juro.2014.01.028.

# Part VIII

# Complications and Outcomes

# 29 Complications in Mini PCNL

Harprit Singh, Alok Kumar Jha, and Haresh G. Thummar

*Nothing worthwhile is ever without complications.*

*— Nora Roberts.*

## 29.1 Introduction

Percutaneous nephrolithotomy (PCNL) is the most widely accepted treatment for large (>2 cm), renal or staghorn, and complex renal stones [1]. Stone-free rates are the best with it, but invasiveness is a concern. There has been a constant effort to better the outcomes and decrease the morbidity of the PCNL.

Miniaturization of the scopes is an effort in this direction. Mini PCNL is defined as a PCNL performed through a track of ≤22 F [2]. There is a belief that a smaller tract means less trauma and damage to renal parenchyma, seamless movement, decreased postoperative pain, and lesser analgesics.

Reduced tracts size, associated with remarkably lesser blood loss or need for blood transfusion, and limited hospital stay [3–11]. As the small tract, hinders the vision, requires more fragmentation and extraction of stones, which results in longer operative time [3, 4, 6, 9]. So, the debate continues between conventional and mini PCNL about the merits of miniaturization. Meta-analysis of these studies showed the risk of bias and confounding risk, due to heterogeneity with respect to tract and stone sizes, so the results are conflicting [3, 4, 6, 7, 10, 12–16].

Complications can occur during renal access, tract dilatation and may include injury to adjacent structures, intra-op bleeding, or infection after the procedure. Knowledge of intrarenal anatomy, selection of appropriate tract, and ability to make multipuncture [17] are prerequisites for safe and successful PCNL.

Fewer access-related complications and better stone-free rates are seen when urologists made the renal access [18].

## 29.2 Uniform Reporting of Complications

Modified Clavien-Dindo classification system (grades 1–5) is the widely recognized approach for uniform reporting and monitoring of complications from PCNL. Clavien score has been shown to have high validity, and higher scores (grade III to V) associated with prolonged hospital stay [19–21] (Fig. 29.1).

There are certain limitations in the current reporting system like auxiliary procedures and staging of the surgery are taken as complications

H. Singh (✉)
Department of Urology, Mercy Hospital, Jamshedpur, Jharkhand, India

A. K. Jha
SSB Heart and Multispeciality Hospital, Faridabad, Haryana, India

H. G. Thummar
Department of Urology, Vedanta Kidney Care, Bhailal Amin General Hospital, Vadodara, Gujarat, India


M. S. Agrawal et al. (eds.), *Minimally Invasive Percutaneous Nephrolithotomy*,
https://doi.org/10.1007/978-981-16-6001-6_29

| | |
|---|---|
| **Grade I** | Any deviation from the normal postoperative course without the need for pharmacological treatment or surgical, endoscopic, and radiological interventions. Allowed therapeutic regimens are: drugs such as antiemetics, antipyretics, analgetics, diuretics, electrolytes, and physiotherapy. This grade also includes wound infections opened at the bedside. |
| **Grade II** | Requiring pharamacological treatment with drugs other than allowed for grade I complications. Blood transfusions and total parenteral nutrition are also included. |
| **Grade IIIa** | Surgical, endoscopic, or radiological intervention that is not under general anesthesia |
| **Grade IIIb** | Surgical, endoscopic, or radiological intervention that is under general anesthesia |
| **Grade IVa** | Life-threatening complication requiring intermediate care or intensive care unit management, single organ dysfunction (including dialysis, brain hemorrhage, ischemic stroke, and subarrachnoidal bleeding) |
| **Grade IVb** | Life-threatening complication requiring intermediate care or intensive care unit management, multi-organ dysfunction (including dialysis) |
| **Grade V** | Death of a patient |
| **Suffix "d"** | If the patient suffers from a complication at the time of discharge, the suffix "d" (for "disability") is added to the respective grade of complication. This label indicates the need for a follow-up to fully eveluate the complication |

**Fig. 29.1** Clavien-Dindoclassification of surgical complications

[22, 23]. Clavien-Dindo classification is not applicable to intraoperative complications [24]. Comprehensive studies are needed to make this classification more adaptive, and applicable to PCNL.

## 29.3 Clinical Anatomy

The kidneys lie in the retroperitoneum, major portion of each is essentially supracostal; the lower pole is mostly subcostal. The longitudinal axis of each kidney is oblique and dorsally inclined, making the upper pole calyces more medial and posterior than the inferior pole [25]. In prone position, posterior calyces of the kidney are at a 30° oblique angle to the vertical plane.

The renal pelvis lies posterior to renal artery and vein. Renal artery normally has four to five branches. Posterior segmental artery is the earliest branch and is located posterior to the renal pelvis. Too medial renal access makes it prone for injury and hemorrhage.

Brödels line is an avascular plane approximately 1 cm from the lateral margin of the kidney on the posterior aspect. Percutaneous access into the collecting system is safest when it is from the fornix of the intended calyx, entry through infundibulum can cause hemorrhage from interlobar or segmental branches of the renal artery [26].

Anterior calyx puncture results in more parenchyma being traversed, makes it more difficult to access the renal pelvis or other portions of the collecting system and may increase the risk of bleeding.

Complete staghorn calculi or when direct access to the PUJ is desired, upper-pole puncture is the most appropriate calyx to work in, which may or may not be supracostal [27, 28].

The medial half of the 12th rib and medial three-quarters of the 11th rib provide attachment to the pleura, while each lung base is located two interspaces higher on full expiration [29].

Supracostal access risks the potential of traversing the pleural space. Higher the renal access more is the chance of thoracic complication. Supra-11th rib punctures (34.6%) than supra-12th rib accesses (9.7%), compared with 4.5% for subcostal access [28]. Access sheath should always remain within the kidney during the supracostal approach.

## 29.4 Complications

Complications can occur at any stage of PCNL [30]. Complications of mini PCNL based on stone size, burden, renal unit, and outcome in children, were reviewed. Mini PCNL for small (<20 mm) or large (>20 mm) renal stones (19.4% vs. 26.9%), complication rate has not been found to be statistically significant and no Grade IV or V complications reported [31].

When simple (mean stone burden 10.18 $cm^2$) and complex (mean stone burden 17.63 $cm^2$) were compared, Grade I, II, III, IV, and V complications were noted in 17.1% versus 16.6%, 4.29% versus 5.58%, 3.82% versus 4.06%, 0.02% versus 0.07%, and 0% versus 0.04% with regard to stone size, respectively.

However, blood transfusion (Grade II) (2.2% vs. 3.2%) and arterial embolization (Grade III) (0.28% vs. 0.67%) were observed more often in patients with complex stones. This can be probably attributed to the larger stone burden of these patients and the consequent need for multiple tracts [32, 33]. Overall, the complication rate of mini PCNL was similar even in patients with a solitary kidney and renal calculi [34].

When mini PCNL performed in children and adults were compared, there was no significant difference in perioperative complication rate [35] but, major complications (Grades IV and V) were not observed in children.

However, intraoperative bleeding was significantly correlated with operative time, stone burden, and sheath size in pediatric patients [36]. When nephrostomy tracts used exceeded 22 F, higher hemoglobin drop (1.6 g/dl vs. 1.1 g/dl) [37] and with multiple nephrostomy tracts, significantly increase in hemoglobin drop and transfusion rate was also noticed in children (2.7 g/dl vs. 2 g/dl and 18.8% vs. 4.5%, respectively) [36]. Mini PCNL remains a safe method; Fig. 29.2 gives an overview of the recently published complication rates [38].

Complications of mini PCNL according to the Clavien system range from 11.9% to 37.9%, whereas conventional PCNL range from 16.2% to 60.3% [22] (Fig. 29.3).

Mini PCNL has an edge over the conventional procedure in terms of a significantly reduced hemoglobin drop (0.53 g/dl and 0.8 g/dL vs. 0.97 g/dL and 1.3 g/dL, respectively) [4, 6] and the need for blood transfusion (1.4% vs. 10.4%) [4]. Analgesic requirement has also been found considerably less in mini PCNL when compared to PCNL (55.4 g vs. 70.2 g tramadol) [6]. Length of stay was significantly shorter after mini PCNL (3.8 days and 3.2 days vs. 6.9 days and 4.8 days, respectively) [6, 10].

| Authors | Years | n (patients) | n (renel units) | Total complication rate (%) | I (%) | II (%) | III (%) | IV (%) | V (%) |
|---|---|---|---|---|---|---|---|---|---|
| Knoll *et al.*[26] | 2010 | 25 | 25 | 28 | 24 | 4 | 0 | 0 | 0 |
| Cheng *et al.* *[39] | 2010 | 69 | 72 | 23.6 | 20.8 | 1.4 | 1.4 | 0 | 0 |
| Zhong *et al.* *[14] | 2011 | 29 | 29 | 37.9 | 10.3 | 17.3 | 10.3 | 0 | 0 |
| Knoll *et al.*[43] | 2011 | 25 | 25 | 16 | 16 | | 0 | 0 | 0 |
| Resorlu *et al.*[33] | 2012 | 106 | 106 | 17 | 17 | | 0 | 0 | 0 |
| Zeng *et al.*[16] | 2013 | 12,482 | 13,984 | 25.9 | 16.8 | 5 | 3.9 | 0.05 | 0.02 |
| Kirac *et al.*[12] | 2013 | 37 | 37 | 16.2 | 2.7 | 13.5 | 0 | 0 | 0 |
| Long *et al.*[12] | 2013 | 163 | 163 | 23.1 | 14.6 | 8.5 | 0 | 0 | 0 |
| Pen *et al.*[36] | 2013 | 59 | 59 | 11.9 | 3.4 | 8.5 | 0 | 0 | 0 |
| Abdelhafez *et al.*[35] | 2013 | 172 | 191 | 23 | 12 | 5.8 | 5.2 | 0 | 0 |

* Randomized controlled trials. I, II, III, IV, V: Grads of complications according to modified Clavien classification system.[50]
PCNL: Percutaneous nephrolithotomy

**Fig. 29.2** Data regarding publication rates of mini PCNL, according to modified Clavien grading system, published in recent series with more than 25 patients

**Fig. 29.3** Comparison of complications between Mini PCNL Versus Conventional PCNL

| CLAVIEN GRADES | MINI PCNL | CONVENTIONAL PCNL |
|---|---|---|
| I | 2.7–20.8% | 4–41.2% |
| II | 1.4–17.3% | 4.5–17.6%, |
| III | 0–10.3% | **IIIa** 0–6.6%, **IIIb** 0–2.8% |
| IV | 0–0.05% | **IVa** 0–1.1%, **IVb** 0–0.5% |
| V | 0–0.02% | 0–0.1% |

CROES multicenter study of 5803 patients undergoing PCNL reported an overall complication rate of 21.5% [39]. Major complications require timely diagnosis and proper treatment and occur at a rate between 1.1% and 7.0% [40].

## 29.5 Bleeding

Renal hemorrhage is the most fearsome complication of mini PCNL and can occur at any point from needle insertion to several weeks postoperatively. Sudden hemorrhage due to injury to the great vessels or main renal vessels is uncommon and occurs in less than 0.5% of cases [41]. Most incidents of great vessel or main renal vessel injury occur during initial percutaneous access.

The posterior calyx that provides the most direct access to the stone should be chosen [42, 43]. The tract should be dilated to the periphery of the calyx under fluoroscopic guidance as proceeding too far medially may result in renal pelvis or hilar vessel injury.

The risk of hemorrhagic complications requiring blood transfusions has been found to be associated with multiple punctures, renal pelvis perforation, surgical inexperience, preoperative anemia, and overall blood loss [44].

Additional risk factors that have been found to be associated with significant blood loss include diabetes, multiple tracts, prolonged operative time, and intraoperative complications [44, 45]. One series reported, upper pole renal access, a solitary kidney, and staghorn calculus all significantly increased the risk of major bleeding [46]. Intraoperatively, bleeding can occur from the nephrostomy tract and can be due to excessive angulation and torque on the kidney [47].

Bleeding with initial percutaneous access and tract dilation is often venous in nature and may arise from the percutaneous tract, renal capsule, or renal parenchyma. Intraoperatively access sheath tamponade the bleeding and postoperatively hemostasis is achieved by collapse of parenchyma upon itself. Minor to moderate bleeding can often be controlled by clamping the nephrostomy [48] digital tamponade [49] or with a balloon dilator or Kaye tamponade catheter, or by placing one's fist over the patient's back and another over the patient's abdomen and applying pressure [50], along with intravenous hydration can also be helpful.

The most common site for significant bleeding is from segmental arteries rather than from small arcuate and interlobular arteries. These small arteries are surrounded by dense parenchymal tissue, can easily be tamponade with nephrostomy [51]. Significant bleeding usually leads to abandoning the surgery due to impaired visualization.

With refinement of techniques and equipment, the overall transfusion rate for PCNL has fallen significantly from 6.9% in the early series, to less than 2% in contemporary reports [38, 52–55]. This is comparable to the rates reported for other percutaneous renal surgeries [41, 48, 52, 56–58].

Significant delayed renal hemorrhage (1–3 weeks) after PCNL occurs in less than 2% of patients [41, 52, 59], usually is secondary to arteriovenous fistula or pseudoaneurysm

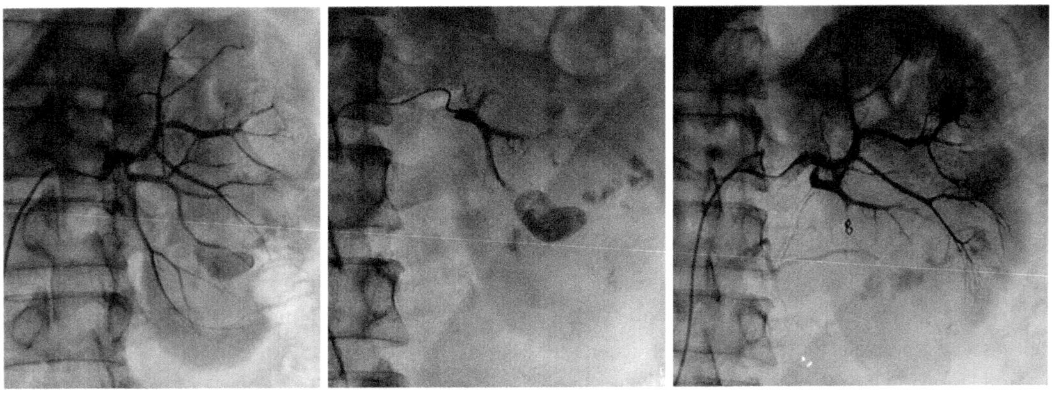

**Fig. 29.4** Pseudo aneurysm, post PCNL with lower calyceal tract causing massive hematuria, superselective angioembolization with proximal Platinum coil

formation and later is more common [48]. Though rare at times this needs intervention.

Arterial injury with subsequent development of arteriovenous fistulas or pseudoaneurysms is a well-known source of bleeding after PCNL. Arteriovenous fistula is formed by a high-pressure leak from a lacerated artery, which is transmitted into a lower-resistance system, such as a vein. Arterial pseudoaneurysms developed when artery is injured, clots off, and then intermittently ruptures often clotting off at variable interval or a connective tissue space [60, 61].

Patient can present with gross hematuria, pain abdomen due to clot colic, or perinephric hematoma or shock.

Suspected cases should undergo angiography with selective angioembolization, which is generally adequate to control the bleed in 92% of the times and this is cost-effective and lifesaving (Fig. 29.4). If conservative measures as well as selective angioembolization fail, open surgical exploration with vascular repair or renorrhaphy or nephrectomy may be used as a last resort [49, 50].

## 29.6 Renal Collecting System Injury

Pelvicalyceal system injury during PCNL occurs in up to 8% of patients. It can occur during initial access or during dilatation, inappropriate choice of guide wire, or overzealous use of rigid nephroscopy. Asserting too hard on a renal pelvic stone during lithotripsy, especially if the pelvis is inflamed or infected or misusing the lithotripter can cause pelvic perforation [61]. Perforation can be intraperitoneal or extraperitoneal. The subsequent extravasation and absorption of irrigation fluid can lead to electrolyte abnormalities, mental status changes, or intravascular volume overload [39, 41, 59, 62–64].

Renal pelvic perforation is usually recognized intraoperatively. Signs of renal collecting system injury include direct visualization of perinephric structures or fat, abnormal hemodynamic parameters, and a decrease in drainage of irrigation fluid [62]. Sudden collapse of distended renal pelvis is a usual sign if the perforation is not visualized directly. Smaller perforations usually heal within 24 to 48 hours and the procedure does not necessarily need to be terminated prematurely [65]. In the case of a large collecting system injury such as at the renal pelvis, the case should be terminated, except it is near completion, in which case the task should be completed at lower irrigation pressure if the patient is doing clinically well [61].

Bigger disruptions including perforation of the renal pelvis require prompt cessation and adequate drainage via a nephrostomy tube, ureteral stent, or percutaneous drain. Depending on the severity of injury, wait for 3 to 7 days before nephrostogram and tube removal [47].

The use of sealants to close the renal collecting system defect is not recommended [66].

There have been reports of massive intra-abdominal collection of extravasated fluid after percutaneous renal surgery [67–70].

At times, perforation is recognized in the post-operative period, flank pain, fever, or abdominal distention and ileus should raise the suspicion for urinary extravasation [41]. It should be treated with drainage of kidney as well as percutaneous drainage of urinoma and abdominal ascites.

Use of fluoroscopy for percutaneous renal access can decrease the risk of renal collecting system injury, isotonic irrigation fluid and open or continuous irrigation systems can reduce intra-operative extravasation and fluid absorption [47].

## 29.7 Thoracic Complications

As the pleura lies in close proximity to the upper pole of the kidney, it becomes an easy target for injury during percutaneous procedure on the kidney, especially if the tract is supracostal. Thoracic complications constitute a significant percentage of overall complications after PCNL with an incidence of 1.8–3.1% [30, 39, 62]. In the CROES study, the upper pole access group had a hydrothorax rate of 5.8% whereas the lower pole access group had a hydrothorax rate of 1.5%. This translated to an odds ratio of 0.4 for lower pole versus upper pole. The odds ratio for access above 11th rib versus above 12th rib was 5.6 [71]. When supracostal access is preferred, it is better to stay lateral to the midscapular line [72] and should be done in expiration to avoid transpleural entry [72, 73], avoid premature withdrawal of the sheath to prevent extravasation in the pleural cavity.

Violation of the pleural space can lead to air (pneumothorax), urine (hydrothorax/nephropleural fistula), or blood (hemothorax) in the pleural cavity. Infection of this can lead to pus formation (pyothorax). Pneumothorax usually occurs due to introduction of external air in the pleural cavity and very rarely due to lung injury. Hydrothorax can result from the accumulation of irrigation fluid during the procedure or urine extravasating from a nephropleural fistula [74]. Rarely serous fluid can accumulate due to reactive effusion.

Hemothorax can be due to accumulation of blood from injured intercostal vessel [75], or from the kidney in the pleural space [76]. Pyothorax or empyema can occur if a sterile hydrothorax gets secondarily infected or infected urine enters the pleural space. Intraoperatively, access sheath should not be taken out during supracostal tract [75].

The diagnosis is made clinically or based on the radiological evaluation. As the venous return gets compromised, narrowing of the pulse width may appear. Decreased airway entry is noted on the ipsilateral side. Intraoperative chest fluoroscopy has been found to be sensitive enough for the detection of pleural air or fluid collection [77]. A contrast study near the end of the procedure can confirm leak of urine into the pleural space [62]. Chest tube can be placed on the operating table if required under the same anesthesia [78].

Post-operatively in the recovery room or ward, if the patient develops pleuritic pain, dyspnea, or falling oxygen saturation then one should suspect pleural injury and proceed for chest X-ray or chest CT scan [62]. Radiography will differentiate pneumothorax from hydrothorax as well as hemothorax. A diagnostic tap can differentiate blood from pus or clear fluid. Clear fluid must be sent for creatinine estimation and a culture. If a nephropleural fistula is suspected then a retrograde pyelogram (RGP) should be done to confirm the diagnosis and look for distal obstruction [75].

Many patients with Pleural injury can be managed conservatively if the volume of air or fluid is low [79]. Those with a significant volume of air or fluid need intervention [30]. The simplest is to place chest tube drainage, a small bore for air and a wider bore for blood or pus. The chest tube is removed with signs of recovery [74]. In case of empyema, tube drainage may not be enough if pus becomes loculated. Such cases require surgical drainage, either Open surgery or Video-assisted thoracic surgery (VATS) [80].

Nephropleural fistula is well diagnosed on retrograde pyelogram and needs chest tube drainage along with a JJ stent and Foleys catheter drainage [81] (Fig. 29.5). Anti-cholinergics may be added to hasten the healing [73, 75]. Sometimes placing a nephrostomy in the lower calyx and early removal

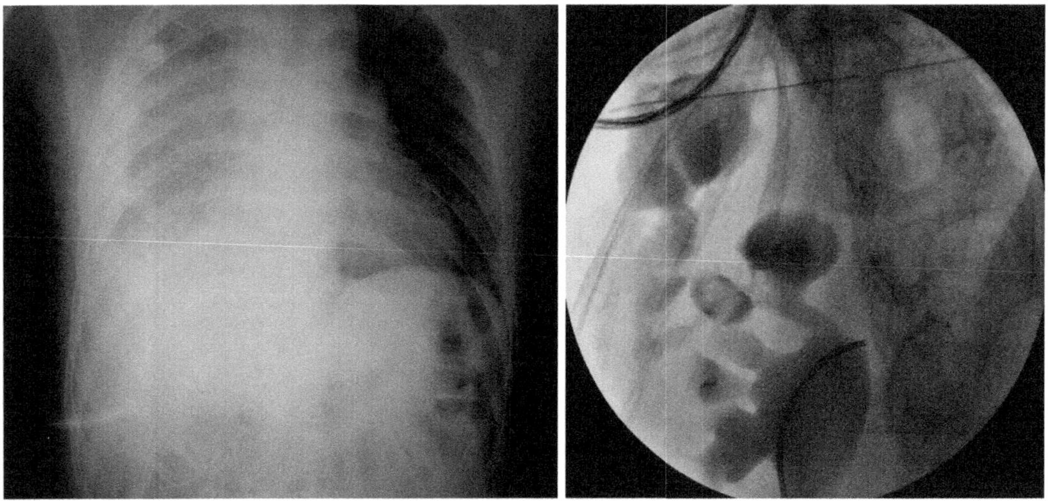

**Fig. 29.5** Chest X-ray, right hydropneumothorax, nephropleural fistula from the upper calyx from a supracostal tract

of supracostal drainage leads to early healing [82]. Use of flexible nephroscope or ECIRS technique to avoid very high supracostal puncture [83].

## 29.8 Colon Injury

Colonic perforation is an extremely rare complication of percutaneous nephrolithotomy (PCNL) occurring in less than 1% of procedures. Ozturk et al. found 36 colonic injuries out of 9996 PCNL patients in one review of literature study with incidence of 0.36% [40].

Colonic injury is due to percutaneous renal access through colon and can be due to various reasons. Early detection, timely intervention, and appropriate care are the keys to successful outcomes.

Risk factors for colonic injury are utmost lateral access to kidney beyond post axillary line, more common on left side with lower pole access, retrorenal colon (0.6–2.0%) [84–88], anatomically distorted kidney due to renal abscess, scoliosis or previous renal surgery, chronic constipation, or dilated bowel loops, ectopic kidney or malrotated kidney or horseshoe kidney [89], more common in elderly [90], thin and lean person with low body mass index (BMI). Patients with high risk should undergo preoperative CT scan [89, 91].

The diagnosis of this injury is usually elusive owing to the variability of symptoms and signs, which can occur immediately or several days after the procedure.

Intraoperatively, one should look for a change in bowel gas shadows pattern while puncturing which may be indirect warning sign of transcolonic needle access. This can be confirmed by colonic enhancement on injection of contrast.

During nephroscopy one can see, air bubbles or bowel contents, sometimes [92] (Fig. 29.6).

In postoperative period, the patient may develop symptoms like abdominal pain and tenderness at local site or maybe generalized, fever, tachycardia, leukocytosis, and ileus [93, 94]. Sometimes symptoms are very obvious like blood per rectum, pneumo-peritoneum, and a gas or feces from percutaneous site or inside nephrostomy tube [84].

Postoperative imaging, either antegrade nephrostogram or CT scan confirming transcolonic passage of the percutaneous nephrostomy (PCN) tube.

Missed colonic injury can lead to abscess formation and nephrocolic or colocutaneous fistula. Peritonitis may also develop from intraperitoneal fecal soiling [92].

Treatment approach depends on the time of identification, extent of injury, clinical status of patient, and spread on bowel content in the peritoneal cavity or localized. Most of the colonic

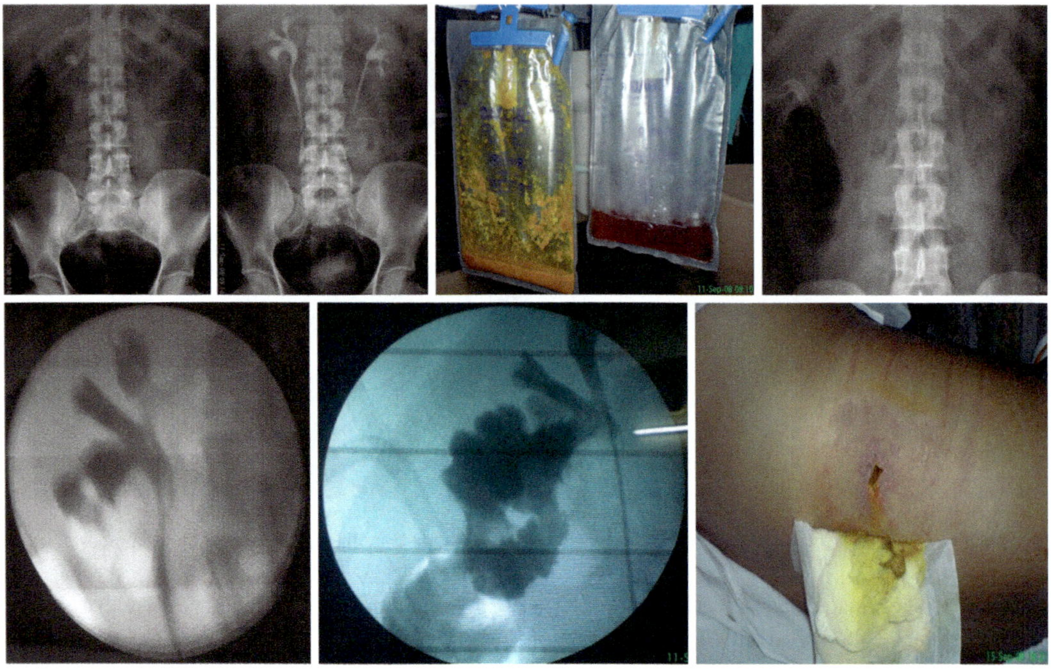

**Fig. 29.6** Colonic injury, right renal pelvic stone, lower calyceal puncture, fecal matter in nephrostomy pulled into the colon, retrograde pyelogram showing nephrocolonic fistula and drain, solid fecal matter from drain site on seventh post-op day (Courtesy- Dr. S K Pal, New Delhi)

injuries due to PCNL are extraperitoneal and respond to conservative treatment [94]. Once identified treatment includes classical triad of antibiotics, bowel rest, and separating bowel from urinary tract. A triple antibiotic usually includes penicillin/cephalosporin group, aminoglycosides (gentamycin/amikacin), and metronidazole (anaerobic organism coverage). Bowel rest is given by giving nothing by mouth, nasogastric tube aspiration, and intravenous fluids for few days. Once stabilized start orally with clear liquids and semisolid as tolerated. If the injury is identified intraoperatively, separation of bowel and urinary tract can be done by drainage of colon (by withdrawing the nephrostomy tube inside colon and working as a colostomy tube) and decompressing urinary tract with PCN (nephrostomy or internal double J stent) and indwelling catheter.

PCN tube withdrawal in the lumen of colonic, allows the medial colonic injury to heal [85, 95]. In postoperative period, after checking with imaging and confirming no renal extravasation, the PCN tube is further withdrawn from colon into pericolonic space to allow drainage of content and lateral colonic injury to heal [85]. Foley's catheter can come out at this point.

The pericolonic drain can be removed after three to seven days depending on clinical status and quality and quantity of drain. Antibiotics should be continued for 5–10 days after drain removal [96].

Intraperitoneal colonic perforation or generalized peritonitis or sepsis warrants open surgical intervention and repair may be required [84]. In case of delayed diagnosis of colonic injury, a general surgical consult is advisable for further expert management.

## 29.9 Visceral Injuries

### 29.9.1 Gall Bladder Injury

It is rare but serious complication of right side PCNL with 8 cases reported till now in literature.

All of them required open exploration and cholecystectomy. It should be suspected if one finds greenish discharge in PCN or signs of peritonitis postoperatively. CT scan is usually diagnostic of this injury and surgical exploration is the answer to avoid its severe complications [40].

## 29.10 Liver and Spleen Injury

It is rare but serious kind of organ injury. Eleven cases of spleen and 1 case of liver injury had been reported [40]. There is minimal risk of spleen injury when puncture is done in expiration above 12th rib but 34% risk when puncture is done above 11th rib so this should be avoided whenever possible. In cases of enlarged spleen and liver, ultrasound guided or CT guided or image access should be tried, lower pole access is preferable [97].

CT scan is the ideal imaging to accurately assess it and is helpful in further management [98]. Disproportionally hemodynamic changes compare to renal bleed should suspicious of these organ injuries.

Usually, conservative management helps unless there is life-threatening hemodynamic instability warranting urgent exploration and splenectomy on left side. Active observation, rest, delayed removal of nephrostomy and novel coagulant down the tract usually helps [40, 99].

Transhepatic percutaneous access is usually without sequelae, and injury to major intrahepatic vessels after track dilation is the greatest risk. If significant bleeding is encountered, balloon tamponade of the path can temporize bleeding and angiographic embolization can be performed [96].

## 29.11 Extrarenal Stone Migration

Extrarenal loss of stone fragments may occur with renal pelvis or ureteral perforation, or through the percutaneous access track. It is rare but must be documented [49]. Extrarenal stone migration occurs due to unwarranted pressure of the probe onto the stone, or an incorrect technique of stone extraction with an Amplatz sheath. Endoscopic retrieval of fragments outside of the urinary tract should not be attempted, as this may only enlarge the perforation [49].

Intraperitoneal [100] and pleural migration [101] of stones has been reported. These rare cases required laparoscopy and thoracoscopy in order to prevent peritoneal and thoracic complications.

## 29.12 Postoperative Persistent Nephrocutaneous Leakage

Percutaneous access tract typically closes within 6–12 hours of nephrostomy tube removal [102]. Urinary leakage persisting >24 h after nephrostomy tube removal called prolonged and usually needs treatment [103]. The incidence of prolonged nephrocutaneous leakage from the tract is between 1.5% and 4.6% [104].

It is advisable to obtain a low-dose CT scan to evaluate for stone fragments in the ureter that may be causing obstruction.

Ureteral stenting is helpful in the majority of cases of prolonged urinary leakage [104]. In addition, a Foley catheter may be inserted for 24 h in order to relieve pressure in the urinary system and promote anterograde drainage of urine [105].

## 29.13 Collecting System Obstruction

Pelvicalyceal system obstruction associated with PCNL is rare, but may result from ureteral avulsion or stricture, transient mucosal edema, blood clot, or infundibular stenosis [106, 107]. Trauma with or without retained stone fragments at ureter or ureteropelvic junction obstruction (UPJ) is also reported [108]. Brief period of obstruction, due to edema or blood clot often resolves without intervention or long-term sequelae. If nephrostomy has been kept, it must be removed after nephrostogram or after a period of clamping to assess clinically for distal ureteral obstruction.

Collecting system obstruction can lead to nephrocutaneous fistulae, hydronephrosis, or hydrocalyx, depending upon early or late formation of the stricture.

## 29.14 Infundibular Stenosis

Infundibular stenosis is a rare complication, 2% of percutaneous nephrolithotomy. It is associated with prolonged operative time, a large stone burden requiring multiple removal procedures and extended postoperative nephrostomy tube drainage, recurrent UTI, open pyelolithotomy, diabetes mellitus, and obesity.

Prolonged inflammatory processes and trauma of the renal mucosa presumably induce fibrosis, scarring, and gradual obliteration of the infundibular lumen. It has been observed within a year of initial percutaneous nephrolithotomy [107, 109–111].

Treatment approach includes endoscopic in majority of cases to open surgical reconstructions or excision with partial or total nephrectomy. If nothing works, one may consider observation provided that the patient is asymptomatic and does not exhibit renal function deterioration [107].

Endoscopic approach to infundibular stenosis either antegrade or retrograde, have the success rate of 60%–80% [112]. Methods are cold knife excision [113], laser ablation [114], balloon dilation [115], or endoscopic formation of a new infundibulum [116].

Salvage strategies included permanent stenting, excision of the dilated portion of the kidney, or heminephrectomy [117].

## 29.15 Renal Dysfunction

Renal dysfunction following PCNL is uncommon and is typically secondary to other operative complications. For example, intraoperative or postoperative bleeding may lead to decreased renal blood flow and transient renal insufficiency, or angioembolization may result in permanent parenchymal infarction [47].

Transient increase in creatinine occurs in less than 1% of patients after PNL [52]. This rate is similar to that of patients undergoing SWL, and not clinically significant [118]. Pre- and postoperative MAG3 studies confirm stable differential renal function at 22 days after PCNL, and the volume of renal scarring in patients with single or multiple percutaneous access tracts amounts to less than 1% of total renal parenchyma [119–122].

## 29.16 Equipment Problems, Energy Sources, Tubes, and Renal Trauma

Aggressive manipulation of the scope and inadvertent misdirection of energy sources can result in damage of either scope or renal trauma. Avoid excessive torque of the miniaturized scopes as they are very fragile, especially when one is operating in a previously operated or inflamed kidney.

We had broken our scope when trying to reach upper calyx from lower calyx in a previously operated because of torque (Fig. 29.7).

Cautious use of pneumatic lithotripsy in an inflamed and edematous renal mucosa as backward moment of fragments might damage it.

Spark from electrohydraulic energy can damage the telescope or collecting system. The probe should always be placed in direct contact with the stone to prevent complications [123].

Ultrasound probe tip becomes very hot, when used for disintegrating stone, risking injury to endothelium. Continuous irrigation helps to cool the tip.

Laser penetration depth is shallow, inadvertent laser discharge on endothelium can lead to bleeding making visualization difficult.

Sometimes we have found pieces of broken nephrostomies, tubes, either due to wear and tear or sometimes get damaged by energy sources they can form a nidus for the stones or sometimes found buried in parenchyma (Fig. 29.8).

Stones fragments that do not easily fit into the amplatz sheath should be further fragmented